GOODALE'S
CLINICAL
INTERPRETATION
OF
LABORATORY TESTS

Edition 7

GOODALE'S
CLINICAL INTERPRETATION OF LABORATORY TESTS

FRANCES K. WIDMANN, M. D.

Associate Professor, Department of Pathology
Duke University School of Medicine
Durham, North Carolina

Assistant Chief, Laboratory Service
Durham Veterans Administration Hospital
Durham, North Carolina

 F. A. DAVIS COMPANY, PHILADELPHIA

Library of Congress Catalog Card Number 72-96970

ISBN 0-8036-9320-6 (Cloth)
ISBN 0-8036-9321-4 (Paperback)

Preface

The four years since this book's last edition have seen still further expansion of laboratory availability. Local laboratories provide tests that heretofore only the most specialized laboratories could do. With the aid of mail and delivery services, individual practitioners have access to every analytical procedure currently in use.

In this seventh edition, I have tried to address that wide range of problems encountered in the usual office or hospital practice. The discriminatory precision of university or other subspecialty practices requires individualized treatment by comparably specialized authorities. The clinician whose patients embody a broad spectrum of disease, and whose responsibilities embrace the entire patient, requires a broad perspective of laboratory service. By discussing widely available tests of proven value, I hope to assist these practitioners in choosing and evaluating diagnostic procedures and interpreting the results. Most users of this book will not perform the tests themselves, so I have omitted technical details except insofar as they are necessary to understand what a procedure can or cannot do. Those technical and nursing personnel charged with performing these procedures will find this book useful in explaining where and how the tests apply to patients' clinical problems.

Edition seven, while resembling edition six in format, embodies much new material. The chapter on serology and immunology has been completely rewritten, to include not only new tests but also enlarged understanding of the body's defenses against external and internal attack. Other chapters completely rewritten since the previous edition are those on microbiologic examinations, on the pathophysiology and laboratory analysis of urine, and on feces, gastric and duodenal analysis, and sputum examination.

No other chapters have been completely replaced, but advances in electrophoresis and immunoelectrophoresis of proteins and analysis and

v

interpretation of serum lipid abnormalities have required extensive new sections. In every chapter, I have tried to include new concepts and procedures as their values have been established. I have deleted those chapters which enumerated selected laboratory findings in selected diseases, because such summaries are available, in greater detail, in the relevant chapters of internal medicine texts. Retained in the clinical discussions which comprise Part 2 are those complex situations in which the fundamental derangements become apparent through changing laboratory values, and in which the combined results of many tests must be coordinated for diagnosis.

The preface to the sixth edition expressed my thanks to many friends and colleagues who assisted me by reviewing manuscripts and offering suggestions. For this edition I would like additionally to express appreciation to Doctors Robert Gutman, Suydam Osterhout, and Peter Zwadyk for reviewing manuscripts, and to Doctors Philip Pratt and George Spooner for encouragement and numerous suggestions. Since their contributions have been modified by the author, the shortcomings of my work should be laid at my door and not at theirs.

Once again, my final word of thanks is to Doctor Raymond Goodale, to whom this book owes its inception, and whose contribution and conception are embodied in the title.

Durham, North Carolina   Frances K. Widmann, M. D.

Contents

Part 1

LABORATORY PRINCIPLES

CHAPTER 1

Hematology Procedures

THE BONE MARROW

DISTRIBUTION

Bone marrow occupies the marrow cavity of all bones, but not every bone contains blood-forming elements. The hematopoietic marrow—the young and adult blood cells and their precursors—is enmeshed and supported by the reticuloendothelial system, and nourished by branches from the arterial supply of the surrounding bone. In fetal life and early infancy, hematopoietic marrow occupies virtually all marrow cavities, and blood is also formed within the reticuloendothelial elements of liver and spleen. Extramedullary hematopoiesis normally ceases very shortly after birth, and the distribution of hematopoietic (red) marrow diminishes during the first few years of life. In older children and adults, red marrow is found principally in the vertebral bodies, the sternum, and the bones of the pelvic girdle. Other bones contain adipose tissue (yellow marrow), but the capacity to produce red and white cells persists. In conditions of physiologic or pathologic stress, the yellow marrow may be activated to hematopoiesis; thus, in severe anemias and in certain hematologic diseases, cell production may recur in marrow cavities normally occupied by inactive tissue, and blood may once again be formed in liver and spleen. Extramedullary hematopoiesis is more common in anemias of childhood than in later life.

The bone marrow forms erythrocytes, granulocytes, monocytes, and platelets. A hypothetical stem cell is thought to differentiate into both red and white cell forms, and to remain capable of circulation and marrow repopulation when suitably stimulated. Under normal conditions, only

3

mature cells enter the blood stream from the marrow, but in pathologic states, a variety of immature cells can be found in the circulating blood.

CONTROL OF HEMATOPOIESIS

Red Blood Cells

The control of erythrocyte production is better understood than control of leukocyte formation. Under normal conditions, a circulating humoral substance called erythropoietin regulates erythropoiesis and thereby controls the total quantity of red cells and red cell precursors available to the body. The kidney appears to be the main source of erythropoietin. In a general way, erythropoietin levels are linked to changes in tissue oxygenation, but the full kinetics of erythropoietin metabolism are still under study. Other factors which may influence the rate of red cell production or hemoglobin synthesis are androgenic hormones, adrenal cortical hormones and the presence of cobalt ions.[19]

White Blood Cells

In experimental studies, substances derived from white cells, from necrotic tissues, and from bacteria have proved to stimulate granulocyte production. It may be, however, that these or similar substances only affect leukopoiesis under pathologic conditions, and the stimulus to normal white cell production is not fully understood. Regulation of the monocyte pool is even more of a mystery since neither the origin nor the function of the monocytes is understood. Lymphocytes enter the blood from lymph nodes, presumably in response to stimuli quite different from those which affect the bone marrow.

MARROW ASPIRATION

To obtain marrow specimens for examination, it is necessary to penetrate the surrounding bone. Various specially adapted needles are used to incise the cortical bone and allow aspiration of the semisolid marrow. Because it is readily accessible, the sternum is a common site for marrow aspiration and one in which functioning marrow is usually present. In sternal puncture, there is always slight risk of penetrating underlying mediastinal structures, and the superior vena cava, the aortic arch, and even the heart itself have occasionally been entered. An additional disadvantage of sternal puncture is that the patient can watch the entire procedure, with emotions ranging from fascination to downright panic. Aspiration from the iliac crest is safer and less traumatic, and offers no particular technical

Table 1. Percentages of Cells in Bone Marrow of Normal Adults*

	Range	Average
Myeloblasts	0.3 to 5.0	2.0
Promyelocytes ("undifferentiated myelocytes," "progranulocytes")	1.0 to 8.0	5.0
Myelocytes		
Neutrophilic	5.0 to 19.0	12.0
Eosinophilic	0.5 to 3.0	1.5
Basophilic	0.0 to 0.5	0.3
Metamyelocytes ("juvenile" forms)	13.0 to 32.0	22.0
Polymorphonuclear neutrophils	7.0 to 30.0	20.0
Polymorphonuclear eosinophils	0.5 to 4.0	2.0
Polymorphonuclear basophils	0.0 to 0.7	0.2
Lymphocytes	3.0 to 17.0	10.0
Plasma cells	0.0 to 2.0	0.4
Monocytes	0.5 to 5.0	2.0
Reticulum cells	0.1 to 2.0	0.2
Megakaryocytes	0.03 to 3.0	0.4
Pronormoblasts (macroblasts)	1.0 to 8.0	4.0
Normoblasts (basophilic, polychromatophilic, and acidophilic)	7.0 to 32.0	18.0

* From Wintrobe, M.M.: Clinical Hematology, ed. 6. Lea & Febiger, Philadelphia, 1967.

problems to the operator, except for some difficulty in applying firm pressure over the site when the procedure is finished. In small children, aspiration is sometimes made from the bones of the leg.

Bone marrow aspiration should be approached as a surgical procedure, with careful attention to maintaining sterility, minimizing tissue damage, and allaying the patient's anxiety. If marrow examination is essential in a patient with a bleeding tendency, every effort should be made to diagnose and treat the hemorrhagic diathesis, and the patient should be scrupulously observed for late complications.

Examining the Specimen

The aspirated marrow can be smeared or imprinted, and a variety of stains, including supravital techniques, can be applied. Fragments of tissue are usually fixed and sectioned. Examination of the marrow includes estimation of cellularity and search for pathogenic microorganisms and neoplastic or inflammatory cellular patterns, as well as evaluation of erythrocyte, leukocyte, and platelet patterns. Sometimes it becomes necessary to obtain an open biopsy of the marrow and overlying bone, but this is usually done when attempts at aspiration have been unsuccessful.

Normal Values

Wintrobe gives normal values in the bone marrow in Table 1, but considerable variation may occur. Abnormal findings are discussed in Chapters 13 and 14, under the individual diseases.

BLOOD AS A WHOLE

FUNCTIONS

The blood must be considered a tissue of complex composition and origin, serving many functions. Both fluid and cellular components are essential; without the fluid medium, cells could not circulate, but without the cells, vascular fluid alone could not maintain life. In addition to transporting cells, the fluid portion of the blood serves to regulate body heat; to maintain the countless cells of the body in adequate hydration; to carry nutritive, protective and regulative substances to all parts of the body; and to transport metabolic waste products of all kinds to the appropriate organs for excretion.

Red cells function principally as shipping containers for hemoglobin. It is the hemoglobin that, in the lungs, actually loads oxygen and unloads carbon dioxide. It transports these gases through the circulatory system and unloads oxygen and carries off carbon dioxide at all sites of metabolic function. The white cells provide various protective functions, and the hemostatic elements of blood help protect the body from the effects of external trauma.

BLOOD VOLUME

The volume of blood circulating through the vascular tree is, in conditions of health, remarkably stable. When blood is lost, the body promptly attempts to restore volume by shifting fluid from the extravascular compartment into the blood. Similarly, if plasma volume is expanded by oral or parenteral fluid intake, the kidney compensates by excreting the excess fluid as dilute urine. The most immediate problem that follows acute volume loss is impaired transport of oxygen to the brain, kidneys, and other vital organs. Slightly less immediate, but still critical, is impairment of pH and electrolyte regulation. It must be remembered that measurement of such values as hemoglobin or sodium ion concentration measures only the quantity of substance in a single aliquot of blood. It does not report on the quantity available to the body as a whole. For example, immediately after loss of 15 per cent of total blood volume and before fluid readjustment has occurred, the hematocrit may be perfectly normal even though oxygen transport is seriously jeopardized.

Indicator Substances

Several methods are available for measuring total blood volume. The earliest technique, as cited by Wintrobe,[35] was to drain all the blood from a cadaver and then measure the result. This method, though accurate, can hardly be adapted for clinical use. Other less drastic methods use the dilution principle to measure circulating blood in the intact organism. If a known quantity of some completely diffusible substance is introduced into a fluid, the final concentration of additive in fluid can be used to calculate the volume in which it is dispersed. The ideal indicator for measuring blood volume should diffuse uniformly throughout the compartment being measured, and it should not enter the cells, or leave the blood stream, or be metabolized or excreted, or merge its identity with other elements in the blood, or be toxic to the patient. Another technical problem in measuring total volume is that distribution of cells and plasma varies in different parts of the body, and expansion of the capillary network can vary with physiologic changes.

A variety of dyes, serum products, and inert substances have been used to measure plasma volume; the red cell compartment has been measured by injecting identifiable compatible cells or by tagging the patient's own hemoglobin with carbon monoxide. At present, the most popular indicators are radioactive isotopes of molecules normally present in plasma or red cells. These are easily identified and quantitated, and if suitable isotopes are chosen, there is virtually no risk from radioactivity. For plasma volume measurement, ^{131}I-labelled serum albumin is popular. This has largely replaced Evans blue dye (T-1824) for plasma determinations. Tagging the patient's own red cells with a radioactive label avoids risk of incompatibility, and di-isopropylfluorophosphate[32] ($DF^{32}P$),^{51}Cr, and glycine-2-^{14}C have all been used.

Normal Values

Normal values differ between males and females, the amount of blood per unit weight being less for females. Since adipose tissue has a sparser blood supply than lean tissue, the patient's body habitus can affect the proportion of blood volume to body weight. Mean normal values for whole blood volume in men and women are given in one study[18] as 75.5 ml/kg and 66.5 ml/kg respectively. Plasma volume averages 44 ml/kg in men and 43 ml/kg in women in the same study.[18] In pregnancy, total volume increases, due largely to increased plasma volume.

Blood volume is usually measured to evaluate acute blood loss following surgical procedures or trauma or to investigate chronic low-grade hemorrhage. It is also useful in certain patients with edema or diminished hematopoiesis. If the blood volume must be measured repeatedly during acute bleeding, there may be technical difficulties from background level of radioactivity and the effects of changing hematocrit, as well as physiologic or pathologic variations in the vascular tree.

RED BLOOD CELLS

Among the laboratory tests most frequently requested is evaluation of the body's capacity to transport oxygen. Oxygen is carried by hemoglobin, and hemoglobin is carried inside the red cells, so several variables can be measured. Three measurements are commonly used: the total concentration of hemoglobin in a blood sample, the number of red cells present in the blood sample, and the volume occupied by red cells in a blood sample.

HEMOGLOBIN DETERMINATION

A number of techniques are used for estimating hemoglobin concentration.

Specific Gravity

Specific gravity methods compare the weight of blood against a solution of known specific gravity, usually copper sulfate. Blood is thicker (and heavier) than water largely by virtue of its protein concentration, and hemoglobin is the most important contributor. The mean normal specific gravity of blood in women and children is 1.053, and in adult men, 1.057. This method provides only a rough-and-ready estimate of hemoglobin value unless a number of finely graded solutions are used. Currently it is most often used as a screening procedure for blood donors since blood can be assumed to be anemic if it lacks required specific gravity. The technique is subject to error if evaporation or contamination changes the specific gravity of the solution or if constituents other than hemoglobin affect the weight of the blood. Abnormal serum proteins are the usual offender, and patients with unusually high protein values, notably from multiple myeloma, occasionally have blood of normal specific gravity despite reduced hemoglobin concentration.

Color Comparison

Visual methods measure light transmitted through a hemoglobin solution. To get intracellular hemoglobin into solution the erythrocytes must first be lysed. The color of the resulting solution can be measured photoelectrically or by visual comparison with prepared standards. Several fairly simple techniques use a minimum of equipment and rely upon the operator's eye to match the test sample and standard. In the Sahli hemoglobinometer, 0.1N hydrochloric acid is added to blood, lysing the red cells and converting hemoglobin to acid hematin. The acid hematin solution is then matched to a single glass color standard. If dilution by a small amount of acid brings the acid hematin solution to that color, the hemoglobin concentration is fairly low. If the acid hematin must be heavily diluted, the initial hemoglobin value is high. Hemoglobin concentrations are read from a calibrated scale based on volume of acid added.

With the Spencer type of hemoglobinometer, the operator compares the light transmitted through a thin layer of hemolyzed blood (oxyhemoglobin) with the light transmitted through a standardized glass wedge at a wave length which approximates that of pure oxyhemoglobin. Both Sahli and Spencer techniques require visual matching, and are subject to human error and fatigue as well as the intrinsic defects of visual discrimination.

Colorimetry

Photoelectric colorimeters or spectrophotometers provide the most accurate color determinations. Their accuracy depends, of course, on the quality of the instrument used, the maintenance of accurate calibration, and careful attention to the wave length of the filter. Hemoglobin must first be converted into a compound susceptible of photometric evaluation, and both oxyhemoglobin and cyanmethemoglobin have been widely used. Cyanmethemoglobin appears to be more stable, to permit more accurate determination, and to measure methemoglobin and carbon monoxide hemoglobin as well as oxyhemoglobin. When large numbers of samples are being tested, or if comparison between samples or between different laboratories is desirable, the cyanmethemoglobin method of hemoglobin measurement appears to be the most satisfactory method presently available. The method can be used on filter-type photometers or narrow-band spectrophotometers, so the necessary equipment is not prohibitively expensive.

HEMATOCRIT

The hematocrit expresses the portion of total blood volume occupied by red blood cells and provides a visual means of estimating the red cell count. Either venous or capillary blood can be used. In the *macro method,* a Wintrobe hematocrit tube 100 mm tall is accurately filled with fluid blood and then centrifuged at 2200 to 2500 g for 30 minutes. The percentage of total volume occupied by red cells, white cells, and plasma can be read directly from the millimeter markings on the tube.

In a *micro method* an uncalibrated tube, approximately 7 cm long and 1 mm in diameter, is filled with blood and is centrifuged at 10,000 g for 5 minutes in a specially adapted centrifuge. The proportions of blood and plasma are calculated from a measuring device. The micro method is rapid, can be used on finger-prick blood samples, and eliminates the need for careful measurement and pipetting, but its very simplicity may diminish the care and skill with which it is performed. When high quality equipment is used, however, a satisfactory degree of accuracy can be obtained by relatively unskilled personnel, and the microhematocrit method is probably the simplest, most reliable, and most informative single test of oxygen-carrying capacity.

ERYTHROCYTE COUNT

A cubic millimeter of normal blood contains between 4.5 and 5.5 million red cells which cannot be individually counted. Both dilution and sampling are necessary for measurement of red cell content, and unavoidable error enters the determination. In the classical technique for counting red cells, the blood is diluted 1:200, and actual evaluation is performed on 0.02 cu mm of this diluted sample. The number of cells counted in the specified volume is multiplied by 10,000 so that every source of error in the entire procedure is multiplied by 10,000 in reporting the count. Manual red cell counts are rarely performed since they require a large investment of time for a relatively inaccurate result. Electronic counting devices are far faster and more accurate than a technician bending over a microscope, but the potential errors of manifold dilution and sampling still obtain.

Normal values for the most important hematologic procedures are given in Table 2.

CORPUSCULAR INDICES

The three tests described above measure, respectively, the quantity of hemoglobin present in 100 ml of whole blood; the proportion of whole blood volume occupied by erythrocytes; and the number of erythrocytes present in one cubic millimeter of blood. By manipulating these data, one can describe the characteristics of individual red cells with an accuracy dependent on the accuracy of the original determinations. The so-called corpuscular indices, or corpuscular constants, describe the red cells in terms of individual cell size (mean corpuscular volume, M.C.V.), the

Table 2. Normal Hematologic Findings*

	Adults		Average Values for Children		
	Average	*Range*	*Birth*	*1 Year*	*10 Years*
Red blood cells in millions/mm³					
Female	4.8	4.0-5.6	5.4	4.5	4.8
Male	5.4	4.5-6.5			
Hemoglobin in Gm per 100 ml					
Female	13.9	12.0-16.0	17.0	11.4	13.0
Male	15.8	14.0-18.0			
Hematocrit in ml per 100 ml					
Female	42	36-47	54	35	39
Male	47	40-54			
Platelets in 100,000/mm³					
Male & Female	3.0	1.5-4.5	2.0	3.0	3.0
White blood cells in 1000/mm³					
Male & Female	7.0	4.0-11.0	17.0	12.0	7.5

* From Damm, H. (ed.): CRC Handbook of Clinical Laboratory Data. Chemical Rubber Co., Cleveland, Ohio, 1965. Used by permission of Chemical Rubber Co.

amount of hemoglobin present in a single cell (mean corpuscular hemoglobin, M.C.H.), and the proportion of each cell occupied by hemoglobin (mean corpuscular hemoglobin concentration, M.C.H.C.).

These indices are calculated by the following formulas:[34]

$$\text{M.C.V.} = \frac{\text{Volume of packed red cells, in cc per 1000 cc blood}}{\text{Red cell count, in millions per cubic millimeter}} \text{ in cubic microns}$$

$$\text{M.C.H.} = \frac{\text{Hemoglobin, in grams per 1000 cc blood}}{\text{Red cell count, in millions per cubic millimeter}} \text{ in micromicrograms}$$

$$\text{M.C.H.C.} = \frac{\text{Hemoglobin, in grams per 100 cc blood} \times 100}{\text{Volume of packed red cells, in cc per 100 cc blood}} \text{ in per cent}$$

The values required by these formulas are not simply the results of standard laboratory tests, since different volumes of blood are used for different indices. The formulas for calculating indices from the reported values are:

$$\text{M.C.V.} = \frac{\text{Hematocrit (as per cent)} \times 10}{\text{Red cell count (always given as millions per cubic millimeter)}}$$

$$\text{M.C.H.} = \frac{\text{Hemoglobin (as grams/100 ml)} \times 10}{\text{Red cell count}}$$

$$\text{M.C.H.C.} = \frac{\text{Hemoglobin (as grams/100 ml)} \times 100}{\text{Hematocrit (as per cent)}}$$

By using these indices, red cell changes in various diseases can be simply described. Anemias are roughly classed as hypochromic or normochromic, depending upon the M.C.H. and M.C.H.C., and as microcytic, normocytic, or macrocytic, depending upon the M.C.V. Red cells are sometimes described as hyperchromic, but this refers to their appearance on a stained blood film rather than to increased hemoglobin concentration. In only one condition does the M.C.H.C. genuinely rise above the normal range of 32 to 36 per cent. This is hereditary spherocytosis, and values to 39 per cent have been reported.[30]

MORPHOLOGY

The morphology and functional capacity of the erythrocytes, as well as their number and size, must often be evaluated. Morphology is best approached through study of a stained smear of peripheral blood. The normal red cell is a nonnucleated, biconcave disk approximately 7 to 8 microns in diameter. When it enters the blood stream from the marrow, all traces of nuclear material have normally disappeared. If immature red cells are released in response to massive erythropoietic stimulation, circulating cells may contain a variety of nuclear remains.

Reticulocytes

Most commonly seen are cells somewhat larger than normal, lacking the normal pale center, and taking more of the basic dye than normal. This gives them a faintly grayish purple hue in a Wright-stained preparation. If the blood is treated with a vital stain, such as brilliant cresyl blue, a delicate tracery of basophilic material can be seen throughout the cell.

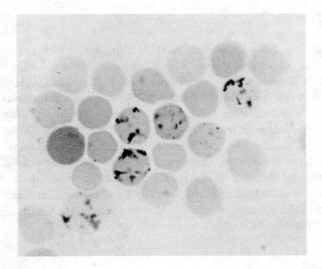

Figure 1. Reticulocytes in blood of patient with a severe hemolytic process. The smear is stained with brilliant cresyl blue; the netlike material cannot be seen on smears stained only with Wright's stain.

These cells are called reticulocytes, from the netlike appearance of the retained material (Fig. 1). Individuals with normal erythropoiesis, in good health, have between 0.5 and 1.5 per cent reticulocytes in their circulating blood. If there is red cell loss through bleeding or hemolysis, erythropoiesis becomes more active, and the number of circulating reticulocytes increases. In conditions of blood loss, absence of an elevated reticulocyte count indicates bone marrow hypofunction.

Nuclear Fragments

Other nuclear remnants may be seen in various conditions. These may take the form of fine or coarse dots, threadlike structures, or twisted rings. Nucleated red cells may be present if the erythropoietic stimulus is great enough to force red cells out of the marrow and into the blood before nuclear extrusion begins. Basophilic stippling is the name given to uniformly distributed, tiny blue dots visible on Wright-stained blood smears in lead poisoning, thalassemia, and other conditions in which normal hemoglobin production is impaired. The larger granules and structures visible in red cells during malarial attacks are not nuclear remnants, but trophozoal structures.

Siderotic Granules

Mature red cells sometimes contain granules of iron-containing substances other than hemoglobin, which become visible if blood smears are stained with Prussian blue reaction. Such cells, called siderocytes, are normally present in small numbers, but become more numerous in hemolytic anemias or following splenectomy. In iron-deficiency anemia, siderotic granules disappear from the cells in both circulating blood and bone marrow. The normal bone marrow contains a modest amount of stored iron. In certain conditions, clusters of siderotic granules may occupy the cytoplasm of erythrocyte precursors, frequently in a perinuclear position. These cells are called sideroblasts, or ringed sideroblasts, and the condition is known as sideroblastic or sideroachrestic anemia (see Chap. 13, Diseases Affecting Red Blood Cells).

Heinz Bodies

Heinz bodies are refractile inclusions that vary in size from 1 to 4 microns and can be demonstrated in erythrocytes with supravital stains. These are thought to consist of denatured hemoglobin[20] and can be induced in blood from patients with glucose-6-phosphate dehydrogenase deficiency.

Several genetically determined hemoglobinopathies are characterized by the appearance of Heinz bodies in circulating erythrocytes following splenectomy. Before splenectomy, these patients with "unstable" hemoglobins, or Heinz body anemia,[9] have sustained hemolysis and splenomegaly. When the spleen is removed, circulating cells show marked variation in size and shape, with numerous inclusion bodies. The shortened life span of such patients is not significantly improved by splenectomy.[20]

Poikilocytosis

Cells that have both diminished hemoglobin content and alterations of morphology may assume a variety of sizes and shapes. The term *poikilocytosis* is used to describe blood in which the red cells take on bizarre shapes, with considerable variety in depth of staining. Among the commonest abnormal cells are target cells or leptocytes (thin cells) in which a central stained area is surrounded by a wide zone of central pallor. The hemoglobin-containing rim is usually thin. These cells may be seen in any hypochromic anemia, but are particularly numerous in blood from patients with

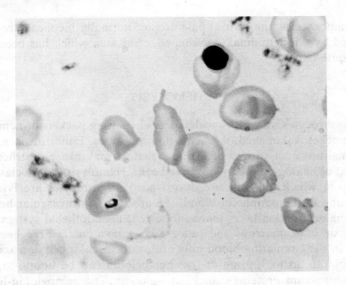

Figure 2. Target cells in blood from patient with thalassemia. Note also retained nuclear fragments and variation in size and shape of the erythrocytes.

hemoglobin C disease, or combined hemoglobin C and hemoglobin S. They are also common in thalassemia (Fig. 2) and in patients with liver disease.

Red cells that are thinner than normal or have decreased hemoglobin content appear as pale, ringlike structures with a wide, central, clear area. Spherocytes are abnormally thick cells that lack central pallor and stain more deeply than normal. Long, crescentic "sickle" forms are seen occasionally on smears of blood taken from a patient with sickle cell disease. Ordinarily the blood must be subjected to reduced oxygen tension to produce the sickle phenomenon, but patients in a sickle cell crisis may have a large proportion of abnormal circulating cells.

Hereditary Oddities

In several hereditary abnormalities, red cells have normal function but abnormal appearance. These must be distinguished from the morphologic abnormalities of various hemoglobinopathies or congenital spherocytosis. The two most notable are ovalocytosis and stomatocytosis, both rare but memorable and both commonly associated with shortened red cell survival. In ovalocytosis, all the red cells have an elongated, elliptical shape. Many patients with this defect have a chronic, compensated hemolytic condition with normal hemoglobin and hematocrit but shortened red cell survival.[16]

In stomatocytosis, the central pale area of normally biconcave red cells is replaced by a longitudinal, bar-shaped, clear area which has been likened to a mouth (stoma).

HEMOLYSIS

Erythrocytes may be considered as circulating packets of hemoglobin. If the packet is damaged, the hemoglobin escapes. Either intrinsic cellular abnormalities or a variety of external factors may cause destruction (hemolysis) of hemoglobin-containing red cells. Hemolysis can be classified by the site in which the cells are destroyed. If erythrocytes are lysed while circulating in the peripheral blood, the process is intravascular hemolysis; when the destruction takes place in the reticuloendothelial system of liver, spleen, or bone marrow, the process is extravascular. Free hemoglobin occurs in the circulating blood only after intravascular cell damage. In 100 ml of blood, up to 100 mg of free hemoglobin can be bound and transported by serum proteins called haptoglobins. The hemoglobin-haptoglobin complex is insoluble, so hemoglobin does not pass the glomerular filter. Once the haptoglobin capacity is exceeded, soluble hemoglobin enters the glomerular filtrate, where it may seriously damage renal tubular epithelium. Following extravascular hemolysis, liberated hemoglobin is degraded by the reticuloendothelial cells and hemoglobin does not appear in either blood or urine.

Intravascular hemolysis is more dangerous but fortunately less common than the extravascular form. It occurs in malarial attacks, in septicemia, and in cases of paroxysmal cold hemoglobinuria. Red cells deficient in glucose-6-phosphate dehydrogenase may undergo intravascular lysis following exposure to certain chemicals. Transfusion of incompatible blood can cause massive intravascular hemolysis if the antibody is strong enough and is of the *complete* or *saline-reactive* type.

Osmotic Fragility

Red cells are biconcave disks which can imbibe a certain amount of fluid without bursting, the amount being dependent on the ratio of volume to surface area. The cell wall acts as a semipermeable membrane, permitting fluid to diffuse in or out, depending on the osmotic gradient between intracellular fluid and the suspending medium. Cells in distilled water are lysed almost immediately because intracellular fluid has a much higher osmotic pressure than water, and large amounts of water enter the cell. Conversely, cells in a concentrated solution will shrivel, since the intracellular fluid loses its water to the more concentrated medium outside. Normal red cells can withstand exposure to saline solutions of 0.5 per cent concentration or greater without hemolysis, while saline solutions of 0.3 per cent or less produce complete hemolysis. Diminished ability to withstand exposure to hypotonic solutions is called osmotic fragility.

For a screening test of osmotic fragility, 0.1 ml of oxalated blood is added to each of two tubes, one containing 1.0 ml of 0.85 per cent saline solution (i.e., normal saline) and the other containing 0.50 per cent saline. After centrifugation, there should be little or no discoloration of the supernatant fluid in either tube. Appearance of a pink tinge in the 0.50 per cent tube suggests increased fragility, and a more detailed test should be performed. In this, as in all other tests of fragility, the patient's blood should be compared against known normal blood tested simultaneously.

Incubation and Quantification. In the quantitative test of osmotic fragility a series of tubes in which the saline concentration goes from 0.10 to 0.85 per cent in graded steps is used, and the degree of hemolysis is measured by colorimetric determination of hemoglobin in the supernatant solution. The test can be made more sensitive by performing it twice, first on freshly drawn blood and then on an aliquot of blood after sterile incubation at 37° C for 24 hours. This period of incubation enhances any tendency toward increased hemolysis, and rather minor deviations from normal can be detected. Both normal and abnormal cells undergo hemolysis more readily after incubation, but the change is more marked in abnormal cells.

Osmotic fragility is increased (i.e., hemolysis occurs at higher concentrations of saline, more nearly approaching the osmotic concentration of plasma) in hereditary spherocytosis, and is decreased (i.e., the surrounding medium more nearly approaches distilled water) in thalassemia, sickle cell anemia, and certain other hemoglobinopathies.

Mechanical Fragility

This test measures the capacity of the red cell to resist mechanical trauma inflicted by glass beads in a rotating flask. The amount of hemoglobin in the plasma after a period of rotation indicates the resistance of the red cells. As in the osmotic fragility test, occult abnormalities can be accentuated by incubating the blood at 37° C for 24 hours. Mechanical fragility is increased in hereditary spherocytosis and in sickle cell anemia as well. Incubation, which lowers the oxygen tension of the cells, markedly enhances the fragility of cells containing hemoglobin S. Cells from patients with autoimmune hemolytic anemia frequently have increased mechanical fragility, especially after incubation.

Hemoglobinopathies

Relatively few of the over 100 known abnormal hemoglobins produce significant hemolytic disease, and of these the group known as *unstable hemoglobins* or Heinz body anemias are numerically insignificant. Hemoglobin S and hemoglobin C, however, are common among the world's black populations and contribute significantly to worldwide morbidity from all causes.

Sickle Cell Preparation. Screening for hemoglobin S employs the physical-chemical properties of the molecular peculiarity. Reducing the oxygen tension of this hemoglobin causes the molecules to assume polymeric configurations known as tactoids or nematic fluid crystals. This occurs whether the hemoglobin is free in solution or confined within cells.

The classic screening test for hemoglobin S is addition of sodium metabisulfite, a powerful reducing agent, to a suspension of cells. The reduced oxygen tension thus created causes affected cells to assume the boat-shaped or crescentic sickle form, whether they contain predominantly hemoglobin S (as in homozygous hemoglobin S disease) or hemoglobin S combined with a normal or other abnormal hemoglobin (heterozygous hemoglobin S + A, hemoglobin S + C, and so forth). The end-point is observed microscopically after 15 minutes, requiring a moderate investment in time, space, and personnel. False negatives are not uncommon, but false positives are extremely rare.

Hemolysate Method. A relatively recent and very rapid screening procedure [26,27] uses the insolubility of the sickled hemoglobin to distinguish between a normal (clear) hemoglobin hemolysate and the abnormal (turbid) solution that occurs with hemoglobin S. Severe anemia, in which the prescribed volume of blood contains insufficient hemoglobin, can cause false negatives. False positives can occur if other protein abnormalities render the solution turbid or if glassware or reagents are contaminated. Distinguishing between clear and mildly turbid solutions only rarely causes difficulty.

Electrophoresis. Accurate delineation of hemoglobin abnormalities requires electrophoresis, combined, when necessary, with other biochemical and genetic studies. Electrophoresis permits distinction between homozygous and heterozygous hemoglobin S, which the above techniques cannot do. No biochemical screening test can presently document hemoglobin C, but electrophoresis readily detects its presence alone or with other hemoglobins. A recently developed screening electrophoretic method[1] may prove fruitful for uncovering a greater variety of hemoglobinopathies than can be detected by hemoglobin S testing alone (see also Chapter 13).

Autohemolysis

When sterile defibrinated blood is incubated for 48 hours at 37° C, relatively little hemolysis normally occurs. The addition of either glucose or adenosine triphosphate (ATP) reduces even this amount of cell damage. Spontaneous hemolysis is increased in hereditary spherocytosis, in certain kinds of congenital nonspherocytic hemolytic diseases, and in some acquired hemolytic conditions. Autohemolysis is strikingly reduced by adding glucose or ATP to red cells in congenital spherocytosis, but in the nonspherocytic hemolytic anemia caused by pyruvic kinase deficiency, glucose does not diminish hemolysis and ATP produces only a slight improvement.[33]

Primaquine Sensitivity

Red cells lacking the enzyme glucose-6-phosphate dehydrogenase (G-6-PD) are subject to in vivo hemolysis when the patient ingests any one of a variety of aromatic compounds. This deficiency affects the normal functioning of the pentose phosphate pathway so that normal oxidation and reduction reactions are impaired. The resulting lack of the reduced coenzyme nicotinamide adenine dinucleotide phosphate (NADP; formerly called triphosphopyridine nucleotide or TPN) impairs the erythrocyte reductase systems. Without glutathione reductase and the methemoglobin reductases, destructive oxidation of cellular elements occurs. Two tests used for uncovering this sex-linked disorder, which is said to affect approximately 10 per cent of American Negro males,[20] are discussed in the next two paragraphs.

Methylene Blue. The most effective procedure[6] challenges the methemoglobin reductase system by oxidizing hemoglobin to methemoglobin with sodium nitrite. Simultaneous addition of methylene blue activates the pentose phosphate pathway to regenerate the reduced coenzyme from the NADP form to NADPH, and permit methemoglobin reductase to restore the oxidized hemoglobin to normal. In red cells which lack glucose-6-phosphate dehydrogenase, the pentose phosphate shunt cannot support methemoglobin reductase activity, and the methemoglobin persists as a muddy grayish brown compound easily distinguished from the clear red appearance of the normal control. A micro method has been adapted[22] for this test, permitting rapid screening of large groups and requiring little equipment or space.

Fluorescent spot test. A recent, rapid, and moderately precise screening test[3] results in the appearance of a fluorescent spot if NADP is reduced to NADPH. Incubating normal blood with NADP and glucose-6-phosphate effects this reduction, but blood from G-6-PD deficient patients cannot produce the fluorescent end-point.

Heinz Bodies. An older procedure[2] induces hemoglobin denaturation by incubating the blood with acetylphenylhydrazine and abundant oxygen. In cells lacking sufficient reducing capacity, large numbers of Heinz bodies can be detected by staining the preparation with crystal violet. This procedure is less reproducible than the methylene blue technique, and preparing readable smears can be somewhat difficult.

Paroxysmal Nocturnal Hemoglobinuria

In a rare condition that affects either sex and intensifies with advancing age, intravascular hemolysis occurs during sleep. The patient, upon awakening, experiences hemoglobinemia and hemoglobinuria.[21] The defect resides in the cells, which are destroyed following transfusion into normal individuals. Normal red cells survive normally if transfused into an affected patient.[11] The defect is demonstrated by incubating 0.05 ml of a 50 per cent suspension of red cells with 0.5 ml of serum acidified by adding 0.05 ml of 0.2N hydrochloric acid. Either normal or patient's serum may be used to produce hemolysis, while normal cells are not destroyed on incubation with the patient's acidified serum. The reaction is complement-dependent, and heating the serum to 56° C abolishes the hemolysis.

Antibodies

Circulating antibodies either sensitize or directly destroy certain specific types of cell. Blood group antibodies can be detected with the indirect Coombs test (see p. 77), and ordinarily cause hemolysis only when incompatible cells are transfused. Some patients with hemolytic anemia appear to have antibodies that react with their own cells. The presence of antibody on the cell surface can be demonstrated by the direct Coombs test (see p. 75).

Donath-Landsteiner Antibody. In a condition called paroxysmal cold hemoglobinuria, intravascular hemolysis may occur if the patient, or one of his extremities, is exposed to cold temperatures. These patients have in their serum a peculiar and characteristic antibody: it requires a cold temperature in order to attach to the cell, but does not destroy the cell in the cold. Hemolysis occurs only when the cell-antibody complex is warmed to 37° C. This behavior is the basis for the Donath-Landsteiner test, in which washed cells, either the patient's or normal cells, are incubated with the suspected serum for 30 minutes at 4° C, and then at 37° C for an hour. Heating the serum to 56° C destroys this activity, which appears to have a blood group specificity directed against an extremely common antigen. Since most cells possess the antigen, most cells will be hemolyzed, but the rare cells which lack the P + P₁ antigen are not affected.[24] Paroxysmal cold hemoglobinuria, the only condition in which this test is positive, is discussed more fully in Chapter 13.

Cold Agglutinins. To be distinguished from the Donath-Landsteiner antibody, which requires sequential exposure first to cold and then to warm temperatures, certain antibodies cause agglutination (rarely hemolysis) of any cells in cold temperatures. Either the patient's own cells or random group O cells can be used to demonstrate the presence of these cold agglutinins. For the test, serially diluted serum is incubated with red cells, one series of dilutions at 4° C and another series at room temperature. Normal serum may, at 4° C, agglutinate group O cells at dilutions as high as 1:32, but will not agglutinate cells at room temperature. The cold agglutinins which accompany certain viral diseases may have titers as high as 1:64,000, and may agglutinate the cells at room temperature as well. Unlike the agglutination produced by blood group antibodies, this type of agglutination can be reversed by warming to 37° C. Reagglutination is induced by returning the cell-antibody mixture to 4° C. Most patients with virus-associated cold agglutinins have no clinical symptoms, but occasionally a hemolytic episode may complicate the pneumonia. The agglutinin does not usually persist beyond several weeks, but some few patients with no history of viral disease persistently have enormous titers of cold agglutinins and may suffer from hemolysis or from peripheral vascular occlusion in cold surroundings.

ERYTHROCYTE SEDIMENTATION RATE

The sedimentation rate measures the speed with which red cells settle in fluid blood, so anticoagulated blood must be used. A column of blood 100 mm high is placed in a tube 1 mm in diameter and is left undisturbed for one hour. This permits direct observation of the rate of fall, and no calculations are needed to express the result in millimeters per hour.

The rate at which red cells settle through a column of fluid blood depends on the concentration of various plasma protein fractions and on the concentration of the red cells. When the proportion of plasma is high and red cell content is low, the cells sediment far more rapidly than in blood with a normal hematocrit. For this reason, it is customary to correct the sedimentation rate for the effect of anemia. The presence of increased quantities of fibrinogen or of abnormal globulins or globulin fractions accelerates the rate of sedimentation. Thus, high sedimentation rates are to be expected in pregnancy, in multiple myeloma, in certain lymphomas, and in the so-called gammopathies, conditions in which abnormal gamma globulins circulate in large quantity. The sedimentation rate rises in response to severe localized or generalized inflammatory processes and when there is a systemic response to tissue necrosis. In chronic inflammatory processes such as tuberculosis and rheumatic fever, Wintrobe[35] believes that the sedimentation rate may be a useful index of the activity of latent tissue reaction. A decreased sedimentation rate occurs in sickle cell disease, in which the cells' abnormal shape and adhesiveness apparently prevent rapid settling through the fluid medium.

WHITE BLOOD CELLS

The cellular elements of blood include, besides the erythrocytes, the leukocytes and platelets. The leukocytes really are white, as the name implies; examination of a centrifuged tube of blood reveals a slightly fuzzy grayish white layer between the packed red cells and the clear yellowish plasma. This "buffy coat" contains the white cells and platelets, and owes its grayish white appearance to the presence of packed white cells.

Three principal types of white cells exist in the body. These are the granulocytes, the lymphocytes, and the monocytes, all of which can be found not only in the blood but also in the fixed tissues. The white cells in the blood probably represent a traveling contingent of constantly changing identity.

GRANULOCYTES

The earliest recognizable bone marrow cell in the granulocytic series is the myeloblast, which probably derives from a stem cell common to the red cell and white cell populations. The myeloblast differentiates through a promyelocytic stage to become a myelocyte, which is the first stage to contain recognizable cytoplasmic granules. These are classified as neutrophilic, basophilic, or eosinophilic, depending upon their reaction with a polychrome stain. The granules increase as maturation progresses through the stages of metamyelocyte and band forms, finally resulting in mature cells with segmented nuclei.

Neutrophils

Mature neutrophilic granulocytes—also called neutrophils or polymorphonuclear leukocytes (PMNs)—are the most numerous of circulating white cells in normal adults. In the blood of young children, neutrophils are relatively less conspicuous owing to the numbers of mature lymphocytes which alter the proportions of circulating cells. Up to 6 per cent of the circulating leukocytes in adults or children may be eosinophils, and basophils are by far the least numerous of the granulocytes.

Neutrophils seem to be the body's first defense in combating infection and other trauma. Neutrophils are thought to be drawn into the peripheral blood and toward the site of injury by products derived from necrotic tissue or bacteria. The process which impels cells to move from one area to another is called chemotaxis. All the granulocytes, as well as monocytes, are capable of active locomotion through vessel walls and through tissue. Neutrophils perform their protective function by phagocytosis—engulfment of particles and especially of bacteria. The neutrophils do not elaborate antibodies, but they transport enzymes which may be functional in phagocytosis. In phagocytizing certain types of bacteria, neutrophils are materially assisted by the presence of circulating antibodies called opsonins, which render the bacteria more liable to engulfment. Eosinophils and basophils are much less active in phagocytosis. There is some evidence that neutrophils must be present at a site of injury in order for lymphocytes, monocytes, and other reparative cells to be attracted subsequently.[28]

Nitroblue Tetrazolium Test. When granulocytes attack bacteria, they phagocytize the organisms into vacuoles, and then destroy the trapped bacteria enzymatically. Releasing lysosomal enzymes into the vacuole requires energy, apparently derived from the hexose monophosphate shunt, and requires active regeneration of the enzymes NADH oxidase and myeloperoxidase.[12] The metabolic activation necessary for successful bactericidal phagocytosis can be monitored by inducing a visible biochemical reaction, the reduction of nitroblue tetrazolium (NBT) to formazan.

Contact with bacteria, or bacterial products, alters granulocyte metabolism in such a way that extracellular NBT can be phagocytized and reduced to blue-black formazan granules within the vacuole. NBT reduction has been incorporated into a test with diagnostic potential in two different situations. Individuals with deficient enzyme systems are unable to mount the lysosomal attack; granulocytes from these patients are unable to phagocytize and reduce NBT after contact with bacterial products which should activate this mechanism. Absence of NBT reduction is a significant feature in diagnosing granulomatous disease of childhood or chronic granulomatous disease, a condition in which deficient bactericidal activity leads to chronic suppurative and granulomatous infections.

IN BACTERIAL INFECTIONS. Of more widespread diagnostic use is the observation that the circulating granulocytes of patients with systemic bacterial infections are already activated to a degree that they will spontaneously reduce NBT.[29] In normal individuals, or those with leukocytosis of nonbacterial origin, fewer than 10 per cent of circulating granulocytes spontaneously reduce NBT. Of granulocytes from infected patients, 15 to 45 per cent develop formazan granules when exposed to NBT. This metabolic change accompanies gram-positive or gram-negative bacterial infections and may occur in malarial and certain fungal infections. The leukocytosis of collagen diseases, advanced carcinomas, pulmonary emboli, and other nonbacterial inflammatory conditions tends to be NBT negative.[25] With tuberculous infections, the response is ambiguous. Pulmonary tuberculosis appears not to give a positive NBT test, but tuberculous meningitis and hematogenous infection do.[14]

Eosinophils and Basophils

The functions of eosinophils and basophils are poorly understood. Eosinophilic granules appear to be a protein core surrounded by phospholipid, while basophilic granules are water soluble and contain a substance which may be heparin. In the mast cells of fixed tissue, there is a similar substance enclosed in similar large granules, and mast cells and basophils appear to be functionally related. Both eosinophils and basophils transport significant amounts of histamine, the eosinophils carrying the larger portion. Despite their frequent temporal and spatial association with allergic phenomena, the role of eosinophils in the etiology or manifestations of allergic reactions is unclear.[4] Nor is it clear why eosinophils disappear promptly from the blood following injection of certain adrenal steroids.

The life span of granulocytic cells has been investigated by many workers, with somewhat divergent results. Clearly, their life is measured in days, rather than weeks or months, but estimates have varied from 24 hours to seven days.[5] Although its physiologic role is a mystery, alkaline phosphatase is found in significant amounts in granulocytes, but is absent from the other circulating leukocytes. Leukocyte alkaline phosphatase increases in reactive leukocytosis and polycythemia vera and decreases in chronic myelogenous leukemia, even though the leukemic cells may be morphologically identical to normal mature granulocytes.

LYMPHOCYTES

The circulating lymphocytes, which comprise 20 to 40 per cent of the white cells in normal adult blood, are only a small percentage of the body's total lymphocyte population. These small, round cells derive from the bone marrow, the lymph nodes, and the thymus. A complicated circulatory pathway exists involving marrow, blood, lymph fluid, lymph nodes, and spleen. Continuous production and destruction exists, although many lymphocytes in the circulation have a life span of months or years. In response to specific immune stimuli, pronounced multiplication can occur, notably in lymph node and splenic follicles, while inflammatory stimuli cause local accumulation of lymphocytes without conspicuous proliferative activity.

Thymus-Dependent Lymphocytes

Lymphocytes, their precursors, and their progeny are the principal effectors of the body's immune response.[17] The two types of immune response, usually described as cell-mediated and humoral, both derive from lymphoid cells, the difference arising from preconditioning of some sort directed by one of two major influences. The thymus bears the brunt of orchestrating the cell-mediated response; lymphocytes under this influence are called thymus-dependent or T-lymphocytes. This group contains the majority of circulating lymphocytes which are also found in lymph nodes in the deep cortical and outermost follicular layers, in the periarteriolar zone in the spleen, and diffusely in other tissues. This population, in its inactive form morphologically indistinguishable from the other major group, is long-lived and remains capable of mitotic activity despite months or years of uneventful circulation.

Antibody-Producing Cells

The other lymphocyte population is designated B-lymphocyte or bursa-dependent. This name derives from analogy with the avian immunologic system in which a specific organ, the bursa of Fabricius, regulates those lymphocytes destined to produce humoral antibodies. In man and other mammals, no discrete organ or site of comparable activity has been identified. The B-lymphocytes appear to be short-lived, with extremely active lymphopoiesis predominantly in the bone marrow,[10] although the differentiation of small uncommitted lymphocyte into antibody-producing plasma cell occurs outside the marrow. B-lymphocytes are found in lymph nodes in the medullary cords, the central follicular areas and the peripheral cortical area, in the red pulp and the follicle centers of the spleen, and in subepithelial lymph follicles in many organs. The lympholytic action of corticosteroids, irradiation, and so forth is probably most active against this pool of short-lived, rapidly proliferating cells.[10]

MONOCYTES

Both origin and function of the circulating monocyte are unclear. A precursor form, the monoblast, is sometimes found in the bone marrow in monocytic leukemia but is not a normal inhabitant of the marrow. Neither production site nor precursor cell has been identified in the tissues, and it may be that monocytes originate in many areas from cells with no morphologic characteristics to distinguish them from a multitude of other round or ovoid cells.

Monocytes are not known to serve any function within the blood, although they constitute a rather stable proportion of circulating white cells in both adults and children. Quite possibly, monocytes exist in the blood only in transit to serve a principal function within the tissues. In the tissue, they are capable of ameboid movement and active phagocytosis. Tissue monocytes, macrophages, participate in both humoral and cell-mediated immune reactions. Epithelioid cells and Langhans' giant cells derive from the monocyte, and the number of circulating monocytes may rise dramatically in tuberculosis.

The life span of the monocyte is probably short, in the same range as the granulocyte, but this too is a subject of controversy.

WHITE CELL COUNT

The white cell concentration is determined by counting cells in a diluted sample. For manual counts, the blood is diluted 1:20, and the volume of diluted blood examined is 0.4 cu mm, so errors of enumeration are magnified by multiplication. The dilution figure for one widely used electronic enumerator is 1:250. To eliminate interference by the far more numerous erythrocytes, the leukocytes must be suspended in diluting fluid which lyses the red cells. Normal values for adults range between 5,000 and 10,000 white cells per cu mm, though values to 4,000 and 11,000 per cu mm may not be significant under most circumstances.

The Differential Count

As important as the total number of leukocytes is the proportion of cell types present. The normal proportions vary with age, as shown in Table 3. The simplest, most productive determination of white cell proportions is the differential white count, performed on a smear of blood one cell layer thick and stained with a polychrome solution containing both basic and acidic dyes. The stain most used is Wright's stain which contains alkalinized methylene blue mixed with eosin. When the stain is carefully applied, the erythrocytes appear pink; the leukocytic nuclei are purplish blue; the cytoplasm shades from blue to faintly pink; and the cytoplasmic

Table 3.   Differential White Counts at Varying Ages
(Values given as per cent of total white cells)*

	Adult	Birth	1 Year	10 Years
Neutrophils	50-75	45-70	20-40	40-60
Lymphocytes	20-45	25-35	50-75	25-45
Monocytes	2-10	2-10	2-10	2-10
Eosinophils	0-6	0-6	0-6	0-6
Basophils	0-1	0-1	0-1	0-1

* From Damm, H. (ed.): CRC Handbook of Clinical Laboratory Data. Chemical Rubber Co., Cleveland, Ohio, 1965. Used by permission of Chemical Rubber Co.

granules show up sharply as lilac, red, and bluish black in neutrophils, eosinophils, and basophils respectively.

A well-prepared, well-stained blood film permits evaluation not only of the relative proportions of white cells, but of the morphology of all cellular elements, and the number and morphology of platelets as well. Meaningful examination becomes impossible if smears are too thick or too thin, unevenly distributed, over- or understained, or excessively acid or alkaline. Smears should not be made from blood to which anticoagulant has been added, for nuclear details and staining characteristics may be markedly altered.

It is customary to count 100 white cells, and report the numbers of each cell present in terms of per cent. Differences in the total white count, however, may alter the significance of counting 100 cells. If the total white count is low, 100 cells is a large proportion of the cells present, and the differential count is probably representative of the actual distribution of cell types. When counts are very high, 100 cells is such a small proportion of the circulating cells that it may not adequately reflect the overall distribution.

It is possible to count the absolute number of eosinophils or basophils per cubic millimeter of blood, using special diluting fluid that destroys the interfering erythrocytes and either destroys or leaves unstained the other white cells. The eosinophil count is sometimes used in evaluating allergic conditions and in the Thorn test for studying the adrenal response to ACTH. The absolute basophil count is rarely done, but it may be useful in evaluating early leukemia and certain types of hypersensitivity states.[31]

CONDITIONS THAT ALTER THE LEUKOCYTE COUNT

The number of circulating neutrophils may rise in response to certain physiologic stimuli, and the total white count may transiently reach values between 20,000 and 30,000 per mm³ without any underlying disease. These physiologic stresses include strenuous exercise, severe emotional distress, paroxysmal tachycardia, and parturition. Such elevation subsides to normal within one or several hours, so the white count should be repeated under relaxed circumstances if the elevated count appears doubtfully significant.

Neutrophilia

The granulocytes respond to stimulation by entering and leaving the blood more promptly than lymphocytes or monocytes. Increased numbers of neutrophils, often including immature forms, occur with infections caused by most gram-positive bacteria and by many gram-negative bacteria, certain viruses, and some rickettsiae. Systemic or localized infections may cause neutrophilia, ordinarily in the range of 15,000 to 40,000 per cu mm but sometimes much higher, depending on the severity of the infection and the resistance of the patient.

Whenever significant tissue or cell damage is present, neutrophilia may occur. This includes such diverse conditions as myocardial infarction, severe burns and other accidents, acute hemolysis, rapid growth or necrosis of malignant neoplasms, and hemorrhage into body cavities. In such cases, the white count rarely exceeds 30,000 per mm^3. Metabolic derangement, from intrinsic causes such as diabetic acidosis or gout or from extrinsic causes like drug or chemical intoxication or insect venoms, may elevate counts to 20,000 to 25,000 per mm^3. Acute external hemorrhage produces a prompt leukocytosis to approximately 20,000 per mm^3. The highest white counts occur with leukemia, especially chronic myelogenous leukemia which causes leukocytosis to 300,000 per mm^3 or higher. Rarely, a reactive leukocytosis may reach levels of 100,000 or more, producing a leukemoid appearance which may be difficult to distinguish from leukemia.

Table 4 lists conditions that are accompanied by neutrophilia.

Neutropenia

Following a variety of stimuli, neutrophils may disappear rather rapidly from the circulation, producing a state of neutropenia (see Table 4). If the lymphocytes are not also affected, a relative lymphocytosis occurs, even though the absolute number of lymphocytes remains unchanged. Neutropenia may be a sudden, idiosyncratic response to some drug or chemical, or it may follow administration of known bone marrow depressants. Certain infections routinely cause neutropenia, especially rickettsial diseases and most viral diseases, including influenza, hepatitis, and many

Table 4. Conditions That Affect Neutrophils*

A. Increased neutrophil counts accompany:
1. Infections: Especially with pyogenic bacteria; either localized, as appendiceal abscess, or generalized, as septicemia.
2. Other disorders associated with acute inflammation or cellular necrosis: Infarction, collagen disease, acute hemolysis.
3. Neoplasms: Leukemia, carcinoma, lymphomas, especially with areas of tissue necrosis and widespread metastases.
4. Intoxications: Drugs; chemicals, especially in poisonings with liver damage.
5. Acute hemorrhage.

B. Decreased neutrophil counts accompany:
1. Infections: Acute viral (rubeola, infectious hepatitis); bacterial (brucellosis, typhoid fever); protozoal (malaria, kala-azar); and overwhelming infections (septicemia).
2. Bone marrow damage: Aplastic anemia or neutropenia due to unknown cause; irradiation; toxic drugs and chemicals (benzol, mustard drugs, antimetabolic agents); drug idiosyncrasy (amidopyrine, sulfonamides, and others).
3. Disorders associated with splenomegaly: Congestive splenomegaly; diseases of the reticuloendothelial system (parasitic diseases, chronic infections, neoplasms); Felty's syndrome.
4. Other disorders: Disseminated lupus erythematosus; anaphylaxis; "aleukemic" leukemia.
5. Nutritional deficiency: Vitamin B_{12}; folic acid.

---

* Adapted, with permission, from Leavell, B.S., and Thorup, O.: Fundamentals of Clinical Hematology, ed. 3. W.B. Saunders Co., Philadelphia, 1971.

exanthems. Typhoid and paratyphoid characteristically cause neutropenia, as does malaria. Sufficiently massive infection by any organism may paralyze the body's responses and produce neutropenia instead of the expected leukocytosis. The more debilitated the patient, the less severe the infection need be to produce this response.

In most conditions of splenic enlargement, there is some degree of neutropenia, sometimes associated with thrombocytopenia as well. Pernicious anemia frequently causes neutropenia, and the remaining granulocytes tend to be large, with excessively segmented and twisted nuclei. Disseminated lupus erythematosus may produce neutropenia, and in some cases of infectious mononucleosis the white count is low.

Eosinophilia

Eosinophilia describes an increase of circulating eosinophils above the normal level of approximately 250 per cu mm, or 2 to 6 per cent of the total white cells. The most notable causes of eosinophilia are allergic conditions, certain skin diseases, and parasitic infestation. A list of common etiologies appears in Table 5. Elevation of the number of eosinophils above 15 per cent in the differential white count is rare, but in pemphigus, acute trichinosis, severe bronchial asthma, and angioneurotic edema higher values are

Table 5.   Conditions That Affect Other Leukocytes*

A. Lymphocytosis may accompany:
   1. Infections
      a. Acute: Infectious mononucleosis, pertussis, infectious lymphocytosis, other viral and bacillary infections.
      b. Convalescence: Especially from viral infections.
      c. Chronic: Tuberculosis, brucellosis, syphilis.
   2. Neoplasms: Lymphocytic leukemia, lymphosarcoma.
   3. Metabolic disease: Hyperthyroidism.
B. Monocytosis may accompany:
   1. Infections
      a. Bacterial: Tuberculosis, subacute bacterial endocarditis, brucellosis, typhoid fever.
      b. Protozoal: Malaria, kala-azar.
      c. Rickettsial: Rocky Mountain spotted fever.
   2. Neoplasms: Monocytic leukemia, Hodgkin's disease, reticuloendotheliosis.
   3. Recovery from infections and agranulocytosis; polycythemia vera.
C. Eosinophilia may accompany:
   1. Allergic reactions: Bronchial asthma, drug reactions, allergic dermatitis, hay fever, angioneurotic edema.
   2. Parasitic infestation: Intestinal (hookworm, tapeworm, ascaris, *Taenia echinococcus*); especially with muscle invasion by trichina.
   3. Skin diseases: Exfoliative dermatitis, pemphigus, dermatitis herpetiformis.
   4. Neoplasms: Metastatic carcinoma, myelocytic leukemia, Hodgkin's disease.
   5. Other diseases: Periarteritis nodosa, eosinophilic granuloma.

* Adapted, with permission, from Leavell, B.S., and Thorup, O.: Fundamentals of Clinical Hematology, ed. 3. W.B. Saunders Co., Philadelphia, 1971.

not uncommon. Following irradiation, mild eosinophilia may be noted, and some degree of eosinophilia may occur with pernicious anemia, periarteritis nodosa, and Hodgkin's disease. Some of the post-streptococcal conditions have been reported to cause eosinophilia, such as scarlet fever, chorea, and erythema multiforme, but not acute rheumatic fever.[35]

A decrease in circulating eosinophils is seldom noteworthy, except in performing the Thorn test for adrenal function (see p. 388). Eosinophils undergo an absolute and relative reduction in most conditions which produce neutrophilia, presumably due to the increased adrenal steroid production that accompanies most conditions of bodily stress.

Basophilia

Basophils normally occupy so small a percentage of the circulating white cells that a decline is scarcely noticeable, while an increase is easily recognized. Relatively few conditions cause basophilic leukocytosis, most notably chronic myelocytic leukemia and polycythemia vera. Other conditions include colitis, myxedema, and Hodgkin's disease,[31,35] while a decrease in the absolute basophil count has been reported in acute allergic reactions, hyperthyroidism, and any stress reaction associated with increased corticosteroid production.[31]

Lymphocytosis

Lymphocytosis occurs in two varieties: relative, in which the total number of circulating lymphocytes is unchanged, but the white count is low due to neutropenia; and absolute, in which the number of circulating lymphocytes increases. Relative lymphocytosis accompanies most conditions mentioned under neutropenia, and may occur in hyperthyroidism.

Absolute lymphocytosis occurs in pertussis and in many of the viral exanthems. Such chronic infections as tuberculosis, secondary or congenital syphilis, or brucellosis may cause a mild-to-moderate lymphocytosis. After many viral infections and sometimes after a bacterial infection with neutrophilia, lymphocytosis may mark the convalescent period. The degree of lymphocytosis is seldom pronounced, except in acute pertussis and in a benign, self-limited condition of unknown etiology called acute infectious lymphocytosis. Very pronounced lymphocytosis is characteristic of chronic lymphocytic leukemia, and a somewhat less marked increase occurs in most lymphomas, although Hodgkins's disease usually produces lymphopenia. Children with rickets or severe malnutrition may maintain their high lymphocyte counts past the age at which childhood lymphocytosis usually disappears.

Lymphopenia

Relatively few diseases cause lymphocytes to disappear, but prompt lymphopenia follows small doses of radiation or of adrenal corticosteroids. Nitrogen mustards affect lymphocytes more promptly than granulocytes. Patients with miliary tuberculosis, systemic lupus erythematosus, or uremia occasionally have low lymphocyte counts.

Monocytosis

An increase in circulating monocytes occurs most frequently in tuberculosis, but monocytes may also increase in some protozoal or rickettsial infections such as malaria and Rocky Mountain spotted fever. Monocytosis may occur with Hodgkin's disease, and with diseases affecting the reticuloendothelial system, such as Gaucher's disease and other lipoidoses. Monocytic leukemia, of course, markedly elevates the number of mature and early monocytes in both the blood and the bone marrow.

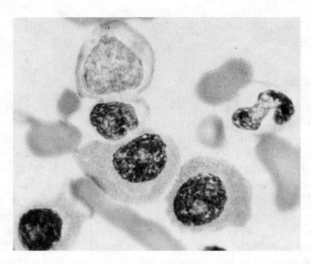

Figure 3.   Atypical immature plasma cells in bone marrow of patient with multiple myeloma.

ABNORMAL WHITE CELLS

Plasma Cells

Plasma cells do not normally circulate, and there are normally only small numbers even in the bone marrow. Demonstration of plasma cells in the blood must arouse suspicion of multiple myeloma, but Wintrobe[35] reports their occasional presence in rubella, serum sickness, and infectious mononucleosis. In multiple myeloma, plasma cells are far more striking in the bone marrow, where they may exhibit many abnormalities of maturation and morphology (Fig. 3). Plasma cell leukemia is a rare condition in which large numbers of plasma cells are present in blood and bone marrow. Plasma cells are virtually absent from the bone marrow in children below the age of five years. Adults with immune globulin deficiencies have very few plasma cells in the marrow.[32]

Atypical Lymphocytes

Atypical lymphocytes are usually associated with infectious mononucleosis (Fig. 4), but may sometimes occur in viral hepatitis, other viral diseases, and allergic conditions. These lymphocytes tend to be larger than normal, with a vacuolated or foamy cytoplasm and a coarse chromatin network in the nucleus. The classical description of these cells was by

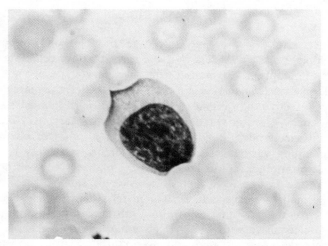

Figure 4.   Atypical lymphocyte in blood from patient with infectious mononucleosis. Note the coarse nuclear chromatin pattern, vacuolated cytoplasm, and cytoplasmic indentation by adjoining erythrocytes.

Downey,[13] who described three types of abnormal lymphocytes distinguished by their size, abnormal cytoplasmic morphology, and a variably immature nuclear chromatin pattern.

The L.E. Cell

The so-called lupus erythematosus cell (L.E. cell) is not a circulating leukocyte, and the blood sample must be manipulated in the laboratory to produce the *L.E. phenomenon.* It is included in this discussion because it is an abnormal cell familiar to those who examine blood smears. The L.E. cell is a polymorphonuclear leukocyte—usually a neutrophil but rarely an eosinophil—that surrounds a round, homogeneous, structureless inclusion body. The inclusion is denatured nuclear protein which is undergoing phagocytosis by the granulocyte. The formation of L.E. cells requires three ingredients: the *L.E. factor,* an abnormal, heat-labile serum protein which alters nuclear protein; a source of nuclear protein; and phagocytic cells to engulf the altered material. The L.E. factor appears in the serum of many patients with lupus erythematosus. The patient's serum, incubated with some exogenous source of nucleoprotein, can induce the L.E. phenomenon in normal granulocytes, for it is the altered protein, rather than the phagocytic cells, that produces the characteristic appearance. Except in special situations, the patient's serum and cells are usually used together to demonstrate the phenomenon.

PLATELETS

Platelets can easily be recognized as particles on examination of stained blood smears. Platelets, not themselves intact cells, are granular fragments of cytoplasm originating from megakaryocytes in the bone marrow. Lacking a nucleus and certain cellular organelles, the platelets are less metabolically active than intact cells and their role in hemostasis depends in part on energy transfer reactions. Platelets consist largely of phospholipids and polysaccharides, but they transport a number of chemical substances including various plasma clotting factors, a variety of enzymes, several clot-promoting factors specific to the platelets, and serotonin. The platelet clotting factors have definite physiologic significance, and hemostatic abnormalities occur with certain platelet deficiencies. The possible physiologic roles of the other transported substances are still under investigation. Platelets share with leukocytes certain antigenic groups, but standardized platelet grouping analogous to erythrocyte grouping is not yet a reality.

The number and morphology of the platelets can be roughly evaluated by examining stained blood films. The phase microscopy method of platelet counting permits fairly accurate quantitation of the circulating platelets. Light microscopic enumeration is also possible but is somewhat less accurate.

Electronic particle counting permits the most rapid and accurate platelet enumeration now available. The coefficient of variation is as low as 4 per cent,[8] and technician effort is reduced to a minimum. The disadvantages include the necessity of removing interfering red blood cells, and of using a hematocrit-based factor to correct the observed plasma platelet count to a whole-blood figure.[7]

A more complete discussion of platelet evaluation is found (p. 360) in the chapter on the hemostatic mechanisms and their abnormalities.

BLOOD COAGULATION

Although a fuller discussion of hemostasis is presented in the section on hemostatic mechanisms, it is appropriate to include a few words about clotting factors here. Various terms and theories abound in the field of blood coagulation, and it is not our intention to exacerbate any controversy. Figure 5 embodies current theory about the clotting processes, using the numerical terminology assigned to the clotting factors by the International Committee for the Nomenclature of Blood Coagulation Factors. A listing and brief description of the individual factors follows. Tests of clotting function are discussed in Chapter 15.

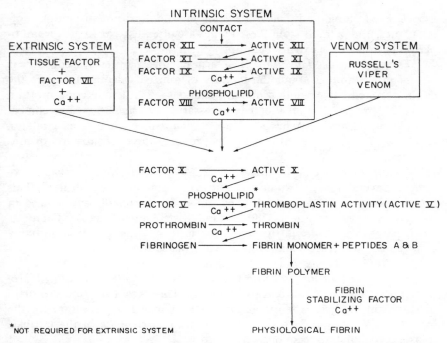

Figure 5. Schema of the intrinsic and extrinsic clotting systems as well as the artificially induced venom system. Note that activation of factor X is the key step in all three systems, and there is only one set of later reactions. (Redrawn, with permission, from Leavell, B.S., and Thorup, O.: Fundamentals of Clinical Hematology, ed. 3. W.B. Saunders Company, Philadelphia, 1971.)

Factor I (almost always called fibrinogen; no other synonyms are currently used). This plasma protein of high molecular weight is synthesized in the liver, and is normally present in the plasma at concentrations of approximately 300 mg per 100 ml. Fibrinogen is hydrolyzed through the proteolytic action of thrombin into polypeptide fragments which recombine to form fibrin.

Factor II (usually referred to as prothrombin). Hepatic synthesis of this protein requires adequate supplies of vitamin K. Prothrombin has a molecular weight of approximately 62,000.[23] It is the inactive precursor of thrombin which is too powerful a proteolytic agent to exist as such in the circulating blood.

Factor III (tissue thromboplastin). Rather than describing a single substance, this term refers to the clot-promoting activity inherent in many tissues. Brain, lung, and placenta are among the most potent clot-promoting tissues, and extracts from these tissues are often used as tissue thromboplastin in tests of the extrinsic clotting system.

Factor IV (ionized calcium). The term Factor IV is never used; there is no misunderstanding about the identity of ionized calcium. It enters the clotting system at several different reactions. A calcium concentration above 2.5 mg per 100 ml blood is necessary for coagulation, but clinical hypocalcemia never reaches this level. Such anticoagulants as oxalates, citrate, and EDTA prevent clotting by reducing the concentration of ionized calcium.

Factor V (proaccelerin, labile factor, Ac-globulin, thromboplastin cofactor). Several synonyms and the numeric designation are all used. This protein disappears rapidly from shed blood. It is probably synthesized in the liver, but is not one of the vitamin K-dependent factors. Factor V participates in both the intrinsic and extrinsic systems, and it is probably consumed in the process since it is absent from serum.

Factor VI. This term is no longer used.

Factor VII (serum prothrombin conversion accelerator, SPCA, proconvertin, pro-SPCA, autoprothrombin I). This is a heat-stable protein produced in the liver when vitamin K is available. It is necessary for the extrinsic (tissue) clotting system, but does not participate in the intrinsic (plasma) coagulation reactions.

Factor VIII (antihemophilic factor or globulin, AHF, AHG, antihemophilic factor A, platelet cofactor I). This protein has a short lifespan in shed blood, and is apparently consumed in the intrinsic clotting process. Its site of origin is unknown. Deficiency of this factor causes classical hemophilia, or hemophilia A.

Factor IX (plasma thromboplastin component, PTC, Christmas factor, antihemophilic factor B, autoprothrombin II). This is another of the vitamin K-dependent proteins synthesized by the liver. Although it participates in the intrinsic clotting system, it is not consumed and remains active both in serum and in plasma after relatively long periods of storage. Factor IX deficiency is Christmas disease, or hemophilia B, a condition clinically identical to classical hemophilia, but distinguished from it by laboratory findings.

Factor X (Stuart factor, Stuart-Prower factor). Another of the vitamin K-dependent factors produced in the liver, this stable protein participates in both the intrinsic and extrinsic clotting systems and appears to be the pivotal substance in activating prothrombin. Following activation, factor X has powerful proteolytic activity. Both aged plasma and serum contain factor X activity.

Factor XI (plasma thromboplastin antecedent, PTA). This highly stable factor is present in small amounts in both plasma and serum. Its nature and site of origin are unknown. One of the plasma procoagulants, it participates only in the intrinsic clotting system.

Factor XII (Hageman factor). Activation of Hageman factor by contact with glass or other surfaces appears to be the first step in the intrinsic clotting system. It is present in small amounts in both plasma and serum. Since congenital deficiency of Hageman factor does not produce a bleeding tendency, its physiologic role is imperfectly understood.

Factor XIII (fibrin stabilizing factor, FSF, fibrinase, Laki-Lorand factor). This was the last of the clotting factors to be discovered and assigned a number, and it apparently performs the last act in physiologic clotting. When fibrinogen is hydrolyzed, the fibrin monomers join by end-to-end hydrogen bonding to form the clot. The enzymatic activity of factor XIII augments the relatively unstable bonds with firm side-to-side linkages, rendering the clot stable and insoluble.

BIBLIOGRAPHY

1. BARNES, M.G., KOMARMY, L., AND NOVACK, A.H.: A comprehensive screening program for hemoglobinopathies. J.A.M.A. 219:701, 1972.
2. BEUTLER, E., DERN, R.J., AND ALVING, A.S.: The hemolytic effect of primaquine. J. Lab. Clin. Med. 45:40, 1955.
3. BEUTLER, E., AND MITCHELL, M.: Special modifications of the fluorescent screening method for glucose-6-phosphate dehydrogenase deficiency. Blood 32:816, 1968.
4. BLATT, H.: Eosinophils in allergy. A brief review. Rev. Allergy 20:650, 1966.
5. BRECHER, G., VON FOERSTER, H., AND CRONKITE, E.P.: "Production, differentiation and lifespan of leukocytes." *In* Braunsteiner, H., and Zucker-Franklin, D. (eds.): The Physiology and Pathology of Leukocytes. Grune and Stratton, New York, 1962.
6. BREWER, S.J., TARLOV, A.R., AND ALVING, A.A.: The methemoglobin reduction test for primaquine-type sensitivity of erythrocytes. J.A.M.A. 180:386, 1962.
7. BULL, B.S.: Aids to electronic platelet counting. Am. J. Clin. Pathol. 54:707, 1970.
8. BULL, B.S., SCHNEIDERMAN, M.A., AND BRECHER, G.: Platelet counts with the Coulter counter. Am. J. Clin. Pathol. 44:678, 1965.
9. CARRELL, R.W., AND LEHMANN, H.: The unstable haemoglobin haemolytic anaemias. Semin. Hematol. 6:116, 1969.
10. CRADDOCK, C.G., LONGMIRE, R., AND McMILLAN, R.: Lymphocytes and the immune response. N. Engl. J. Med. 285:324, 1971.
11. DACIE, J.V., AND MOLLISON, P.L.: Survival of transfused erythrocytes from a donor with nocturnal hemoglobinuria. Lancet 1:390, 1949.
12. DOUGLAS, S.D.: Analytic review: disorders of phagocyte function. Blood 35:851, 1970.
13. DOWNEY, H., AND McKINLEY, C.A.: Acute lymphadenosis compared with acute lymphatic leukemia. Arch. Intern. Med. 32:82, 1923.
14. FEIGIN, R. D.: NBT test in the diagnosis of febrile patients. N. Engl. J. Med. 285:347, 1971.
15. GAGON, T.E., ATHENS, J.W., BOGGS, D.R., AND CARTWRIGHT, G.E.: An evaluation of the variance of leukocyte counts as performed with the hemocytometer, Coulter, and Fisher instruments. Am. J. Clin. Path. 46:684, 1966.
16. GEERDINK, R.A., HELLEMAN, P.W., AND VERLOOP, M.C.: Hereditary elliptocytosis and hyperhaemolysis. A comparative study of 6 families with 145 patients. Acta Med. Scand. 179:715, 1966.

17. GOWANS, J.L.: Immunobiology of the small lymphocyte. Hosp. Pract. 3:34, 1968.
18. GREGERSEN, M.I., AND RAWSON, R.A.: Blood volume. Physiol. Rev. 39:307, 1959.
19. GERNEY, C.W.: Erythropoietin and erythropoiesis. Ann. Intern. Med. 65:377, 1966.
20. HARRIS, J.W., AND KELLERMEYER, R.W.: The Red Cell, rev. ed. Harvard University Press, Cambridge, 1970.
21. HARTMAN, R.C., AND JENKINS, D.E.: Paroxysmal nocturnal hemoglobinuria: current concepts of certain pathophysiologic features. Blood 25:850, 1965.
22. KNUTSEN, C.A., AND BREWER, G.J.: The micro-methemoglobin reduction test for glucose-6-phosphate dehydrogenase deficiency. Am. J. Clin. Path. 45:82, 1966.
23. LAMY, F., AND WAUGH, D.F.: Certain physical properties of bovine prothrombin. J. Biol. Chem. 203:489, 1953.
24. LEVINE, P., CELANO, N.J., AND FALKOWSKI, F.: The specificity of the antibody in paroxysmal cold hemoglobinuria (PCH). Transfusion 3:278, 1963.
25. MATULA, G., AND PATERSON, P.Y.: Spontaneous in vitro reduction of nitroblue tetrazolium by neutrophils of adult patients with bacterial infection. N. Engl. J. Med. 285:311, 1971.
26. NALBANDIAN, R.M., HENRY, R.L., NICHOLS, B.M. ET AL.: Molecular basis for a simple, specific test for S hemoglobin: the Murayama test. Clin. Chem. 16:945, 1970.
27. NALBANDIAN, R.M., NICHOLS, B.M., CAMP, F.R., JR. ET AL.: Dithionite tube test—a rapid, inexpensive technique for the detection of hemoglobin S and non-S sickling hemoglobin. Clin. Chem. 17:1028, 1971.
28. PAGE, A.R., AND GOOD, R.A.: Studies on cyclic neutropenia: a clinical and experimental investigation. Am. J. Dis. Child. 94:623, 1957.
29. PARK, B.H., FIKRIG, S.M., AND SMITHWICK, E.M.: Infection and nitroblue-tetrazolium reduction by neutrophils. Lancet 2: 532, 1968.
30. PRICHARD, R.W.: A reason for a high M.C.H.C. Letter to the Editor. Am. J. Clin. Path. 45:751, 1966.
31. SHELLEY, W.B., AND PARNES, H.M.: The absolute basophil count. J.A.M.A. 192:108, 1965.
32. STEINER, M.L., AND PEARSON, H.A.: Bone marrow plasmacyte values in childhood. A morphologic correlation in developmental immunology. J. Pediatr. 68:562, 1966.
33. TANAKA, K.R., VALENTINE, W.N., AND MIWA, S.: Pyruvic kinase (PK) deficiency hereditary nonspherocytic hemolytic anemia. Blood 19:267, 1962.
34. WINTROBE, M.M.: The size and hemoglobin content of the erthrocyte. J. Lab. Clin. Med. 17:899, 1932.
35. WINTROBE, M.M.: Clinical Hematology, ed. 6. Lea and Febiger, Philadelphia, 1967.

CHAPTER 2

Serology

Serology is the study of serum, specifically of serum proteins with immunologic activity. These immunologically active proteins are termed antibodies or, in more general terms, immunoglobulins. Circulating antibodies are not the only manifestation of immune processes, and serologic testing must not be considered the only suitable tool for immunologic investigation.

CELL-MEDIATED IMMUNITY

The human organism, like other vertebrates, can respond to antigenic stimuli in two distinct fashions: by producing antibodies or by developing cell-mediated immune mechanisms. Study of this latter phenomenon has been relatively recent. Until the 1930s and 1940s, virtually all experimental immunology concerned antibodies, although the peculiar properties of the immune response to tubercle bacilli had long been observed. We now know that cellular immune mechanisms have specificity comparable to that of circulating antibodies. Examples of this cell-mediated immunologic activity are tissue reactivity of the tuberculin type, the protective responses against many fungal and some bacterial invaders, and the organism's response to transplanted tissue.

TESTS FOR SPECIFIC SENSITIVITY

The most common clinical tests involving cell-mediated immunity are the skin tests for tuberculosis, for such fungi as Histoplasma and Coccidioides, and for certain viruses, notably mumps. In these tests, the appropriate antigen is introduced into the patient who reacts in a visible, predictable fashion if he has previously had experience with the organism. This principle is comparable to the search for specific bacterial antibodies as an index of previous exposure. The question at issue is, "Has the patient had sufficient prior exposure to the organism to induce an immune response?" This kind of skin testing is relatively insensitive, is not amenable to subtle differentiation among antigens, and may have clinical effects, either desirable or undesirable, in the patient.

More discriminating tests for the presence of specific cell-mediated immunity are becoming available in specialized laboratories. Under appropriate conditions, a specific antigen can induce cellular alterations or induce measurable reactions when added to cultured lymphocytes of a patient sensitized to that antigen. Variants of these techniques are used in evaluating organ transplants, since the patient's immune response can be tested in vitro against several potential donors to select the one whose tissues evoke the least response.[76]

TESTS FOR IMMUNE COMPETENCE

There is a second question that can be answered about cell-mediated immunity, "Has the patient the capability to mount any cell-mediated immune response?" This question has diagnostic importance in evaluating diseases which affect the immune system, such as Hodgkin's disease, lymphoproliferative disorders, and congenital immunodeficiency syndromes. Both in vivo and in vitro tests are feasible. The patient can be exposed to antigenic material such as halogenated nitrobenzenes, which reliably evoke a visible cell-mediated reaction in normal individuals. If the patient's response is diminished or absent, his cellular immune system is assumed to be impaired. More elegant are techniques in which cultured lymphocytes are exposed to powerful stimulators of lymphocytic activity; phytohemagglutinin is most widely used. Up to 75 per cent of lymphocytes from immunologically normal individuals undergo transformation to blast forms, but cells from patients with impaired cell-mediated responses will respond only minimally.[10] These and other tests, only recently developed, are expensive and exacting, but do open avenues for studying cell-mediated immunity, which has hitherto eluded experimental scrutiny.

HUMORAL IMMUNITY

Circulating antibodies, in contrast, are easily obtained and fairly easily studied. Antibodies are immunoglobulins produced in response to an antigenic stimulus, which react specifically with the responsible antigen. The immunoglobulins are serum proteins, heterogeneous in certain physical and chemical characteristics, but having a common structural pattern with several universally present subunits, and manifesting considerable similarity in reactivity. In normal human serum, the combined immunoglobulins contribute 0.6 to 2.0 Gm of protein per 100 ml, all at the slower moving end of the electrophoretic spectrum. The rate of migration is variable, however, depending on the class of immunoglobulin. Further heterogeneity is observed when the electrophoretically separated immunoglobulins are allowed to react with broad-spectrum antibody mixtures, in the techniques of immunoelectrophoresis.

IMMUNOGLOBULIN CHARACTERISTICS

All immunoglobulins consist of two pairs of polypeptide chains joined by disulfide bonds. Chemical and enzymic cleavage techniques reveal that one pair, the light chains with molecular weight of approximately 25,000, form part of all immunoglobulin classes. The other, heavier (molecular weight approximately 50,000) pair of polypeptide chains is unique to each class. The classes are termed IgA, IgD, IgE, IgG, and IgM, the common element Ig denoting immunoglobulin identity, while the variable letters refer to the heavy chains, designated respectively alpha, delta, epsilon, gamma, and mu. The biologic activities are also distinctive. Very little is known about IgD. IgA exists in bodily secretions at far higher concentrations than in serum; it is thought that respiratory and gastrointestinal tract surface immunity depends on this immunoglobulin class.[68] Although very little IgE circulates, it appears to play an important role in fixed tissue responses, and is active in skin sensitization, asthma, and other atopic reactions.[33] We need consider at length only IgG and IgM.

Antibody Production

The immune activity in which IgG and IgM participate can be briefly summarized as follows. Antigen, defined here as a specific substance foreign to the host and of suitably large molecular weight, enters the immunologically competent organism. The raw antigen undergoes some form of processing or recognition procedure, thought to be mediated by macrophages. The altered antigen then interacts with certain members of the small lymphocyte population capable of producing antibody. In mammals, the nature and location of the agency which confers on lymphocytes the antibody-producing capacity is unknown, although its function is analogous to that of an organ in birds identified as the bursa of Fabricius. Without this *bursal equivalent* influence, mammalian lymphocytes do not evolve into antibody-producing cells. Lymphocytes which have been exposed, early in the life of the organism, to the *bursal equivalent* respond to antigen with enormous protein production, resulting in successive structural changes by which the cells eventuate as plasma cells. It is the plasma cell which manufactures antibody, the immunoglobulin which circulates and can be measured.

The general pattern of antibody production and behavior is that, shortly after antigen introduction, specific antibodies of the IgM class appear. IgG antibody of the same specificity develops somewhat later. IgG production tends to persist longer than IgM. To a considerable extent, persistence of circulating IgM suggests that the eliciting antigen is still present, while IgG production may continue after the antigen has disappeared from the organism. Immunologic responsiveness depends upon innumerable factors, including the nature of the antigen, its mode of introduction, the genetic constitution of the host and the ongoing health of the host. For these reasons, any summary such as the foregoing will be incomplete and inapplicable in a variety of specific situations, but it provides a useful framework for later discussions of individual serologic tests.

Combining Sites. All antibodies have the capacity to combine specifically with the eliciting antigen. This combination depends upon the configuration of antigen and antibody, and very minor spatial or chemical changes may alter reactivity. The amino acid sequence of the N-terminal end of the heavy chains confers specificity, but combination with antigen is markedly enhanced by the participation of the N-terminal end of the light chain.[31] All antibody molecules have at least two combining sites, presumably reflecting the paired structure of the molecule. IgM molecules, which are thought to have five pairs of heavy chains and five pairs of light chains, appear to have five combining sites.[31]

Cross-Reactivity. Naturally antigenic materials tend to be complex molecules, with many individually definable chemical groupings. Antibodies may unite with small portions or large portions of the molecule, and a single antigenic material can provoke several distinct antibodies. Although antibodies can be exquisitely specific, they may also react with antigenic sites somewhat different from the eliciting antigen. The tendency for an antibody to unite with chemical groupings other than the inciting antigen is called cross-reactivity. Likelihood of cross-reactivity tends to correspond with degrees of similarity between nonidentical antigens. Species relatedness often influences cross-reactivity; for example, rabbit antibodies to human proteins cross-react better with proteins from other primates than with dog protein. However, rather unpredictable cross-reactions may occur, such as the antibodies to human red cell antigens which also combine with bacterial or protozoan antigens.

Antigen-Antibody Interaction. The union between antigen and antibody, although firm and specific, is reversible. Individual antibody molecules detach from the antigen and are replaced by other molecules if the mixture is at equilibrium. If the physical conditions of the antigen-antibody mixture are altered, the equilibrium can be changed. Temperature and ionic strength of the medium are particularly important in determining activity, and individual antibody molecules may differ in physical reactivity despite identical specificity. Each antibody molecule has a fixed number of combining sites, but there is no uniformity in the number of combining sites an antigen may have. Individual antigen molecules may have between 10 and 200 combining sites,[31] and the reacting antigenic material may consist of complex particles or aggregates containing many molecules. While the reaction between antigen and antibody may be specific and uniform, the in vitro and in vivo results of this reaction can vary with the condition of the antigen and the physical or physiologic conditions in which the reaction occurs.

Classical serologic categories define antibodies as precipitins, agglutinins, complement-fixing antibodies, lysins, opsonins, antitoxins, and neutralizing antibodies. To some extent, these varieties of visible end-points result from variations in the nature of the antigen and the circumstances of the reaction, although in other cases the antibodies are, indeed, of different sorts. Precipitation describes the formation of an insoluble complex when soluble antigen combines with its antibody. Agglutination describes the aggregation of particles on whose surface is antigen which reacts with antibody. The antibody may be the same; the physical state of the antigen determines the end-point of the reaction. If an initially soluble antigen is aggregated or fixed to the surface of a carrier particle, the detection procedure will change from precipitation to agglutination, using the same serum.

Complement. One extremely important influence on both biologic and in vitro behavior is serum complement. This is a complex of proteins, mostly globulins, which can combine sequentially to produce such effects as cell lysis, leukocyte chemotaxis, histamine release, and surface alterations of cells. Individually inactive, the cofactors serially unite when a suitable antigen-antibody reaction triggers the first step. The antigen-antibody reaction occurs first; subsequent complement activation depends on the nature of the antibody. Some antibodies have the property of *fixing* complement (i.e., initiating the first steps of complement combination) and others do not. The capacity to bind complement is independent of the antibody specificity, and does not affect the interaction of antibody with antigen. In the absence of complement, an antigen-antibody reaction may occur and precipitation or agglutination or no visible effects may ensue. The same reaction, in the presence of complement, can initiate independent effects deriving specifically from complement activity. Without the prior occurrence of antigen-antibody reaction, the complement cofactors would be inert. Both IgG and IgM antibodies have complement-fixing capacity, but the larger, multivalent IgM molecules tend to have greater individual effectiveness. While two IgG molecules must be attached to antigenic sites quite near to each other on a cell before complement fixation occurs, a single IgM attachment can activate complement.

TYPES OF REACTIONS

Agglutination

With this quick background to antibody behavior, we can discuss the principles of some commonly used serologic tests. Most tests use, as endpoints, some feature of precipitation, agglutination, or complement fixation. The agglutination procedures are, perhaps, the simplest. If the antigen is part of the surface of a particle, such as a red blood cell or a bacterial cell, combination with the specific antibody produces visible clumping. In serologic testing, the question at issue is: "Does the patient's serum contain antibodies against the pertinent antigen?" Provided a suitably standardized, convenient form of the antigen is available, the answer depends on whether or not the patient's serum agglutinates the particles.

Rough quantitation is achieved by diluting the serum and observing the highest dilution at which agglutination occurs. Serial dilutions may be two-fold, ten-fold, or other combinations. The highest dilution at which reaction occurs is called the titer of the antibody, 1:4 or 1:10,000 or whatever. Changing serum antibody levels are reflected as changes in titer, but dilution techniques and the innate sensitivity of the test are important in evaluating whether changing titers are significant.

Agglutination When Antigen Is Soluble. Even if the antigen is natively nonparticulate, agglutination reactions can be used. This requires attaching the antigen to a carrier, most often plastic particles of uniform size or red blood cells treated to retain adsorbed material. This technique is especially useful for detecting antibodies against serum proteins. The proteins themselves are soluble, but, suitably purified, they can be adsorbed onto treated red cells, or latex particles. This permits extremely sensitive testing. Precipitin testing can measure antibody concentrations no lower than 10 μg of nitrogen per ml, but with an agglutination end-point, antibody may be detected at levels of 0.001 μg of antibody nitrogen per ml or below.[31] IgM antibodies more readily produce agglutination than IgG.

Precipitation

Precipitation occurs when soluble antigen and soluble antibody combine to form an insoluble complex. Precipitation can be induced in fluid media or in agar gel. The simplest approach is, in a narrow, clear tube, to layer the antigen-containing material over the antibody-containing fluid, and observe formation of opaque precipitate at the interface. Proportions of antibody to antigen are critical for precipitation, so this approach may require trial dilutions before the optimum end-point is reached. The problem of proportions can be solved by permitting the reactants to diffuse through a gel, so that antigen and antibody can find their own optimum; precipitation will occur as an opaque line wherever the proportions are right in the gel. This diffusion technique has many applications, since a variety of antigens and antibodies can diffuse through agar.

Single Diffusion. Diffusion tests performed in a test tube are called one-dimensional, since antigen and antibody move vertically only. In two-dimensional diffusion tests, the reactants move in any direction through a flat agar surface. One reactant may be incorporated into the gel. When the other reactant is added at a single site, it diffuses through the medium until optimum proportions are reached and precipitation occurs in a ring around the site of application. The concentration of the diffusing material can be inferred from the size of the reaction zone, since the material in the gel is uniformly distributed. If the gel contains a measured amount of purified, specific antibody, the diameter of the reaction zone reflects the concentration of antigen in the test material. The reaction zone of the material under test can be compared against zones resulting from known concentrations of a standard, and very accurate quantitation of proteins is thereby possible. This technique, called single, radial diffusion, is used primarily for quantitating known materials, rather than for identifying unknowns in a test system.

Double Diffusion. In double diffusion, both antibody and antigen travel through a neutral gel medium. For qualitative testing, the antibody and the antigen are placed in wells located suitably distant from each other. The advancing fronts diffuse toward one another and precipitation occurs where optimum concentrations meet. With a known antibody, unknown sera can be tested for the presence of antigen; conversely, the presence of antibody in an unknown serum will be demonstrated if a known antigen is used. The end-point is the presence or absence of a precipitin line. The intensity of the precipitin line and its location relative to the application points of antigen and antibody roughly reflect the concentration of the reactants. The sensitivity of this technique can be enhanced by altering the properties of the suspending gel, thereby affecting the diffusion of the materials.

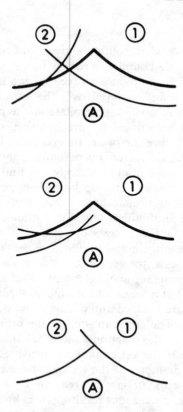

Figure 6. In these three examples, a multispecific antiserum is in well A and different unknown serum samples are in wells 1 and 2. *Top,* Both unknowns have two different antigens that react with antibody A. The symmetrical arcs that meet precisely indicate a single, identical reactant in both unknowns. The diverse shape and locations of the other arcs indicate complete dissimilarity between the other reactants. *Middle,* Samples 1 and 2 contain the same reactant. Sample 1 contains no other antigens recognized by antibody A, but Sample 2 has two additional reactants. *Bottom,* The reactants in these two unknowns are very similar since the arcs have similar shapes and locations. The extending *spur* shows that the reactants are not identical.

     Another application of immunodiffusion is the determination of whether apparently similar materials are immunologically identical. With a single antiserum, several unknowns can be placed equidistant from the antibody. The shape and location of the resulting precipitin lines are specific for various antigens, so the lines from several unknowns can be directly compared (see Fig. 6).

     Immunoelectrophoresis. Immunodiffusion can be combined with electrophoresis in the procedure called immunoelectrophoresis. If a mixture of proteins is placed in an electrical field, each protein will migrate according to its intrinsic charge. Electrophoresing a protein mixture on an agar strip separates the major groups of proteins present. Subsequent addition of suitable antibody produces precipitin arcs wherever antigenically distinct proteins are located. The intensity and size of the precipitin arcs will reflect the concentration of antigen in the area of reaction. The added antibody may be monospecific or may react with several different proteins. Adding monospecific antibody permits approximate quantitation of an individual protein in a complex mixture. When more than one antibody is used, the relative amounts and interactions of various proteins can be observed.

Complement Fixation

In agglutination and precipitation tests, the end-point results directly from the combination of antigen with antibody. Sometimes the antigen-antibody reaction must be documented indirectly. The classic example of this is the complement fixation test. We have already stated that some antibodies activate complement when they combine with antigen. The complement system, once set in motion, can produce such diverse effects as lysis of red blood cells, opsonization of bacteria, and leukocytic chemotaxis. Red blood cell lysis (hemolysis) is an end-point easily observed and readily measured, so it is most often employed as the visible end-point documenting some nonvisible antigen-antibody reaction.

The principle of complement fixation tests is as follows. Complement activation, initiated by an antigen-antibody reaction, produces hemolysis. The steps need not occur simultaneously. Complement can be added to cells already coated with antibody, and hemolysis ensues. The visible end-point, hemolysis of cells known to be coated with antibody, indicates that complement was present in the final medium. If complement is not present in the added material, hemolysis fails to occur. The end-point indicates whether or not complement was added. The presence or absence of complement, in these tests, depends upon whether or not an independent, complement-fixing antigen-antibody reaction had previously occurred.

For example, if antirubella antibodies combine with a soluble, purified rubella antigen, complement will be fixed, resulting in an antigen-antibody-complement complex. This entire complex is soluble, so no visible change occurs in the reaction mixture. The complement, once bound into the complex of antigen and antibody, is no longer free to participate in other activities. In short, the complement initially present is "fixed" when the rubella antibody reacts with its antigen. If antibody-coated, potentially hemolyzable red cells are added to the medium containing the antigen-antibody-complement complexes, the cells do not lyse because no complement is available. On the other hand, if the test serum had had no rubella antibodies, the original antigen-antibody reaction would not have occurred, the original complement would still be available, and the coated cells would promptly hemolyze when placed in the medium. The end-point, hemolysis of previously sensitized red cells, indicates whether or not the rubella antigen-antibody reaction has occurred. If the cells lyse, we know the reaction has *not* taken place, because there is still complement available for hemolysis. Failure of lysis indicates that the antigen-antibody reaction *did* occur, because the complement has been used up.

Uses and Sensitivity. Complement fixation tests can demonstrate the presence of either antigen or antibody in the unknown material. The known reagent must be a specific antibody if the presence of antigen is under test, or a purified known antigen if the presence of antibody is in question. In either case, an exogenous source of complement is used, usually prepared from guinea pigs, since species origin is not critical. The indicator system, the sensitized red cells, is also standardized—often sheep red cells coated with a rabbit anti-sheep-cell antibody. The test is performed sequentially. First the serum to be tested is incubated with the known reactant, either antigen or antibody. Then an appropriate concentration of complement is added; in some procedures, complement is included in the primary incubation phase. The last step is the addition of sensitized indicator cells, and the visible end-point is the degree of hemolysis.

Complement fixation tests can detect very low concentrations of antibody, as long as the antibody is one which activates complement and a suitable antigen preparation is available. The test is technically exacting, since the proportions of antigen, antibody, and complement affect the fixation step and the proportion of complement to sensitized cells affects the occurrence of visible lysis.

Potential Problems. Another problem with complement fixation tests is that some serum samples are anticomplementary, i.e., they block the activity of complement by their simple presence, whether or not the antigen-antibody reaction has occurred. Serum with anticomplementary activity will give spurious positive results, since the end-point, complement-mediated hemolysis, will always be absent. A control must accompany each test, wherein the unknown serum is incubated with complement without added antibody or antigen, and sensitized cells are added afterward. If hemolysis fails to occur in this tube, the results of the test, when both antigen and antibody are present, can have no validity. Anticomplementary activity can result from pathologic or physiologic peculiarities of the patient, or may develop if the serum sample becomes contaminated.

Hemagglutination Inhibition

Analogous to complement fixation is hemagglutination inhibition, in which the occurrence of an antibody-antigen reaction is demonstrated by its prevention of an expected visible effect. Many viruses, or the products of viral cultures, have the capacity to agglutinate mammalian red blood cells. This does not, apparently, depend on antigenic specificity of the cell surfaces, and is not an antibody-mediated agglutination. This hemagglutinating property of a given virus is neutralized by antibodies specific for the virus. In the test system the question is, "Does the patient's serum contain antibodies against the specific virus?" There must be a pure, active culture of the virus at issue, and the test conditions must be standardized so the unmodified culture preparation visibly agglutinates the red cell suspension. Addition of serum containing virus-neutralizing antibody will abolish agglutination, so a positive test result is the *absence* of agglutination. The antibody can be roughly quantitated by diluting the test serum to a point at which it no longer inhibits agglutination. One problem is that some serums may contain complex proteins which inhibit virus activity without being specific antibodies.

Fluorescence Microscopy

Still another means for demonstrating antigen-antibody interaction is fluorescence microscopy. After a fluorescent dye, usually fluorescein, has been attached to appropriately selected immunoglobulin molecules, the location of the antibody on a slide or in a tissue section is clearly signaled by localized fluorescence. Since the dye can be attached to an enormous range of antibodies, the applications of this technique are wide. One problem is that nonspecific fluorescence may occur in the tissue or slide preparation, but this can usually be corrected with suitable adsorption or suitable controls or both.

Direct Test. In direct fluorescence tests, the fluorescent label is bound to some purified, specific antibody. The antibody is then incubated with the unknown material on a slide. The question asked in this technique is, "Does the unknown material contain the antigen for which the antibody is specific?" If antigen is present, the labelled, known antibody attaches to it,

DIRECT IMMUNOFLUORESCENCE
(TO LOCALIZE ANTIGENS)

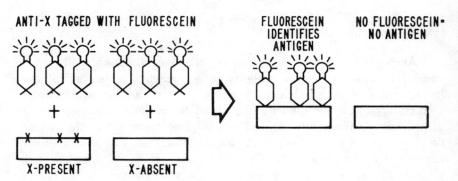

Figure 7.   In direct immunofluorescence, a single, specific labelled antibody identifies the presence or absence of that one antigen in the unknown material.

producing localized fluorescence. If antigen is absent, no antibody is bound, and all the fluorescent material comes off in the rinse (see Fig. 7).

Indirect Test. Sometimes the antigenic specificity is known, and the question at issue is, "Does the unknown material contain antibody directed against the known antigen?" Answering this requires a two-step procedure. In the first phase, the unknown serum is incubated with a slide containing the antigen, which need not be in a highly purified form. Fixed bacterial cells or frozen sections of tissue are eminently suitable forms of antigen. If the serum under test contains the antibody, immunoglobulin molecules will bind with material on the slide, but no visible effect signals that reaction has occurred. To demonstrate that antibody molecules have attached themselves to the prepared antigen, fluorescent antiglobulin serum is added. This binds to and serves to localize the immunoglobulins fixed from the test serum. If the unknown did not contain antibodies to the antigen on the slide, there will be no globulins on the slide to react with the fluorescent antiglobulin serum (see Fig. 8).

The indirect fluorescence technique has more applications than direct fluorescent staining, since the only specific antibody required is an antiglobulin serum. A host of antibodies may be present in a serum sample; by using suitable separate antigen preparations, the different antibody activities can be identified, using only the single fluorescent antiglobulin reagent. In the direct technique, a well characterized, purified single antibody must be prepared and labelled, and the approximate location of the antigen in the test material must be known.

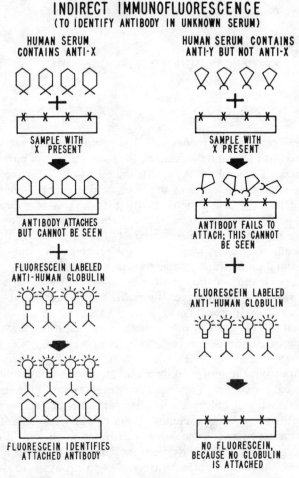

INDIRECT IMMUNOFLUORESCENCE
(TO IDENTIFY ANTIBODY IN UNKNOWN SERUM)

HUMAN SERUM
CONTAINS ANTI-X

HUMAN SERUM CONTAINS
ANTI-Y BUT NOT ANTI-X

SAMPLE WITH
X PRESENT

SAMPLE WITH
X PRESENT

ANTIBODY ATTACHES
BUT CANNOT BE SEEN

ANTIBODY FAILS TO
ATTACH; THIS CANNOT
BE SEEN

FLUORESCEIN LABELED
ANTI-HUMAN GLOBULIN

FLUORESCEIN LABELED
ANTI-HUMAN GLOBULIN

FLUORESCEIN IDENTIFIES
ATTACHED ANTIBODY

NO FLUORESCEIN,
BECAUSE NO GLOBULIN
IS ATTACHED

Figure 8. In indirect immunofluorescence, a variety of different antigens can be used to seek antibodies in unknown serums. Labelled antiglobulin serum will signal any human globulin that attaches to the prepared test system.

Other Techniques

Other immunologic techniques are available to measure antigen-antibody interactions in test materials not readily adaptable to the kinds of procedures outlined above. Some of these include mixed agglutination, and a variety of procedures which measure the consumption, or removal, of antibody from a previously quantitated serum. Although enormously useful in immunologic research, these are not in general use for serologic diagnosis.

SPECIFIC IMMUNOLOGIC PROCEDURES

SEROLOGIC TESTS FOR SYPHILIS

Ever since Wassermann recognized that complement-fixing antibodies were associated with syphilitic infection, the laboratory has played a large part in the diagnosis of syphilis. Adequate diagnosis and effective treatment are important in all three stages of the disease to prevent spread of infection and avoid harm to the patient. In the primary phase, which is from initial contact to the disappearance of the chancre, both the blood and the local lesion are infective; in the secondary phase of mucocutaneous rash, the exudate from the lesion teems with spirochetes. The dangers in the latent and tertiary phases are to the patient rather than to his contacts. Since both primary and secondary stigmata disappear spontaneously and produce no visible lasting damage, the patient may unwittingly or intentionally overlook their appearance.

Differential Diagnosis. The differential diagnosis in the primary phase includes chancroid, granuloma inguinale, lymphogranuloma venereum, and herpes progenitalis. Dark-field demonstration of characteristic spirochetes in smears from the lesion confirms the diagnosis of syphilis, but this exacting technical procedure is not always available or reliable. Even small doses of penicillin taken before the chancre appears can seriously impair dark-field identification of spirochetes in the primary lesion.[50] If material from the moist mucocutaneous secondary lesions is subjected to dark-field examination, organisms can readily be seen. The rash tends to be nonpruritic and evanescent, so the patient rarely goes to a physician during this phase. In the differential diagnosis of secondary syphilis, the absence of pruritis and the frequently symmetrical distribution of the rash on the extremities help in distinguishing the rash from pityriasis rosea, drug eruptions, psoriasis, or lichen planus of the mucous surfaces. The tertiary manifestations of syphilis may be legion, leading to the classic description of syphilis as "the great imitator."

Wassermann-Type Reactivity

Wassermann's original observation of complement-fixing activity directed against treponema-infested fetal liver suggested antibody specificity against the organism. Subsequent observations that reactive serums gave similar results against uninfected liver and against extracts of other tissues cast doubt on the identity of this activity as an antibody. The antigen has been characterized as a complex lipid present in many mammalian tissues but particularly accessible from mammalian heart. Present day tests use an alcoholic extract of beef heart as the source of cardiolipin, with added lecithin and cholesterol.

Doubt as to the nature of serum reactivity is reflected in the various terms used to describe it—Wassermann antibody, cardiolipin antibody, or Wassermann reagin. Reagin, as used in this sense, must be distinguished from the skin-sensitizing antibodies to which the term is also applied. The reacting elements have been identified as 19S and 7S immunoglobulins[69] and the pattern of reactivity follows that of antibody production. All the pathogenic treponemas evoke the Wassermann antibody, which develops shortly after infection, and tends to parallel the level of tissue reaction to the organism. It confers no protective effect, however, and, despite the fact that the cardiolipin antigen with which it reacts is widespread throughout the human body, it seems to cause no tissue effects. Both complement fixation and flocculation techniques are useful in demonstrating Wassermann-type reactivity.

Complement Fixation. In complement fixation tests, the suspected serum is incubated with cardiolipin reagent, permitting the antigen-antibody interaction to bind complement and remove it from the reaction mixture. A sheep blood indicator is then added which hemolyzes in the presence of free complement. If the sheep cells fail to hemolyze, complement is seen to be absent; its absence testifies to the prior occurrence of an antigen-antibody reaction. The complement fixation procedure is technically exacting, and may give inaccurate results if the serum has anticomplement activity, if the numerous reagents lose their standardized potency, or if the glassware or reagents are contaminated by alcohol, detergents, or contact with certain ionic solutions. Nevertheless, many laboratories get excellent results from routine use of the Kolmer and Kolmer-Reiter protein tests, descendants of Wassermann's original complement fixation procedure.

Flocculation Procedures. A second test for reagin is induction of flocculation. If reagin-containing serum is added to an even suspension of cardiolipin reagent, coarse flocculation occurs. This is the basis for the Kahn, Mazzini, and Venereal Disease Research Laboratory (VDRL) tests, and for a variety of rapid-screening procedures such as the Rapid Plasma Reagin test (RPR), Unheated Serum Reagin test (USR), and the plasmacrit procedure (pct.). Like the complement fixation tests, flocculation tests require careful standardization and rigid adherence to the directions for the specific procedure. Flocculation tests are much less expensive and require less time and technical skill than the complement fixation procedures.

PROBLEMS FROM NONSPECIFIC TESTS. Despite their undoubted usefulness in syphilology, nonspecific tests for reagin have two serious drawbacks. (1) During the primary phase, when infectivity is high, reagin tests are usually negative, and (2) conditions other than syphilis frequently cause a positive reaction, called a biologic false positive (BFP). The most frequent offenders in this respect are malaria and leprosy, but biologic false positives cause more difficult diagnostic problems when they accompany less well defined disease entities. Although biologic false positives occasionally follow infectious disease or immunization procedures, most are associated with diseases of uncertain etiology, such as infectious mononucleosis, systemic lupus erthematosus, thyroiditis, hepatitis, and periarteritis nodosa.[58]

Treponemal Antibodies

Treponemal infection also evokes specific antibodies, but until fairly recently these have been difficult to demonstrate. The Treponema pallidum immobilization test (TPI)[47] employs the observation that specific antibodies, when incubated with living treponemas, cause markedly reduced spirochetal motility. This procedure is specific for treponemal antibodies, but becomes positive only late in primary infection and is only moderately sensitive. Its principal drawback, however, is the expense and difficulty of the procedure, and the problems inherent in maintaining live cultures of the organism. Very few laboratories now devote the effort and expense necessary for the TPI test, when other satisfactory tests are available.

Fluorescent Treponemal Antibody Test (FTA). Currently considered the most sensitive, specific, and reliable test for treponemal antibodies is a fluorescent antibody technique in which serum is incubated with a spread of killed organisms, and antibody attachment is documented by subsequent application of fluorescent antihuman globulin serum.[14] The original procedure proved extremely sensitive, even early in primary infection, but gave an undesirably large number of false positives. Specificity has been greatly enhanced, with little reduction in sensitivity, by absorbing the serum under test with protein from the Reiter treponema, which shares group-reactive antigens with T. pallidum and so removes nonsyphilitic anti-treponemal activity.[32] The fluorescent treponemal antibody-absorbed procedure (FTA-ABS) is more expensive and exacting than the nonspecific reagin procedures, but is well within the reach of general laboratories and can be adapted for automated performance.

The FTA-ABS has proved extremely useful in differentiating biologic false reactors to nonspecific tests from patients with syphilitic exposure. Positive results on nonspecific tests should be confirmed with a treponemal test, unless syphilis is clearly present, and even then the documentation provides a valuable record against which subsequent specimens may be checked. The Wassermann antibody develops later and recedes earlier than the antibody detected on FTA-ABS, so the fluorescent test is the procedure of choice in suspected early lesions or late tertiary phases. When the differential diagnosis includes neurologic manifestations of tertiary syphilis, the FTA-ABS is far more reliable than any other available procedure[27,45] and some workers believe it can reliably be applied to cerebrospinal fluid testing.[18] Occasional patients with lupus erythematosus,[38] hyperglobuline-mia,[45] and other apparently nonsyphilitic conditions[4] may give positive results on FTA-ABS testing, but the incidence is well below 1 per cent.

FEBRILE AGGLUTININS

An early serologic procedure still in use is the agglutination test for bacterial antibodies, the so-called *febrile agglutinins*. In this technique the patient's serum is reacted with a standardized suspension of specific killed-bacterial cultures. The test is a direct one; if the patient has antibodies against the organism, agglutination occurs. The antigens are available in commercial preparations, and can be used on slides or in tube dilution procedures. Slide tests are customary for screening, and can be done without detailed serial dilutions. Instead, decreasing volumes of serum are added to constant volumes of the antigen suspension, so the final concentration of serum in the several mixtures approximates doubling dilutions from 1:20 to 1:320. Greater precision, of course, results from test tube dilutions, and the antigens can then be incubated with the serum under standardized conditions.

Agglutination tests are performed most often against salmonella, brucella, rickettsia, and tularemia antigens. In all these diseases, culturing the organism from the patient would provide absolute proof of infection. These agents, however, tend to be elusive clinically or difficult to grow. In the absence of direct documentation, the agglutination tests offer indirect evidence of infection by documenting development of specific antibodies. The presence of antibody, however, indicates only prior experience with the agent or with something that cross-reacts with it; it does not prove ongoing infection. If the antibody is one known to subside rapidly after eradication of the organism, then a single serum specimen with high titered antibody suggests recent or active infection. Better proof of recent biological activity is demonstration that the antibody titer is rising during or shortly after the suspected illness. A rise in titer between two or more samples drawn several weeks apart provides excellent, though often retrospective, diagnostic information.

Widal Test for Salmonella

The earliest bacterial agglutinin test was the Widal test, employing two Salmonella paratyphi and two Salmonella typhi antigens. The battery of antigens now used has grown. The salmonellae are flagellated organisms, and both the somatic (O) and flagellar (H) portions are antigenic. Exposure by infection or vaccination induces agglutinins to the H antigen, which persist long after the organism has disappeared. H agglutinins also tend to rise after nonspecific stimuli, so a markedly elevated, or a sharply rising curve of O-agglutinin activity has greater diagnostic significance. Both H and O antibodies do cross-react with antigens of other enteric bacteria,[65] so the test is not truly specific. Salmonella typhi has a surface antigen, called Vi, which also stimulates agglutinin production.

Early in a salmonella infection, while organisms can still be cultured from feces or blood, agglutinin titers may be negative. Detectable antibodies begin developing within a week of onset and reach a high level at about four weeks. The O agglutinins should return to insignificant levels within a year, unless continuing infection or a carrier state is present. Antibodies to the Vi antigen subside even more promptly than the O agglutinins, so a high level of Vi antibody strongly suggests ongoing or fairly recent infection. Persistence of Vi antibodies indicates a carrier state. The usual battery of enteric antigens includes O antigens for Salmonella groups A, B, C, D, and E, and the H antigens for S. paratyphi groups A, B, and C and S. typhi group D. The Vi antigen of S. typhi may also be included.

Interpretation. Significant agglutinin titers are generally considered 1:80 or above, although H agglutinins may remain that high in some vaccinated individuals. To be significant, a changing titer should cover a four-fold dilution (e.g., 1:40 to 1:160, or 1:80 to 1:320), since a two-fold change is only a single dilution. Up to 1.4 per cent of normal individuals may have significant salmonella antibodies.[74] Elevated levels may also occur in patients with generalized increases in gamma globulins, notably those with liver disease,[55] and narcotic addicts.[71] Patients whose humoral antibody production is impaired from congenital deficiencies, immunosuppression, or general debility, will fail to produce febrile agglutinins despite documented infection. Infected patients who receive prompt, effective antibacterial therapy may recover without producing antibodies.

Tularemia and Brucellosis

Agglutination tests are important in the diagnosis of tularemia and brucellosis. The organisms P. tularensis and the Brucella species are very difficult to isolate from patient material at all phases of the diseases, so serologic diagnosis, although indirect, may be essential. Only Brucella abortus is used, since antigens from all three of the pathogenic brucellae cross-react. Unfortunately, some cross-reaction may occur among P. tularensis, B. abortus, and Proteus OX-19 antigens, but when a single serum reacts with all three, the highest titer tends to indicate the significant pathogen. The tests are performed in the same manner as the Widal procedure, with slide testing used as a screening test for more accurate, but time-consuming, tube dilutions. Tularemia antibodies usually appear within two weeks of onset, peaking at approximately eight weeks, and high levels often persist after recovery. Brucella agglutinins may also persist. Complement-fixing Brucella agglutinins can also be identified. Since these ordinarily disappear within a year after successful treatment of the disease,[36] they are more reliable in following this chronic, relapsing disease than the agglutinins.

Weil-Felix Test

The Weil-Felix reaction uses cross-reactivity as the basis for diagnostic inference. Serum is tested against antigens from the bacterium Proteus, but the infections under scrutiny are caused by rickettsiae. In several varieties of typhus, the patient develops agglutinins which manifest activity against certain strains of Proteus. If rickettsial antigens and the technical facilities for complement fixation or hemagglutination tests are available, the specific rickettsial antibodies can also be identified, but Proteus agglutination is far more generally available.

The nonmotile strain Proteus OX-19 is most widely used, because patients with epidemic typhus, murine (endemic) typhus, and Rocky Mountain spotted fever (tick-borne typhus) characteristically develop strong agglutinins to this strain. Weak agglutination of Proteus OX-2 may also occur, but OX-K antigens are not agglutinated. The opposite picture occurs in scrub typhus (tsutsugamushi), in which OX-K is strongly agglutinated, but neither OX-19 nor OX-2 is reactive. Agglutinins tend to occur at or after the tenth day of illness,[52] while a diagnostically significant four-fold rise in titer requires several weeks. The diagnostic agglutinin level is considered to be 1:160 or 1:320, while rickettsial complement fixation titers are significant at 1:8. Specific Proteus infections may confuse results of Weil-Felix testing, since these, too, induce anti-Proteus agglutinins, and anamnestic elevations may occur with cross-reacting bacterial infections. Antibiotic therapy may abort or delay antibody production. Infections with those rickettsial species causing Q fever and rickettsial pox do not produce a positive Weil-Felix test.

RUBELLA

The rubella virus would hold little interest for clinicians were it not so destructive to the conceptus in early pregnancy. The native disease is mild, self-limited, and has few sequelae, except for offspring of pregnant women infected in the first trimester. Intensive work on characterizing the virus and its antibodies aims ultimately to prevent infection of pregnant women, and meanwhile to document when infection occurs and how vaccination can modify infection patterns. Serologic tests for rubella can identify susceptible subjects, those without antibodies; can diagnose infection, by seroconversion; and help monitor the levels of immunity in infected and vaccinated populations.

Antibody Development

Native infections occur via the respiratory tract. Both viremia and virus shedding from the throat occur in the latter half of the incubation period, permitting ample opportunity for person-to-person spread. As the rash appears, antibodies circulate and the viremia clears, although respiratory tract shedding may continue for another week.[30] The virus is complex, its variety of antigenic sites provoking antibodies of various serologic characteristics. Unfortunately, it is not clear which antibodies confer protection. The hemagglutinating antibodies are first to appear, and persist the longest. Complement-fixing antibodies occur latest, one to three weeks after the rash, and disappear soonest. Neutralizing antibodies, several precipitating antibodies, and those demonstrated by fluorescence techniques are intermediate in development and disappearance.

The hemagglutination inhibition test (HI)[44,63] is in widest use, partly because it is rapid and reproducible and partly because the antibodies it identifies are the most widely distributed. Titers of 1:8 or above signify that an individual, at some time, has had rubella infection. Because HI antibodies persist with relatively little decline for many years, a single determination gives little dynamic information. Titers below 1:8 indicate susceptibility; titers above 1:64 reliably accompany resistance; a four-fold rise in titer between two consecutive samples is considered seroconversion, indicating recent infection.

Antibody Distribution

Between 60 and 80 per cent of American adolescents and young adults give serologic evidence of prior rubella infection.[19,30,53] During epidemics, virtually all susceptibles contract apparent or subclinical disease; reinfection in those with relatively low titers is by no means uncommon.[19] Reinfection rarely produces clinical disease, and the rapid antibody response probably prevents significant viremia.[12]

Antibody levels following vaccination are significantly lower than those after native infection, and reinfection rates are far higher.[2,12] An interesting qualitative difference is that wild infection leads to appearance of precipitating antibodies, while vaccination with most of the strains widely used at present does not.[42] Still to be answered is the critical question of whether reinfection following vaccination produces fetus-damaging viremia. Large scale vaccination programs and detailed serologic and virologic investigations will continue to be necessary before *rubella syndrome* can be expected to disappear.

PRIMARY ATYPICAL (MYCOPLASMAL) PNEUMONIA

Serologic diagnosis of primary atypical pneumonia is changing with the recognition that this disease is due to infection with Mycoplasma pneumoniae (Eaton agent, pleuropneumonia-like organism, PPLO). This organism can be cultured from throat swab specimens during the acute illness.[67] Specific antibody tests can now be performed, since cultured organisms are available to provide antigens. These are not, however, widely available, whereas the disease is widely disseminated, especially among children and young adults. Several older, nonspecific serologic procedures are diagnostically useful in conjunction with clinical and epidemiologic considerations.

Cold Agglutinins

Most normal serums have the capacity to agglutinate, or to attach to normal group O human red cells at 4° C. Often special techniques are needed to demonstrate this activity, which probably has anti-H specificity and is usually of very low titer. In perhaps half of patients late in the first week of atypical pneumonia, this cold agglutinating activity increases markedly. The agglutination is readily reversed when the antibody-red cell agglutinates are warmed to 37° C, unlike the behavior of many cold-reacting antibodies directed against specific blood group isoantigens.

The test is easily performed. The patient's serum is diluted with saline, and then added to a suspension of group O human red cells. After overnight refrigeration, the tubes are examined for agglutination, and then warmed to reverse the agglutination. An even easier bedside screening procedure has been adapted.[24] Chilling a small quantity of citrated whole blood for approximately one minute will induce visible agglutination of the patient's own cells, if the cold agglutinin titer is 1:64 or above.

Interpretation. In mycoplasmal pneumonia, cold agglutinin titers rise to 1:32 or above, but the reasons for this activity are by no means clear. The height of the titer roughly parallels the severity of the disease, although extremely high titers and a transient hemolytic process occasionally follow otherwise uncomplicated episodes of pneumonia. Cold agglutinins may also accompany adenovirus infections, and sometimes occur with malaria or vascular disease. The agglutinin tends to disappear within four to six weeks, unlike the specific anti-mycoplasmal antibodies which persist for months.[16]

Streptococcus MG Antibody

Late in the course of M. pneumoniae infection, or shortly after recovery, approximately 40 per cent of patients develop antibodies which agglutinate suspensions of killed streptococcus MG. This nonhemolytic streptococcus was originally isolated from patients with primary atypical pneumonia, but it is probably not etiologically significant and can exist in many individuals without causing illness. Significantly elevated titers begin at 1:20 and, as with other antibodies, a four-fold or greater rise between two serum samples is presumptive evidence for the disease. The appearance and disappearance of cold agglutinins and streptococcus MG antibodies correlate poorly with each other, and the relation of either one to the course of the disease is somewhat unpredictable.

Mycoplasmal Antibodies

Positive diagnosis of M. pneumoniae infection is possible when these highly fastidious organisms are grown from throat swabs on media specially enriched with serum and other nutrients.[20] Serologic diagnosis is less demanding, and permits retrospective epidemiologic studies. Antibodies demonstrable by complement fixation, immunofluorescence, or metabolic tests reliably follow infection within two to three weeks, affording more accurate diagnosis than the nonspecific serologic tests described above. These antibodies may persist for as long as two years, and reinfection has been documented in patients known to possess antibodies.[66] Hemagglutination-inhibiting antibodies also occur, but follow a different pattern of appearance[13] and may be reactive with some other determinant of these rather puzzling organisms.

ANTISTREPTOLYSIN O (ASO) TEST

Documenting the presence of antibodies usually results in retrospective diagnosis, since the acute illness tends to be over before significant antibodies develop. In testing for antistreptolysin O (ASO) the goal is to document an infection that is no longer present. The post-streptococcal illnesses, rheumatic fever and glomerulonephritis, develop approximately 3 weeks or 10 to 14 days, respectively, after the acute illness. Streptococci are ordinarily easy enough to culture, but by the time symptoms occur, the streptococcus has disappeared. Since the differential diagnosis of rheumatic fever and post-streptococcal glomerulonephritis often includes many other conditions, documenting recent streptococcal infection becomes highly significant.

Cultures of most group A streptococci produce an enzyme capable of hemolyzing human or rabbit red blood cells. Following streptococcal infection, most patients develop a variety of fairly short-lived antibodies against the bacterial antigens and by-products, including one which neutralizes streptolysin in vitro. The test is performed by incubating increasingly diluted serum with a constant volume of streptolysin O and fresh red blood cells. Normal serum at low dilutions may contain hemolysin-neutralizing activity, since streptococcal exposure is extremely widespread. Test results are reported in Todd units, the reciprocal of the highest serum dilution which completely prevents hemolysis.

Interpretation. Values to 166 Todd units have little acute significance, but values of 250 or higher indicate recent streptococcal infection, as does a rising titer in two samples a week apart. Values above 500 are frequently found with acute rheumatic fever or glomerulonephritis. Hemolysed serum cannot, of course, be used for the test.

An elevated or rising ASO level does not identify the strain or the location of the infecting organism, nor does it indicate whether the infection is past or ongoing. The antibody rises within one or two weeks of infection, and remains elevated for a variable period of weeks to months. When symptoms suggest rheumatic fever, a high ASO level confirms that recent streptococcal infection has occurred, thus making the diagnosis more probable. The same symptoms with persistently low ASO levels, in an immunologically competent individual, would have to be ascribed to some other cause. ASO elevations follow nearly any streptococcal infection, not only those which produce post-streptococcal disease. A persistently high titer over several months suggests an ongoing infection, which should be located and treated if at all possible.

C-REACTIVE PROTEIN

Not every serum protein which reacts with bacterial products is a specific antibody. Patients suffering from a variety of nonpneumococcal disorders often possess an alpha globulin which precipitates the C-polysaccharide of pneumococcus. This reactive property is called C-reactive protein, a noncommittal descriptive term. First noted in the serum of patients with pneumococcal pneumonia, it has subsequently been found in patients with active streptococcal and other infections, rheumatic fever, lupus erythematosus, myocardial infarction, some kinds of carcinoma, or in any situation characterized by inflammatory reaction.

Significance. C-reactive protein (CRP) has been described as an "acute phase reactant," since it appears within 12 to 24 hours of the onset of inflammation, and subsides within a few days of correction. Although extremely sensitive, the test offers practically no specificity, since it cannot discriminate among the various possible inciting causes. The test is valuable more for prognosis than diagnosis. In rheumatic fever, for example, successful treatment of an inflammatory episode will cause the CRP to disappear, so persistently elevated CRP indicates smoldering activity. Reappearance of the CRP, in a disease characterized by exacerbations and remissions, heralds a flare-up.

Technique. Present day tests for C-reactive protein do not use the patient's serum to precipitate the pneumococcus C antigen. Instead, the presence of CRP is demonstrated immunologically, using rabbit antiserum active against human C-reactive protein. When antiserum and test serum are mixed in a capillary tube, visible precipitation occurs. In another technique the antiserum is attached to latex particles, which agglutinate in the presence of serum containing CRP. By diluting the serum for agglutination testing, one can roughly quantitate the CRP level, while the amount of precipitate serves as a rough guide to quantity in the capillary tube procedure.

RHEUMATOID FACTOR

Rheumatoid arthritis is a disease of puzzling and complicated etiology, which may present several serologic peculiarities. Many, though not all, patients with this disease have circulating immunoglobulins with activity directed against human immunoglobulin G. This anti-IgG activity is sometimes called rheumatoid factor (RF), although there is probably not just one such immunoglobulin, and the relation of the antibody to the disease is far from clear. In most patients, the antibody is an IgM molecule reactive against all human IgG molecules, including their own, and against IgG from other mammals. A few anti-IgG rheumatoid factors are, themselves, IgG. Some have antigenic specificity, recognizing the so-called Gm groups which are antigenically active portions of gamma heavy chains.

Despite the name, rheumatoid factor occurs in a variety of other diseases, notably lupus erythematosus, sarcoidosis, cirrhosis, leprosy, and macroglobulinemia. All these diseases share the finding of generally increased serum globulin levels, but anti-IgG activity occurs only sporadically in these conditions. Conversely, patients with well documented rheumatoid arthritis may be hypoglobulinemic, and lack both rheumatoid factor and other globulins as well.[31] Although RF is not the sole efficient cause of the tissue changes in rheumatoid arthritis, its localization in plasma cells of chronically inflamed joints and nodules, and its presence, with complement, at sites of tissue destruction raise a host of tempting speculations.

Technique. Various tests are available for RF activity in serum. The simplest procedure uses whole human serum and latex particles coated with IgG. A slide method can be used for screening, with tube titration for quantitation. This test is neither as sensitive nor as specific as more complex procedures using tanned red cells from human or other species and gamma globulin from rabbits. Variations involving serum inactivation, adsorption, or fractionation can improve sensitivity, but require additional time and technical skill for accurate performance. In a well standardized latex test, titers of 1:100 or 1:160 are considered positive, and approximately 70 per cent of adult patients with rheumatoid arthritis will be seropositive.[11,73] Some patients with adult rheumatoid arthritis are persistently seronegative, and most patients with the juvenile form of the disease are negative.[7]

Interpretation. False positives are fairly common, as many as 5 per cent of the general population having low levels of anti-IgG activity in their serum.[72] This reflects on the poor specificity of the serologic phenomenon, not on the technique of the test. Patients with chronic infections or hyperglobulinemia of other causes may develop anti-IgG activity, and the aging process itself seems to predispose to seropositivity.[28] Chronic interstitial pulmonary fibrosis and nodular pulmonary silicosis produce RF activity in up to 50 per cent of patients.[11] Although normal individuals may occasionally present with an elevated RF titer,[73] such a finding should prompt careful search for incipient rheumatoid disease or other covert chronic illness.

ANTINUCLEAR ANTIBODIES

The L. E. Cell

True autoantibodies are those immunoglobulins which react with components present in the patient's own tissue as well as material of other mammalian species. Hargraves' initial description of the *L.E. cell*, in 1948,[26] focused attention on the peculiar serologic features in patients with lupus erythematosus, and work has progressed apace since then. Production of the L.E. cell is an in vitro process which occurs in two stages: interaction of the serum factor with nuclei so altered or slightly damaged that nuclear antigen is accessible; and engulfment of this altered nuclear material by phagocytic cells, usually neutrophils. Both IgG and IgM antinuclear antibodies can produce alterations in the nucleoproteins, but only IgG antibodies initiate the complete, biphasic process of L.E. cell production.[46] This antibody has been shown to react with a DNA-histone nucleoprotein, but it is by no means the only antinuclear antibody produced by patients with this very complex disease.[21] The L.E. cell test is probably the most frequently performed test for the presence of antinuclear antibodies because it is widely available and requires a minimum of equipment or reagents. It is fairly sensitive, giving positive results in perhaps 80 per cent of active cases of lupus,[9] but is not specific and cannot be quantified.

Immunofluorescence

A widely used, versatile technique to show antinuclear activity is indirect immunofluorescence, in which the patient's serum is reacted with frozen sections of mammalian kidney or liver as a source of nuclei. Globulin localization, if the serum contains antinuclear antibodies, is demonstrated with fluorescein-conjugated antihuman globulin serum. Serums with antinuclear activity produce several different patterns of fluorescent labelling suggesting activity directed against specific nuclear elements. The four major patterns are: homogeneous fluorescence of the entire nucleus; fluorescence of speckled areas throughout the nucleus, perhaps less pronounced at the periphery; nucleolar fluorescence with no reaction to the remaining substance; and peripheral staining, most pronounced around the rim.[64]

The identification of patterns, let alone interpretation of these patterns, remains fraught with pitfalls. When carefully performed, indirect immunofluorescence testing for antinuclear antibodies gives 95 to 99 per cent positive results in active lupus erythematosus,[9,59] thereby constituting the most reliable diagnostic procedure for this disease. Serums can be diluted as an index of antibody strength, but staining patterns sometimes change with dilution, and the test remains essentially qualitative.

Agglutination of DNA

As with so many other tests, agglutination techniques have been applied to the study of antinuclear antibodies. Tanned red blood cells can be coated with antigen prepared from calf thymus, a substrate considered suitable for measurement of anti-DNA activity. DNA antigen has also been adsorbed onto latex particles. Since patients with rheumatoid factor may appear positive with this procedure, a latex particle RF test should be run concomitantly as a control. With this test system, quantitation by serial dilutions gives good results, and agglutinating titers of 1:8 or above are highly correlated with lupus erythematosus.[35] Serum anti-DNA activity tends to wax and wane as the disease exacerbates and remits, with the correlation especially close between DNA antibody and renal involvement.[60]

Other Autoantibodies. Immunofluorescence techniques permit rather rapid screening for the presence, in serum, of globulins reactive with antigens from specific tissue sites. Human antibodies exist which react with a variety of mammalian tissues, including human organs. These include antibodies active against, among others, gastric parietal cells,[57] several different elements of thyroid tissue,[61] glomerular basement membranes,[70] the striations in skeletal muscle,[51] and against the cytoplasm of smooth muscle.[34] The pathogenetic role of these *autoantibodies* is the subject of enormous debate, so their use as diagnostic tests is still an unsettled question. Tests for thyroid antibodies are well established in evaluating thyroid disease (see Chap. 16), but the others have largely investigational applications. It is tempting to assign significance to gastric antibodies in pernicious anemia, to colonic mucosal antibodies in ulcerative colitis, and to striated muscle antibodies in myasthenia gravis. Less coherent is the association between antibodies to smooth muscle and the presence of chronic active hepatitis. Unless some antigenic cross-reactivity is postulated between normal smooth muscle and normal or abnormal liver tissue, the conjunction appears fortuitous, yet up to 40 or 50 per cent of patients with chronic active hepatitis have serum activity against this antigen.[75] When L.E. cell or antinuclear antibody tests are also positive, the incidence goes even higher.

SEROLOGIC TECHNIQUES IN LIVER DISEASE

Hepatitis-Associated Antigen

Immunologic testing is used to recognize an antigen in serum, closely associated with hepatitis of the long-incubation period type (serum hepatitis, MS-2, hepatitis B). This antigen, variously called Australia antigen, Au (1), hepatitis-associated antigen (HAA), serum hepatitis antigen (SH), and HB Ag, circulates during the prodromal period and early clinical illness, usually disappearing as the disease clears or somewhat earlier. The hepatitis patient whose serum contains HAA can reliably be said to have long-incubation period hepatitis. Using this marker, many investigators[5,22,23,29] have shown that nonparenteral spread can occur with this disease which was formerly considered a blood-borne condition, although contagion is far less frequent than with short-incubation period, "infectious" hepatitis.

Techniques. The test most widely used for HAA is counter-immuno-electrophoresis, or immuno-osmoelectrophoresis. At pH of 8.6, the antigen migrates toward the anode, while the antibody, which is at a pH close to its isoelectric point and therefore very weakly charged, moves toward the cathode because of endosmotic forces in the suspending medium. Early studies used two-dimensional immunodiffusion, but this technique proved too time-consuming and insufficiently sensitive for large scale use. Complement fixation techniques are sensitive and susceptible to automation, but subject to the drawbacks of all complement fixation techniques. Hemagglutination and radioimmunoprecipitation techniques are extraordinarily sensitive, and are being used in increasing numbers of laboratories.

Significance. Blood containing HAA carries a 40 to 70 per cent risk of causing hepatitis if transfused, and transfusion facilities screen all donor bloods to ensure that only HAA-negative blood is used. HAA can also be found in many patients with chronic active hepatitis[25,48] whether or not prior acute hepatitis has occurred. HAA is found frequently in renal dialysis patients, in institutionalized patients with Downs' syndrome, and in some patients receiving immunosuppressive medication. A small number of seemingly healthy individuals have circulating HAA. Some of these prove, on liver biopsy, to have smoldering hepatic disease,[62] but some do not.[17,56] Most give no history of acute illness. It may be that very low-dose infection is more likely to produce a carrier state than large-dose exposure, which produces acute illness and subsequent antigen clearing.[8]

Because antigenemia is transient and sometimes unpredictable, failure to demonstrate HAA does not prove a patient's hepatitis to be the short-incubation period type. By the time a patient presents with clinical illness, the antigen may already have disappeared, or it may be present at levels below the sensitivity of the test. Short-incubation period, or "infectious," hepatitis is always HAA negative; efforts to identify comparable antigenic markers for the epidemic form of hepatitis have not been conclusive.[3,15]

Anti-HAA Antibodies. The antibodies first used to demonstrate the hepatitis-associated antigen came from patients who had received multiple transfusions, usually hemophiliacs. Antibodies can also be raised in nonhuman species, and both human and nonhuman antibodies are in current use. It appears that there are several different antigenic components to the *hepatitis-associated antigen,* although a single common element appears to be present in all the antigen-antibody reactions described.[37,41,43]

For some time it appeared that HAA infection or exposure did not, in most patients, lead to antibody production. Since most virus infections produce prompt antibody response, it was puzzling that complement fixation and counter-electrophoresis techniques so rarely documented antibodies in patients recovering from hepatitis. Only patients receiving multiple transfusions, such as hemophiliacs and those with thalassemia, consistently had demonstrable antibodies.

It now appears that the problem was one of detection rather than production. Radioimmunoprecipitation and passive hemagglutination techniques have shown that most patients do develop antibodies after infection, and antibody incidence in various populations parallels expected levels of exposure to the hepatitis virus.[39,40,54] These tests are not yet in sufficiently wide use to make serodiagnosis of hepatitis standard procedure.

Alpha Fetoprotein

Another serum element demonstrable in liver disease by immunologic means is alpha fetoprotien, also called fetulin or alpha fetoglobulin. This globulin is produced by the normal fetal liver, but disappears from the circulation in the first week or so of life.[1] In only one disease is it found in adult serum, hepatocellular carcinoma. This provides the basis for a simple, fairly specific test for an otherwise often difficult diagnosis.[49] The globulin can be precipitated, on an immunodiffusion plate, by anti-alpha fetoglobulin raised in rabbits. The incidence rate seems to vary with the population tested. In those Negroid and Oriental populations in which hepatoma is frequent, between 70 and 90 per cent of patients may have positive tests, while in Caucasians the rate is much lower. Counter-immunoelectrophoresis permits detection of far smaller quantities than does immunodiffusion, but even so the incidence is only 50 per cent.[6] A positive test strongly indicates hepatoma, but absence of the protein does not rule out the diagnosis.

BIBLIOGRAPHY

1. ABELEV, G.I.: Production of embryonal serum α-globulin by hepatomas: review of experimental and clinical data. Cancer Res. 28: 1344, 1968.
2. ABRUTYN, E., HERRMAN, K.L., KARCHMER, A.W. ET AL.: Rubella vaccine comparative study. Nine-month follow up and serologic response to natural challenge. Am. J. Dis. Child. 120:129, 1970.
3. AJDUKIEWICZ, A.B., FOX, R.A., DUDLEY, F.J. ET AL.: Immunological studies in an epidemic of infective, short-incubation hepatitis. Lancet 1:803, 1972.
4. ALLISON, M.J., DALTON, H.P., AND ESCOBAR, M.R.: An evaluation of the VDRL and FTA-ABS in a general hospital laboratory. Am. J. Clin. Path. 51:420, 1969.
5. ALMEIDA, J.D., KULATILAKE, A.E., MACKAY, D.H. ET AL.: Possible airborne spread of serum hepatitis virus within a haemodialysis unit. Lancet 2:849, 1971.
6. ALPERT, E., HERSHBERG, R., SCHUR, P.H., AND ISSELBACHER, K.J.: α-fetoprotein in human hepatoma: improved detection in serum and quantitative studies using a new sensitive technique. Gastroenterology 61:137, 1971.
7. ANSELL, B.M., HOBOROW, J., ZUTSHI, D. ET AL.: Comparison of three serological tests in adult rheumatoid arthritis and Still's disease (juvenile rheumatoid arthritis). Ann. N.Y. Acad. Sci. 168:21, 1969.
8. BARKER, L.F., AND MURRAY, R.: Acquisition of hepatitis-associated antigen. Clinical features in young adults. J.A.M.A. 216:1970, 1971.
9. BARNETT, E.V., AND ROTHFIELD, N.: The present status of antinuclear antibody serology. Arthritis Rheum. 12:543, 1969.
10. BLOOM, B.R.: In vitro approaches to the mechanism of cell-mediated immune reactions. Adv. Immunol. 13:101, 1971.
11. CATHCART, E.S.: "Serologic techniques." In Cohen, A.S. (ed.): Laboratory Diagnostic Procedures in the Rheumatic Diseases. Little, Brown & Co., Boston, 1967.
12. CHANG, T.W., DESROSIERS, S., AND WEINSTEIN, L.: Clinical and serologic studies of an outbreak of rubella in a vaccinated population. N. Engl. J. Med. 283:246, 1970.
13. CORDERO, L., FLOREY, C. DU V., AND HORSTMANN, D.: Persistence of antibodies to Mycoplasma pneumoniae following naturally ocurring infections. Am. J. Epidemiol. 88:428, 1968.
14. DEACON, W.E., FALCONE, V.H., AND HARRIS, A.: A fluourescent test for treponemal antibodies. Proc. Soc. Exp. Biol. Med. 96:477, 1957.
15. DEL PRETE, S., DOGLIA, M., AJDUKIEWICZ, A. ET AL.: Detection of a new serum-antigen in three epidemics of short-incubation hepatitis. Lancet 2:579, 1970.
16. DENNY, F.W., CLYDE, W.A., JR., AND GLEZEN, W.P.: Mycoplasma pneumoniae disease: clinical spectrum, pathophysiology, epidemiology, and control. J. Infect. Dis. 123:74, 1971.
17. DUDLEY, F.J., FOX, R.A., AND SHERLOCK, S.: Relationship of hepatitis associated antigen (H.A.A.) to acute and chronic liver injury. Lancet 2:1, 1971.
18. ESCOBAR, M.R., DALTON, H.P., AND ALLISON, M.J.: Fluorescent antibody tests for syphilis using cerebrospinal fluid. Am. J. Clin. Pathol. 53:886, 1970.
19. EVANS, A.S., NIEDERMAN, J.C., AND SAWYER, R.N.: Prospective studies of a group of Yale University freshmen. II. Occurrence of acute respiratory infections and rubella. J. Infect. Dis. 123:271, 1971.
20. EVATT, B.L., DOWDLE, W. R., JOHNSON, McC., JR., AND HEATH, C. W.: Epidemic mycoplasma pneumonia. N. Engl. J. Med. 285:374, 1971.
21. FRIOU, G.J.: Antinuclear antibodies: diagnostic significance and methods. Arthritis Rheum. 10:151, 1967.
22. GARIBALDI, R.A., HATCH, F.E., BISNO, A.L. ET AL.: Nonparenteral serum hepatitis. Report of an outbreak. J.A.M.A. 220:963, 1972.
23. GARIBALDI, R.A., RASMUSSEN, C.M., HOLMES, A.W., AND GREGG, M.B.: Hospital-acquired serum hepatitis. Report of an outbreak. J.A.M.A. 219:1577, 1972.
24. GRIFFIN, J.P.: Rapid screening for cold agglutinins in pneumonia. Ann. Intern. Med. 70:701, 1969.

25. GROB, P.J., JEMELKA, H.J., AND MÜLLER, J.W.: B, A and SH antigen in chronic hepatitis. Gastroenterology 61:91, 1971.
26. HARGRAVES, M.M., RICHMOND, H., AND MORTON, R.: Presentation of two bone marrow elements: the "tart" cell and the "L.E." cell. Mayo Clin. Proc. 23:25, 1948.
27. HARNER, R.E., SMITH, J.L., AND ESRAEL, C.W.: The FTA-ABS test in late syphilis. J.A.M.A. 203:545, 1968.
28. HEIMER, R., LEVIN, F.M., AND RUDD, E.: Globulins resembling rheumatoid factor in serum of the aged. Am. J. Med. 35:175, 1963.
29. HERSH, T., MELNICK, J.L., GOYAL, R.K., AND HOLLINGER, F.B.: Nonparenteral transmission of viral hepatitis type B. (Australia antigen-associated serum hepatitis). N. Engl. J. Med. 285:1363, 1971.
30. HORSTMAN, D.M.: Rubella: the challenge of its control. J. Infect. Dis. 123:640, 1971.
31. HUMPHREY, J.H., AND WHITE, R.G.: Immunology for Students of Medicine, ed. 3. F.A. Davis Co., Philadelphia, 1970.
32. HUNTER, E.F., DEACON, W.E., AND MEYER, P.E.: An improved FTA test for syphilis: The absorption procedure (FTA-ABS). Public Health Rep. 79:410, 1964.
33. ISHIZAKA, K.: The identification and significance of gamma E. Hosp. Pract. 4:70, 1969.
34. JOHNSON, G.D., HOLBOROW, E.J., AND GLYNN, L.E.: Antibody to smooth muscle in patients with liver disease. Lancet 2:878, 1965.
35. JOKINEN, E.J. AND JULKUNEN, H.: DNA haemagglutination test in the diagnosis of systemic lupus erythematosus. Ann. Rheum. Dis. 24:477, 1965.
36. KERR, W.R., McCAUGHEY, W.J., COGHLAN, J.D. ET AL.: Techniques and interpretations in the serological diagnosis of brucellosis in man. J. Med. Microbiol. 1:181, 1968.
37. KIM, C.Y., AND TILLES, J.G.: Immunologic and electrophoretic heterogeneity of hepatitis-associated antigen. J. Infect. Dis. 123:618, 1971.
38. KRAUS, S.J., HASERICK, J.R., AND LANTZ, M.A.: Fluorescent treponemal antibody-absorption test reactions in lupus erythematosus. N. Engl. J. Med. 282:1287, 1970.
39. LANDER, J.J., GILES, J.P., PURCELL, R. H., AND KRUGMAN, S.: Viral hepatitis, type B (MS-2 strain). Detection of antibody after primary infection. N. Engl. J. Med. 285:303, 1971.
40. LANDER, J.J. HOLLAND, P.V., ALTER, H.J. ET AL.: Antibody to hepatitis-associated antigen. J.A.M.A. 220:1079, 1972.
41. LE BOUVIER, G.L.: The heterogeneity of Australia antigen. J. Infect. Dis. 123:671, 1971.
42. LE BOUVIER, G.L., AND PLOTKIN, S.A.: Precipitin responses to rubella vaccine RA 27/3. J. Infect. Dis. 123:220, 1971.
43. LEVENE, C., AND BLUMBERG, B.S.: Additional specificities of Australia antigen and the possible identification of hepatitis carriers. Nature (Lond.) 221:195, 1969.
44. LIEBHABER, H.: Measurement of rubella antibody by hemagglutination inhibition. II. Characteristics of an improved HAI test employing a new method for the removal of non-immunoglobulin HA inhibitors from serum. J. Immunol. 104:826, 1970.
45. MACKEY, D.M., PRICE, E.V., KNOX, J.M., AND SCOTTI, A.: Specificity of the FTA-ABS test for syphilis. J.A.M.A. 207:1683, 1969.
46. McDUFFIE, F.C.: Twenty years of the lupus erythematosus cell. Ann. Intern. Med. 70:413, 1969.
47. NELSON, R.A., AND MAYER, M.M.: Immobilization of Treponema pallidum in vitro by antibody produced in syphilitic infection. J. Exp. Med. 89:369, 1949.
48. NIELSEN, J.O., DIETRICHSON, O., ELLING, P., AND CHRISTOFFERSEN, P.: Incidence and meaning of persistence of Australia antigen in patients with acute viral hepatitis: development of chronic hepatitis. N. Engl. J. Med. 285:1157, 1971.
49. O'CONER, G.T., TATARINOV, Y.S., ABELEV, G.I. ET AL.: A collaborative study for the evaluation of a serologic test for primary liver cancer. Cancer 25:1091, 1971.
50. OLANSKY, S.: The diagnosis of early syphilis. Med. Ann. D.C. 35:367, 1966.
51. OSSERMAN, K.E.: "Muscles (myasthenia gravis)." in Miescher, P.A., and Müller-Eber-

hard, H.J. (eds.): Textbook of Immunopathology. Grune & Stratton, Inc., New York, 1969.

52. PETERS, A.H.: Tick-borne typhus (Rocky Mountain spotted fever). Epidemiologic trends, with particular reference to Virginia. J.A.M.A. 216:1003, 1971.

53. PLOTKIN, S.A.: Rubella: epidemiology, virology and immunology. II. The virology of rubella. Am. J. Med. Sci. 253:356, 1967.

54. PRINCE, A.M., SZMUNESS, W., WOODS, K.R., AND GRADY, G.F.: Antibody against serum-hepatitis antigen. N. Engl. J. Med. 285:933, 1971.

55. PROTELL, R.L., SOLOWAY, R.D., MARTIN, W.J.: Antisalmonella agglutinins in chronic active liver disease. Lancet 2:330, 1971.

56. REINICKE, V., DYBKJAER, E., POULSEN, H. ET AL.: A study of Australia-antigen-positive blood donors and their recipients, with special reference to liver histology. N. Engl. J. Med. 286:867, 1972.

57. ROITT, I.M., AND DONIACH, D.: "Gastric autoimmunity." in Miescher, P.A., and Müller-Eberhard, H.J. (eds.): Textbook of Immunopathology. Grune & Stratton, Inc., New York, 1969.

58. SCHEPERS, G.W.H.: Laboratory diagnosis of venereal disease. Med. Ann. D.C. 35:357, 1966.

59. SCHUR, P.H.: A.N.A. N. Engl. J. Med. 282:1205, 1970.

60. SHARP, G.C., AND IRVIN, W.S.: Hemagglutinating antibody to DNA and to the extractable nuclear antigen in systemic lupus erythematosus. Arthritis Rheum. 11:116 (abst.), 1968.

61. SHULMAN, S.: Thyroid antigens and autoimmunity. Adv. Immunol. 14:85, 1971.

62. SINGLETON, J.W., MERRILL, D.A., FITCH, R.A. ET AL.: Liver disease in Australia-antigen-positive blood-donors. Lancet 2:785, 1971.

63. STEWART, G.L., PARKMAN, P.D., HOPPS, H.E. ET AL.: Rubella virus hemagglutination inhibition test. N. Engl. J. Med. 276:554, 1967.

64. TAN, E.M.: Relationship of nuclear staining patterns with precipitating antibodies in systemic lupus erythematosus. J. Lab. Clin. Med. 70:800, 1967.

65. TAYLOR, K.B.: Immunological mechanisms of the gastrointestinal tract. Gastroenterology 51:1058, 1966.

66. TAYLOR-ROBINSON, D., SOBESLAVSKY, O., JENSEN, K.E. ET AL.: Serologic response to Mycoplasma pneumoniae infections. I. Evaluation of immunofluorescence, complement fixation, indirect hemagglutination, and tetrazolium reduction inhibition tests for the diagnosis of infection. Am. J. Epidemiol. 83:287, 1966.

67. THOMAS, L.: Mycoplasmas as infectious agents. Annu. Rev. Med. 21:179, 1970.

68. TOMASI, T.B., JR., AND DECOTEAU, E.: Mucosal antibodies in respiratory and gastrointestinal disease. Adv. Intern. Med. 16:401, 1970.

69. TURNER, T.B.: "Syphilis and the treponematoses." In Mudd, S. (ed.): Infectious Agents and Host Reactions. W.B. Saunders Co., Philadelphia, 1970.

70. VERNIER, R.L., FISH, A.J., AND MICHAEL, A.L.: "The immunologic basis of renal disease." In Kagan, B.M., and Stiehm, E.R. (eds.): Immunologic Incompetence. Year Book Medical Publishers, Chicago, 1971.

71. VOGEL, H., CHERUBIN, C.E., AND MILLIAN, S.J.: Febrile agglutinins in narcotic addicts. Am. J. Clin. Path. 53:932, 1971.

72. WALLER, M.: Methods of measurement of rheumatoid factor. Ann. N.Y. Acad. Sci. 168: 5, 1969.

73. WALLER, M.: Present status of rheumatoid factor. Crit. Rev. Clin. Lab. Sci. 2:173, 1971.

74. WEIL, A.J., AND SAPHRA, I.: Incidence of antibodies to Salmonellae among the population of the Bronx, N.Y. J. Immunol. 74:485, 1955.

75. WHITTINGHAM, S., MACKAY, I.R., AND IRWIN, J.: Autoimmune hepatitis: immunofluorescence reactions with cytoplasm of smooth muscle and renal glomerular cells. Lancet 1:1333, 1966.

76. ZMIJEWSKI, C.M., AND FLETCHER, J.L.: The preoperative assessment of histocompatibility. Arch. Int. Med. 123:514, 1969.

CHAPTER 3

Blood Banking

Every time a blood transfusion is given, living red cells that originate in one individual are given to another who uses them as though they were his own. The technique of classifying blood for transfusion appears easy. Most bloods are designated briefly, using one or two letters and the notation "positive" or "negative." Classification into ABO group and description as Rh positive or Rh negative afford sufficient information that transfusion is feasible. Yet it is probable that the red cells of each individual are unique, characterized by a particular combination of antigens specific to his cells. Immunohematology is the study of these antigens and their associated antibodies. Transfusion therapy and understanding of hemolytic disease of the newborn are the most important clinical results of research in immunohematology.

IMMUNOLOGIC PRINCIPLES

The study of blood groups and blood banking must begin with blood group antigens. These antigens reside in or on the surface of the red cell stroma, and an enormous variety is known to exist. Their structure is determined genetically. Most blood group antigens are combinations of carbohydrate and amino acid units[28] and many can be identified very early in fetal life.

Antigens are identified when they react with an antibody. Antibodies are globulins that combine, in a highly specific manner, with the corresponding antigen. This definition is somewhat circular since the antibody is defined by the antigen and the antigen is defined by the antibody. Both entities do, however, have objective existence. Antibodies can be separated and characterized by physical and chemical, as well as immunologic, means, and a number of antigens have had their chemical formulas determined. Nevertheless, the terminology and specificity of antibodies and antigens are mutually dependent.

IMMUNIZING EVENTS

Without getting too involved in complexities of immunologic theory, we might briefly define the term *antigenic stimulation* or *immunizing event.* This is the introduction, into a susceptible individual, of substances capable of provoking an antibody response. In immunohematology this means that red cells containing a particular antigen enter an individual whose cells lack that antigen. People do not ordinarily form antibodies to antigens they already possess. If red cells containing some other antigens enter the circulation, the individual's immune mechanisms can identify the "foreign" antigens and may produce antibodies against them.

Red cells can enter the circulation by blood transfusion. During pregnancy and parturition, fetal cells may enter the maternal blood stream. Rarely, intramuscular injections of red cells have stimulated antibody production. The antibody or antibodies produced after such exposure are called immune antibodies and are frequently, though not always, IgG molecules. Antibodies that exist without any apparent immunizing event are called naturally occurring and are almost always IgM molecules.

AGGLUTINATION

In blood banking, the visible end-point of most antigen-antibody reactions is agglutination. Agglutination requires that the antigen be on the surface of a particle, in this case the red cell. When antibody unites with the surface antigen on several particles, a visible aggregate is formed. Red cells are sufficiently large particles that agglutinates of even a few cells can readily be perceived.

Agglutination occurs in two phases. First the antibody must recognize, and attach to, its specific antigen. This attachment is reversible, but the antibody-antigen union reaches an equilibrium at a speed dependent upon constants intrinsic to the specific antibody, and influenced by temperature, pH, and ionic strength of the suspending medium. This union of antigen with antibody need not result in agglutination. All antibodies have at least two combining sites, but both sites may attach to antigens on the same cell, or one site may remain unoccupied. If, however, adjacent cells are sufficiently close to one another, a second antigen-antibody reaction may occur, whereby the immunoglobulin molecule attaches to another cell, forming a physical link between the two cells. Figure 9 shows a schematic

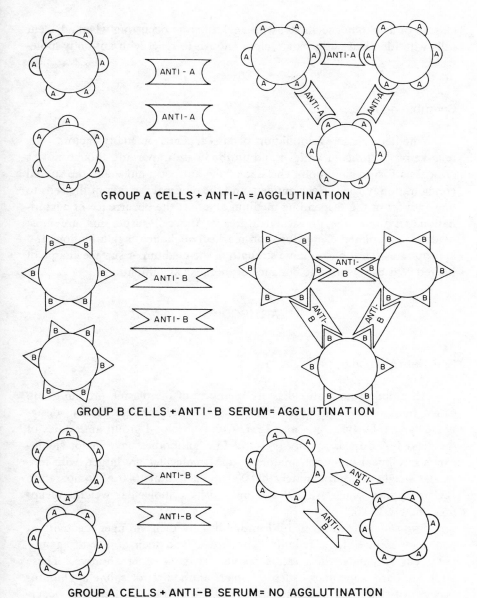

GROUP A CELLS + ANTI-A = AGGLUTINATION

GROUP B CELLS +ANTI-B SERUM= AGGLUTINATION

GROUP A CELLS + ANTI-B SERUM= NO AGGLUTINATION

Figure 9. Agglutination occurs when the antibody combines with its specific antigen on the cell surface.

version of antibody specificity, with agglutination occurring when adjacent cells with identical antigens are close enough to react with antibody molecules.

Contributing Factors

Whether or not agglutination occurs depends on many factors. The relative proportions of antigen and antibody are important, though not as critical as for precipitation. The size of the antibody molecule, the spatial configuration of the surface antigen, and the physical relation of the cells to one another in the suspending medium all affect the occurrence of agglutination. Of these, the physical features of the cell suspension are most readily manipulated. Centrifugation markedly enhances agglutination, and appropriate alterations in ionic strength of the medium or surface charge of the red cells can be used to enhance or diminish agglutination.

ANTIBODIES

Complete Antibodies

All blood group antibodies are members of the plasma protein group called immunoglobulins. Five immunoglobulin classes are known, designated IgA, IgD, IgE, IgG, and IgM. Although blood group antibodies of the class IgA do exist,[18] only IgG and IgM antibodies have major significance in clinical immunohematology. IgM molecules are larger, with molecular weight of approximately 900,000 and length of 1000 Å, compared to IgG molecules which are 250 Å long and have molecular weights of approximately 150,000.

Two salient features of IgM antibodies are their stronger reactivity at cool temperatures than at body temperature, and their ability to agglutinate cells suspended in a saline medium without other additives. These antibodies are sometimes called *complete* antibodies, or *saline agglutinins* because of this latter characteristic. They are also called *naturally occurring,* because most antibodies which occur with no prior identifiable immune stimuli such as transfusion, pregnancy, or deliberate inoculation are of this class. Most IgM antibodies are complement-binding. IgM molecules do not cross the placenta from mother to fetus.

Immune Antibodies

The IgG antibodies behave rather differently from the larger IgM proteins. Unlike the complete antibodies, IgG molecules ordinarily fail to agglutinate red cells suspended in saline. If the suspending medium is altered by adding serum albumin or changing the ionic composition, the red cells may be brought close enough together for the IgG molecules to cause direct agglutination. Frequently, however, the IgG antibodies attach themselves to the red cell surface but do not agglutinate the cells. This behavior was first described as "blocking." The antibody, by attaching to the antigens, prevents subsequently added complete antibody from uniting with the antigen and agglutinating the cells. To demonstrate this blocking effect, it is necessary to have a strong complete antibody of the same specificity.

Antiglobulin Serum

The work of Coombs, Mourant, and Race,[7] in 1945, made the detection of incomplete antibodies vastly simpler, permitting the discovery of many new antigens and antibodies. Following their work, the use of antihuman globulin serum (Coombs' serum) has been of enormous importance. Antiglobulin serum is used according to the following principles. Blood group antibodies are globulins. Blood group antibodies formed by human beings are human globulins. Introduction of human globulin into certain animals (rabbits, guinea pigs, goats, etc.) causes them to form antibodies against the general antigenic category of human globulins. In this case human globulin (the human blood group antibody) is the antigen; the animal serum is the antibody.

The Coombs Test. Various procedures of purification and absorption permit preparation of specific antisera against subdivisions of the globulin category, such as IgG globulins, or IgM, or a number of other fractions, but the principle of all tests is the same. The antibody to human globulin reveals the presence of the corresponding globulin antigen. In the case of incomplete antibodies, the IgG molecules attach themselves to the red cell antigens. The antibody molecules bristle on the cell surface but do not agglutinate the cells. If Coombs' serum is added, the antiglobulin antibodies attach to the IgG antibodies on the cell surface; by attaching to two molecules simultaneously, they cause the coated red cells to agglutinate Fig. 10). The red cells coated with incomplete antibody are said to be sensitized and addition of antiglobulin serum (Coombs' serum) demonstrates that sensitization has occurred. Sensitization cannot occur unless the red cells possess the antigens for which the incomplete antibody is specific.

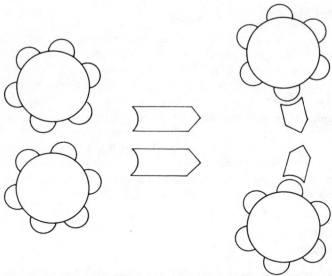

**CELLS WITH ANTIGEN + INCOMPLETE ANTIBODY = COATED
CELLS THAT ARE NOT AGGLUTINATED**

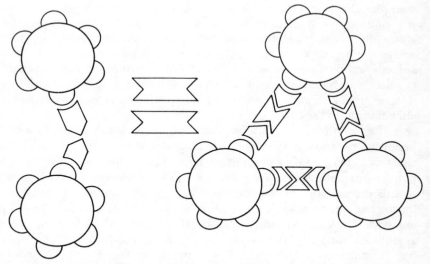

COATED CELLS + ANTI-GLOBULIN SERUM = AGGLUTINATION

Figure 10.   In the Coombs antiglobulin procedure, antibody is detected on the cell surface by addition of an antihuman globulin serum which unites the antibody molecules and causes the red cells to agglutinate.

DIRECT COOMBS TEST. Several circumstances exist in which it is desirable to know whether sensitization has occurred. The direct Coombs test is done on an unmodified sample of the circulating red cells to see whether antibody has attached to the cells in vivo. Such in vivo sensitization characterizes autoimmune hemolytic anemias and may also occur after transfusion of incompatible blood (see p. 91) and in hemolytic disease of the newborn. Performance of the direct Coombs test requires only addition of Coombs' serum to a washed sample of red cells. If the cells are coated with antibody, they will agglutinate when antiglobulin serum is added. The test is called direct because only one step is needed—addition of antiglobulin serum directly to the washed cells.

ANTIBODY-SCREENING TEST. Antiglobulin serum can also be used to investigate whether or not a serum sample contains antibodies other than those of the ABO system. This is sometimes called an indirect Coombs test. An antibody's existence becomes apparent only after combination with an antigen. If the antibody is of the IgG or incomplete type, there may be a problem in demonstrating that the reaction has taken place, since the red cells do not agglutinate when incomplete antibody combines with red cell antigens. The antiglobulin serum can be used to demonstrate antibody attached to the cell surface.

The antibody-screening test requires a suspension of red cells which contain a large number of previously identified antigens. The serum sample is incubated with the red cells under optimum conditions for antigen-antibody interaction. After incubation the cells are washed and antiglobulin serum is added. If the serum contains an antibody to one of the antigens present on the cells, antiglobulin serum will agglutinate the sensitized cells. Absence of agglutination indicates that the serum was free of antibodies to those antigens known to be present. The end result of the direct and indirect Coombs tests is the same—addition of antiglobulin serum to cells which, if sensitized, are agglutinated. The difference is that the direct Coombs test investigates in vivo sensitization, whereas the indirect Coombs test demonstrates whether or not a serum sample contains antibodies.

Neither the direct antiglobulin test nor the antibody-screening test specifies which particular antibody and antigen is involved. Enormous numbers of both are known to exist, and can be identified with suitable applications of the above-mentioned techniques.

INHERITANCE OF BLOOD GROUPS

Red cell antigens are genetically determined. Although their composition is not fully elucidated, the antigens appear to derive specificity from characteristic linkages of carbohydrate groups and peptides. Recent work[29] suggests that genetic control is exerted through the enzymes that mediate these structural linkages. The study of blood groups is a satisfying genetic exercise for there are very few recessive genes. In most blood group systems the allelic genes are codominant; that is, each gene signals its presence by determining a specific antigen. Some genes, however, are amorphs. Amorphs are genes which have no phenotypically recognizable effect, and their presence will be masked if the opposite chromosome contains an active allele. Only when the amorphic gene is present on both chromosomes does the effect become apparent, namely the absence of a particular antigenic configuration.

The nature of an amorphic gene is best illustrated in the ABO system. Human red cells generally fall into one of four major groups—A, B, AB, or O. Cells that are group A possess the A antigen; cells that are group B possess the B antigen; cells that are group AB possess both A and B antigen; and cells that are group O possess neither A nor B. The gene controlling the group O characteristic is an amorph; it does not produce a specific antigen of its own, but when it is present, an *A* or *B* gene cannot occupy the site. Only one *A* or *B* gene is necessary for A or B antigens to be present on the cell. The individual with an *A* gene on one chromosome and a *B* gene on the other will have group AB red cells. Only when two *O* genes are present will the red cells be group O, for then there is no active gene to mediate the necessary sugar linkages.

Blood group antigens are wonderful tools for the geneticists, for the phenotypic effect of each gene is easily identified. Although there are, inevitably, certain complexities about interaction and expression, the presence of individual genes can be demonstrated with considerable certitude, and the distribution and inheritance of genes can be traced by relatively simple technical procedures. Inheritance of all the blood groups has been found to follow mendelian laws, so blood group studies are useful in anthropologic and genetic studies and also in considering paternity problems.

THE ABO SYSTEM

ANTIGENS AND ANTIBODIES

Grouping the red cells into the major ABO categories is relatively simple. The red cells are tested for the presence of the A and B antigen using appropriate antisera. An individual's ABO group is further identified by the presence in the serum of naturally occurring antibodies directed against the antigens *not* present on his own cells. The ABO system is

Table 6.   The ABO System

Individual's Blood Group	Antigens on Red Cells	Antibodies in Serum	Frequency,* as percent of Total Population	
			Caucasians in New York City	American Negroes
O	neither	anti-A anti-B	45	49
A	A	anti-B	37	27
B	B	anti-A	13	20
AB	A and B	neither	5	4

* From Technical Methods and Procedures of the American Association of Blood Banks, ed. 5, 1970.

unique in this respect. Although red cells contain myriad antigens, the serum normally contains only the A and B antibodies; a few persons have naturally occurring antibodies with some other specificity.

The origin of the naturally occurring ABO antibodies has not been fully explained. A variety of plant, animal, and bacterial substances are antigenically similar to the A and B antigens, and exposure to these substances may stimulate production of the naturally occurring antibodies. There are certain flaws in this theory, but no completely satisfactory explanation has evolved. Regardless of etiology, the fact remains that group A individuals have anti-B antibody in their serum; group B individuals have anti-A. Persons whose red cells are group O have both anti-A and anti-B, and those with group AB cells have neither antibody in the serum (see Table 6).

IMMUNE ANTIBODIES

The naturally occurring antibodies, also called isoagglutinins, are of the IgM type. They cause prompt agglutination of cells suspended in saline, i.e., act as complete antibodies; they are unable to cross the placental barrier; and they have a sedimentation constant of 19S. Certain group O individuals also have anti-A and anti-B antibodies that are IgG. These antibodies do not agglutinate cells in vitro until antiglobulin serum is added. Since the IgG antibodies have the same specificity as the IgM components, these antibodies are overlooked unless special procedures are used to identify them. The IgG isoantibodies are sometimes called "immune" anti-A or anti-B because their action is similar to that of IgG antibodies which are known to be antigenically induced, but in most of the group O individuals no immunizing event can be identified. Ordinarily the presence of immune antibodies in group O blood causes no trouble, but they have been implicated in some transfusion reactions when group O blood is given to a group A or group B recipient. Because IgG molecules can cross the placenta, maternal anti-A or anti-B may enter the fetal circulation and produce hemolytic disease of the newborn (see p. 95).

SUBGROUPS OF A

One further complexity of the ABO system deserves mention. In approximately 20 per cent of group A individuals, the red cells give a reaction slightly weaker than normal with standard typing sera. These cells are called group A_2, and there are qualitative as well as quantitative differences from the more frequent A_1 antigen. Individuals who are A_2 may have naturally occurring anti-A_1, so initial tests appear to reveal a group A individual with an antibody against his own group of cells. By the use of sera that agglutinate only A_1 cells and leave the A_2 cells unaffected, bloods can readily be classified as A_2. A patient with an anti-A_1 antibody can only receive A_2 blood, since cells with the A_1 antigen are incompatible.

The ABO system is far more complex than this introduction indicates, but for practical clinical purposes, a summary discussion is sufficient. A few further complexities will be included in the section on transfusion therapy.

THE RH SYSTEM

Landsteiner and his colleagues discovered the presence of ABO antigens simply by mixing cells and serum from different individuals and observing the consequent agglutination. With none of the other blood groups could this be done, for no other antibodies occur spontaneously in the serum of large numbers of people.

DISCOVERY

The Rh system was discovered by Landsteiner and Wiener[15] in 1940 when they used a rabbit antiserum prepared against the cells of rhesus monkeys and tested the anti-rhesus cell serum against human cells. Using this antiserum, they discovered that approximately 85 per cent of the white population possesses a red cell antigen which the other 15 per cent lacks. Since this antigen appeared to be the same as the one on the rhesus monkey cells, the antigen was called Rh. It subsequently developed[16] that

Table 7.   Comparative Nomenclature in the Rh System
The Most Common Individual Rh Factors on Red Cells

Rh-Hr Terminology	CDE Terminology
Rh₀	D
rh′	C
rh″	E
hr′	c
hr″	e

the anti-rhesus cell serum recognizes an antigen somewhat different from the antigen now called Rh, but this does not affect the work on the Rh system.

TERMINOLOGY AND CONTROVERSY

The "rhesus factor" originally described is only part of a very large, complicated system of related red cell antigens, but it is by far the most important member of the group. Whenever the unmodified term *Rh factor* is used, it refers to this antigen, and the term *Rh positive* means that a red cell possesses that one antigen. Two terminologies are in current use for the Rh antigens, of which the major ones are listed in Table 7. The original Rh factor is called Rh₀ in one usage and D in the other. The terminology employing variants of the letters r and h was first used by Wiener, and the one using the letters C, D, and E was introduced by English workers in the early 1940's.

There has been considerable controversy over the preferred terminology and the theoretical principles behind each usage. The controversy centered on proposed genetic mechanisms of antigen determination. The original English theory, propounded by Fisher, proposed the existence of three sets of genes, each with two alleles. These genes were C and c, D and d, and E and e. The assortment of antigens on an individual's red cells would be determined by the selection of these genes inherited from the mother and those from the father. However, Wiener[30] maintained that the different antigens were not separable and that genetic transmission involved a single gene for a "package" of antigenic groups, which he termed an agglutinogen. Thus, in Fisher's terminology a person whose red cells were agglutinated by anti-Rh₀(D), anti-rh′(C), and anti-hr″(e), but not by anti-rh″(E) or anti-hr′(c), would have the genotype DCe/DCe, while in Wiener's terminology the genotype would be R^1R^1 and the existence of the R^1 gene would determine the presence of the antigens Rh₀(D), rh′(C), and

Table 8.   Comparative Nomenclature in the Rh System
The Most Common Genes in the Rh System

Rh-Hr	CDE	Frequency*
R^1	DCe	0.4076
r	dce	0.3886
R^2	DcE	0.1411
R^o	Dce	0.0257

* These figures are for an English population and are taken from Mollison, P. L.: Blood Transfusion in Clinical Medicine, ed. 4. F. A. Davis Company (Blackwell Scientific Publications), 1967.

hr"(e). Table 8 lists the most common genes of the Rh system, using both terminologies.

Subsequent discovery of variant antigens and failure to discover an antigen allelic to Rh_o(D) have obliged modification of both theories. It is now agreed that a single gene determines the inheritance of the Rh antigens, embodying not only the major antigens but a variety of minor and combination antigens as well. More than 30 different Rh antisera have been identified, each defining a specific antigen.

ANTIGENIC STRENGTH

There are five major antigens in the Rh system. Rh_o(D), the first to be discovered, is the most important in clinical situations; members of the 15 per cent of the population who lack this antigen can, if exposed to cells containing the antigen, be easily stimulated to form an anti-Rh_o(D) antibody. Since the Rh antibodies are rarely present without a prior immunizing event, a single transfusion of Rh positive blood into an Rh negative individual causes no difficulty. If the patient forms an antibody, however, any subsequent transfusion of Rh positive blood would cause a serious transfusion reaction. Rh_o(D) is said to be a "strong" antigen because a single injection of Rh positive blood stimulates antibody formation in 50 to 75 per cent of the Rh negative recipients.[18] Antibodies, once formed, may persist for years, so a seemingly innocuous Rh incompatible transfusion might not cause trouble until many years later if a second transfusion then became necessary.

The four other major antigens in the Rh system are far less likely to stimulate antibody production, the next strongest antigen being only one twenty-fifth as likely to provoke antibody production in a negative recipient.[9] The others are weaker still, and in ordinary transfusion practice no effort is made to ensure compatibility of any of the Rh factors except $Rh_o(D)$. All the other Rh antigens were identified when the defining antibody was discovered in a patient's blood. None of the other Rh antibodies have been prepared by deliberate immunization of laboratory animals.

The complexities of the Rh system have a special fascination for geneticists and immunohematologists. For the clinician the Rh system becomes important in two situations—in transfusion therapy and in hemolytic disease of the newborn. In each situation it is almost always $Rh_o(D)$ that causes difficulty, although a respectable number of problems involve hr'(c), and occasionally anti-rh"(E) is the offender. In the sections on transfusion therapy and on hemolytic disease of the newborn, the ways in which these problems can best be identified and avoided will be discussed.

OTHER BLOOD GROUPS

The red cell surface contains many antigens in addition to those of the ABO and Rh systems. These antigens assume clinical importance when antibodies to one or several of them cause transfusion problems or hemolytic disease of the newborn. Certain red cell antigens provide useful genetic markers for the anthropologist and the geneticist.

As new antibodies are found and new antigens defined, problems of classification arise. There are at present several large groups under which many individual antigens are subsumed. Still other antigens appear to be independent of the larger systems and are classified as separate types. Many antigens originally considered independent are found later to be related to larger systems, usually on the basis of genetic studies in populations or families possessing the significant trait.

THE KELL SYSTEM

Of greatest clinical importance is the Kell system. Anti-Kell, the defining antibody, was discovered in 1946, a short time after the Coombs antiglobulin technique was introduced. The Kell (K) antigen is present in approximately 10 per cent of the Caucasian population. Kell is highly antigenic; its introduction into a Kell negative individual is very likely to call forth an antibody. Second after the Rh antibodies, anti-Kell is the antibody most frequently incriminated as a cause of clinical difficulties. Other antigens in the Kell system have been named Cellano (k), Penny (Kp^a), Rautenberg (Kp^b), and Peltz (Ku), and the Sutter antigens (Js^a and Js^b). Most antibodies to these antigens are of the incomplete, Coombs reacting variety.

THE MNSs SYSTEM

Another complex group of antigens and antibodies is subsumed in the MNSs system. M and N antigens were discovered in 1927 by Landsteiner and Levine who developed rabbit antisera to human blood cells. Naturally occurring anti-M and anti-N have been found and may cause crossmatching difficulties. At least sixteen different antibodies recognize antigens which are part of the MNSs system, but aside from naturally occurring anti-M or rare anti-N and occasional immune anti-S and anti-s, the antibodies are rarely of clinical significance.

THE P SYSTEM

The P system was discovered by Landsteiner and Levine in the same series of rabbit immunization studies that produced the MN system. Subsequent complexities have inevitably followed. P antibodies are rare but are naturally occurring, and some have been found to equal or surpass anti-A and anti-B in hemolytic power.

THE LEWIS SYSTEM

The Lewis system, discovered by Mourant in 1946, differs from other systems in that the primary antigen is a soluble substance adsorbed onto the red cells from the plasma. Inheritance of Lewis blood groups is related to inheritance of the secretor trait, whereby individuals have a water soluble form of the ABO antigens in their serous fluids. Naturally occurring and immune Lewis antibodies have been found, and their behavior, both in vivo and in vitro, is often unpredictable.

OTHER SYSTEMS

Other blood group systems first discovered through clinical problems with immune antibodies are Duffy (Fy), Kidd (Jk), and Lutheran (Lu). Many other antigens and antibodies are known, but their natures remain obscure. Some antigens occur in the vast majority of the population, with antibodies arising only in the extremely rare individual who lacks the antigen. These are called "public" antigens. Still other antigens have been found in members of only one or a few families and are called "private" antigens.

TRANSFUSION THERAPY

The physician, ever mindful of the maxim *primum non nocere* (the most important thing is to cause no harm), must continually weigh the probable benefits of each blood transfusion against the many known risks. Hemolytic transfusion reaction—that is, infusion of incompatible blood—is fortunately rare, but when it occurs is dramatic, dangerous, and occasionally fatal. The less dramatic dangers are more common: induction of febrile or allergic reaction; transmission of infectious disease, notably hepatitis; or stimulation of antibody production which might complicate later transfusions or childbearing. Since there are, at present, no effective means of predicting or preventing some of these problems, every transfusion must be considered potentially dangerous.

CROSSMATCH PROCEDURES

To prevent reactions from incompatible transfusions, a variety of increasingly sophisticated procedures are used. These are collectively termed the crossmatch; and before blood is administered, a meticulous crossmatch should be performed. Crossmatching involves subjecting the serum and cells of both donor's blood and patient's blood to conditions optimal for antibody activity. The first step in selecting blood for transfusion is determining the recipient's ABO group and Rh type; in this case, reference is made only to the presence or absence of Rh_o (D). Ordinarily, only blood of that group and type is considered for transfusion. Since antibodies may react in several ways and different types of antibodies require different temperature and different suspending media, several different tests must be performed to ensure that dangerous antigen-antibody reactions will not follow infusion of the donor blood.

Major and Minor Crossmatch

The two possible combinations of antigen and antibody are: the donor's antibody and the patient's cells, and the patient's antibody and donor's cells. Since the volume of patient's blood is larger than the volume of transfused blood, the ratio of antibody to antigen is far greater when the patient's antibody is directed against donor cells than when the donor blood contains an antibody against the patient's cells. The combination of the patient's serum and donor's cells is called the *major crossmatch*. It is of major importance because donor cells, entering a blood supply which contains an effective antibody, may be rapidly destroyed. The combination of donor's serum and patient's cells is called the *minor crossmatch* because the volume of entering antibody, as each drop of blood enters the circulation, presents only a minor problem relative to the large number of circulating cells.

In many blood banks, the minor crossmatch is omitted. Instead, each donor's blood is tested with the antibody-screening test (see p. 77) to ensure that no antibodies other than those of the ABO system are present. If the antibody-screening test is negative, it is unlikely that a significant reaction would occur between the donor's blood and the patient's red cells. The major crossmatch, however, is indispensable, and every unit of donor blood must be tested against the serum of the patient who is to receive it.

Techniques

Once the donor blood has been shown to be free of unexpected antibodies, the crossmatch involves testing the patient's serum against the donor's cells at room temperature in a saline medium, at 37° C in a high protein medium, and after the addition of antiglobulin serum. Incubation in a saline medium at room temperature enhances activity of the complete IgM antibodies. These tend to be naturally occurring and most often involve the Lewis, MN, or P systems, although rarely a naturally occurring Rh antibody may be encountered. Incubation at 37° C in a high protein medium permits agglutination by some of the stronger incomplete antibodies, while subsequent addition of antiglobulin serum reveals the presence of antibodies that sensitize but do not agglutinate the cells. If the donor blood has not been tested for antibodies, a parallel set of tests is run on the donor serum and patient's cells.

Emergency Release

The complete crossmatch is time-consuming, but blood cannot safely be transfused before the entire procedure has been completed. In some emergencies, the physician may consider the risk of delaying transfusion to be greater than the risk of possible incompatibility. In these cases, blood is released on an emergency basis, but in most blood banks the physician must certify his acknowledgment of the risk involved and his opinion that the patient's welfare is best served by taking the unavoidable risk.

Group O as Universal Donor. Whenever possible, transfused blood should be the same group and type as the patient's, and this can usually be determined quite rapidly. Occasionally the physician may consider even this brief delay dangerous, and as a last resort group O blood is sometimes given without any testing. Group O red cells, containing neither A nor B antigens, will not be damaged by whatever isoagglutinins the patient has.

Group O blood does carry a risk, however, since it contains anti-A and anti-B. Ordinarily these antibodies are unlikely to harm the group A or group B patient's red cells, but if so-called immune (7S or IgG) anti-A or anti-B is present in high concentration, hemolysis may occur. Unless the blood has been tested for absence of these immune antibodies, administration of randomly selected group O blood to unselected patients may have serious consequences.

Group AB Recipients

Blood of a group other than the patient's is often used for group AB recipients. Since less than 5 per cent of the population is group AB, this blood is difficult to obtain in large quantities, and the AB patient who needs massive transfusion may find himself without the necessary blood supply. Fortunately, people whose cells are group AB have neither anti-A nor anti-B in their serum, so cells of any type can enter the circulation without being destroyed. In practice, many group AB patients receive group A blood and suffer no ill effects. The anti-B in the donor's group A blood is rapidly diluted and neutralized before the patient's cells are damaged. Group B blood could be used but is usually in short supply. Since there is always the risk of immune anti-A and anti-B in group O blood, group O is seldom used for AB patients, and it offers the additional deterrrent of containing both anti-A and anti-B.

Prevention of Rh Sensitization

Despite the care taken to avoid it, it occasionally happens that an Rh negative individual receives Rh positive blood. Rarely, this is necessary if no other blood is available in an emergency; more often it follows cases of typing or transfusion error. The previously unsensitized recipient will sustain no immediate ill effects, but 69 to 82 per cent of Rh negative persons who receive Rh positive blood can be expected to develop anti-Rh_o(D). [21,22] Sensitization is particularly disastrous in females who expect subsequently to bear children, and in individuals who may need emergency transfusions at some later date.

Recent work[17,21,22] has shown that intramuscular injection of purified anti-Rh_o(D) shortly after infusion of up to 500 ml of Rh positive whole blood can prevent primary sensitization. The dose recommended is 20 μg anti-Rh_o(D) globulin for each milliliter of red cells transfused. Since the volume of infused cells is usually known, the appropriate dose can readily be calculated. Antibody injection appears to shorten the survival of the circulating Rh positive cells, but not to cause intravascular hemolysis. In one study of 20 experimental subjects, circulating, antibody-coated\ Rh positive cells were present in the circulation for 7 to 28 days, while the mean bilirubin elevation 60 hours after transfusion was 1.8 mg/100 ml.[21]

Limitations. This prophylaxis offers great promise in preventing a serious complication of a readily identifiable transfusion mishap. It will not prevent susceptible individuals from developing antibodies to the myriad foreign antigens they receive with every transfusion. Except for $Rh_o(D)$ and the ABO antigens, no others are routinely tested. These antigens are so variably immunogenic, and the combination of donor and recipient antigens in any one transfusion is so complicated, that there is no reasonable expectation of extending this technique to other antigens.

TRANSFUSION HAZARDS

Transmission of Disease

Hepatitis. Perhaps the most serious complication following compatible transfusion is transmission of hepatitis. Viral hepatitis has traditionally been subclassified into *1,* the serum variety, spread by blood transfusion and parenteral inoculation, and *2,* the infectious form, spread by fecal-oral transmission. Discovery of the Australia antigen, or hepatitis-associated antigen (HAA), has permitted refinement of epidemiologic study so the types of hepatitis and modes of transmission are being clarified. The long incubation period disease, previously called serum hepatitis, is associated with positive tests for HAA, but this disease can be transmitted by nonparenteral means as well. The bulk of post-transfusion hepatitis has been of this type, so the current practice of transfusing only HAA negative blood should markedly reduce hepatitis incidence. Since virus suspensions too dilute for present detection techniques can transmit hepatitis,[1] universal HAA testing cannot be expected to eradicate the disease. In addition, the other kind of hepatitis, which seems never to give a positive HAA test, can also follow blood transfusion,[11] so the problem is not yet solved.

AUSTRALIA ANTIGEN. The Australia antigen, so-called because it was first identified in an Australian aborigine,[2] is a largely protein macromolecule which may be a fragment of the virus itself but which is, at the very least, very closely associated with the virus. Patients with long incubation period hepatitis very frequently have blood-borne antigen early in the disease, often before chemical abnormalities or clinical symptoms occur. The test, then, is extremely useful for diagnosing early or prodromal hepatitis. While most patients with HAA positive hepatitis recover and become HAA negative, some have persistent antigenemia and evidence of smoldering disease, and a few are persistently HAA positive with no identifiable abnormalities at all. Many asymptomatic carriers of HAA give no history of clinical hepatitis at any time.

The HAA test can be done by immunoelectrophoresis, by complement fixation, by radioimmunoassay, or by hemagglutination inhibition. The essential feature is to have a strong antibody capable of identifying the antigen, which seems to have at least several separable specificities. Most transfusion services use an immunoelectrophoretic technique to screen donors. Blood positive for HAA carries a 40 to 70 per cent risk of transmitting hepatitis, and the incidence of HAA positive donors ranges from 0.1 per cent of largely voluntary donors to levels of 2 to 5 per cent in donor populations containing many drug addicts, alcoholics, and individuals living in crowded and unhygienic surroundings.[2]

Malaria. Malaria can be transmitted following red cell transfusions, even from donors in seemingly good health. Suppressive medication may prevent expression of clinical illness without eradicating the parasite, so prospective donors who have visited or temporarily lived in endemic areas should not give blood until 36 asymptomatic months after discontinuing prophylaxis.[6] Lifelong residents of heavily endemic malarial areas can have infective blood without any history of identifiable illness, and following illness, there is no certainty that the parasite disappears. For these reasons, transfusion services in nonmalarial areas do not accept blood from individuals who have ever had malaria, or who are natives of endemic areas. Despite these precautions, malaria should be remembered as a post-transfusion complication, particularly in the recently transfused patient who develops spiking fevers with no apparent etiology.

Syphilis. Viable treponemas can transmit syphilis following transfusion of freshly drawn blood. In the primary luetic episode, the serologic test for syphilis may be negative while organisms are in the blood stream, and are potentially infectious after blood is drawn. After storage at 4° C for 48 to 72 hours, organisms become nonviable, so whenever possible, blood should be quarantined for this period before transfusion.

Febrile Reactions

The most common untoward reaction to transfusion is a febrile response, with body temperature sometimes rising to 104° F or higher. In some cases, febrile reactions appear to result from leukocyte incompatibility. Following multiple transfusions, some patients develop antibodies to white cell antigens, and fever can result from administration of granulocytes containing these antigens. When leukocyte antibodies are proven or suspected to be present, transfusion should be with fresh blood from which the white cells have been removed.[12]

Most febrile reactions cannot be diagnosed so easily. Occasionally it is possible to demonstrate antibodies to certain serum protein allotypes;[8] but patients with known Gm antibodies may not have febrile reactions, and febrile reactions frequently occur in patients without antibodies. The possibility remains that the donor blood may contain other substances to which the patient is sensitive, but this has not been documented. Patients with Hodgkin's disease, various lymphomas, and liver disease seem particularly prone to febrile reactions; and if transfusion must be continued or repeated, the patient may benefit from antipyretic, antihistamine, or steroid therapy.

Urticarial Reactions

Urticarial reactions commonly follow transfusion in "atopic" individuals, but fortunately anaphylactic reactions are rare. Patients who complain of itching or wheals during or after a transfusion usually respond well to antihistamines, although in some cases it may be advisable to give steroids before beginning transfusion therapy. Whenever febrile or allergic reactions are anticipated, the medication should be injected into the patient, not into the bottle of blood.

Hemolytic Reactions

The unmodified term *transfusion reaction* usually refers to destruction of incompatible red cells, that is, red cells that contain an antigen against which the patient has an antibody. As crossmatching techniques have become more sensitive, this type of reaction has become less frequent, although even a compatible crossmatch cannot guarantee against the subsequent occurrence of a hemolytic reaction.

Errors of Identity. It must be emphasized that most transfusion reactions result from carelessness in identifying blood samples or in checking patients' identity. Casual errors, rather than inadequate crossmatching techniques, cause the vast majority of transfusion disasters. Mistakes can occur anywhere in the complicated series of events leading up to transfusion. Patients have been misidentified; tubes of blood have been mislabelled; bottles of blood have been mislabelled; crossmatches have been done on samples that were not from the correct container of blood; transfusionists have infused blood without checking the identity of the patient or the numbers on the blood label; labels have fallen off and been replaced on the wrong bottle. The list of mishaps is long and frightening. For this reason, every hospital and every blood bank has a series of rules and crosschecks to prevent or discover this type of error, and only with rigorous attention to these safeguards can transfusion therapy be considered.

Investigating the Hemolytic Reaction. If a hemolytic reaction is suspected, certain steps should be taken to investigate the event. The first step is to discontinue the infusion if all the blood has not been given. Blood remaining in the container should be cultured to be sure contamination has not occurred. As transfusion equipment has been improved, contamination has become increasingly rare, but prompt culture is still advisable. The remaining blood should be returned at once to the blood bank even if only a few drops remain in the plastic or glass container, along with some blood drawn from the patient at the time the reaction is suspected. Without a post-transfusion sample, adequate investigation is impossible.

CHECKING THE CROSSMATCH. Upon receiving the post-transfusion blood sample and the remaining donor blood, the laboratory personnel perform a number of tests. The patient's pre-transfusion sample—the one that was used for the crossmatch—is checked against the post-transfusion sample to be sure the ABO group and Rh type are the same. The blood remaining in the container is similarly checked against the sample used for crossmatching to be sure the sample truly represented the container's contents. The crossmatch procedures are repeated, using the blood in the container and *both* the pre- and post-transfusion samples from the patient.

CHECKING FOR ANTIBODIES. These procedures are done to check the crossmatching technique. To document whether a reaction has, in fact, occurred, the post-transfusion sample is subjected to several other tests. A direct Coombs test is done to determine if any cells are coated with antibody. The serum is examined for the presence of free hemoglobin. Since hemoglobin is normally present only in red cells, the presence of hemoglobin in the serum suggests that red cells have been damaged and their contents liberated.

CHECKING FOR HEMOGLOBIN. It is also advisable to check the patient's urine for the presence of free hemoglobin. The serum haptoglobins can bind a certain quantity of hemoglobin (100 to 150 mg per 100 ml), but if more than that amount is present, the unbound hemoglobin crosses the glomerular filter and enters the urine. Hemoglobin tests should be done on the supernatant fluid of a centrifuged sample, for hematuria from any cause gives a positive reaction in tests on uncentrifuged urine or on the cellular sediment.

If hemolysis has occurred, the serum bilirubin rises within several hours to levels proportional to the amount of liberated hemoglobin. Most incomplete antibodies cause hemolysis in the spleen and liver rather than directly in the circulation, so the plasma hemoglobin level may not be a good index of the amount available for conversion to bilirubin.

OBSERVING THE PATIENT. The clinical symptoms of a hemolytic reaction vary with the condition of the patient, the nature of the antibody, and the quantity of blood received. Although we cannot, in this discussion, consider all the manifestations, it must be emphasized that the initial clinical signs of transfusion reaction may be quite minimal in an anesthetized patient. The anesthetized patient is unable to complain of pain at the infusion site, or back or chest pain, and temperature change may be masked by the operative manipulation. In such cases, falling blood pressure or a rapidly developing coagulation defect may be the critical sign, and this may be rather late in developing.

HEMOLYTIC DISEASE OF THE NEWBORN

PATHOPHYSIOLOGY

In hemolytic disease of the newborn (HDN), antibody crosses the placenta from the mother to the infant whose cells are hemolyzed. The antibody is directed against an antigen absent from the mother's cells and present on the fetal cells. By far the commonest offender is anti-Rh_o(D) in Rh negative women, but any of the immune (7S or IgG) antibodies is capable of crossing the placenta, including immune anti-A and anti-B from a group O mother. Although scattered cases occur due to various minor group antibodies, the vast majority of cases are due to anti-Rh_o(D), followed by immune anti-A or anti-B, and modest numbers arise from anti-hr' (c), anti-rh"(E), and anti-Kell.[10]

In Utero Hemolysis

All the pathologic problems of hemolytic disease of the newborn arise from the primary immunologic reaction causing red cell hemolysis. The maternal antibody crosses the placenta quite early in pregnancy, and since the erythrocyte antigens develop quite early, the fetus must fight a chronic hemolytic condition throughout gestation. Depending on the severity of the process, the fetus frequently maintains adequate oxygen-carrying capacity by markedly increasing erythropoiesis. If the hemolytic process outstrips the erythropoietic response, progressive anemia develops and the fetus may succumb in utero. Fetal death appears to result from anemia, cardiac failure, hypoproteinemia, and edema, a syndrome known as hydrops fetalis.

Bilirubin Disposal

In infants with successful erythropoietic response, a variable degree of anemia may exist at birth. Many, but not all, infants with HDN are anemic at birth, but jaundice, if present, is relatively mild. Hemolysis takes place in liver and spleen, not in the circulating blood. Bilirubin from the liberated hemoglobin readily crosses the placenta for excretion through the mother's biliary system. Although amniotic fluid may be discolored by bile pigments, the bilirubin does not remain in the infant's circulation, and jaundice is absent or minimal at birth. After birth, bilirubin continues to form, but the pathway for maternal disposal is disrupted.

In the normal course of bilirubin excretion in adults, unconjugated bilirubin goes to the liver, where it is conjugated with glucuronic acid and other substances and subsequently excreted in the bile. Conjugation depends upon the enzyme glucuronyl transferase, and the newborn's liver contains very little of this essential enzyme. In the premature infant, the enzyme is still more deficient, so that bilirubin excretion is seriously impaired. The normal infant is not seriously embarrassed by this enzyme deficiency, but the infant with HDN faces mounting quantities of bilirubin and no way to excrete it. The other serious problem he faces is anemia.

Neonatal Problems

Although separation from the placenta removes the infant from the original source of antibody, an ample supply of antibody usually remains in the circulation to maintain the hemolytic process well into the newborn period. The child with HDN has enormous numbers of reticuloctyes and nucleated red cells in the circulating blood, reflecting the bone marrow's efforts to compensate for red cell destruction; hence the other name for this condition—erythroblastosis fetalis. Even if no antibody can be demonstrated in the infant's serum, his red cells are coated with the antibody, and are susceptible to destruction on successive trips through the liver and spleen. As the coated red cells are destroyed, bilirubin accumulates even if erythropoiesis is adequate to meet the child's oxygen-carrying needs.

Accumulation of bilirubin poses a more serious threat than anemia. Bilirubin, in its unconjugated form, is toxic to the developing cells of the central nervous system, especially the neurons. Levels of unconjugated bilirubin above 20 mg per 100 ml may cause irreversible neuronal damage, resulting in mental or motor retardation of children with HDN who survive the newborn period. Some fortunate infants appear to have unusually high levels of glucuronyl transferase; in some children with HDN the jaundice is severe, but a large proportion of the bilirubin is conjugated. The level of unconjugated bilirubin, rather than total bilirubin, determines the prognosis.

EXCHANGE TRANSFUSION

Treatment of HDN must accomplish several goals. It is necessary to reduce the concentration of bilirubin, to treat the anemia, and to prevent further hemolysis which aggravates both problems. All these goals are achieved by exchange transfusion. In this procedure, successive aliquots of the child's blood are withdrawn and replaced by blood compatible with (i.e., not liable to destruction by) the antibody. Complete exchange is never possible, since the antibody-containing jaundiced blood cannot be totally removed and totally replaced by fresh compatible blood. Allowing for the inevitable mixing, however, a significant portion of the coated cells, the antibody, and the bilirubin can be removed by a single exchange transfusion. If the condition is especially severe, more than one exchange transfusion may be necessary.

Selection of Blood

Blood for exchange transfusion must be compatible with the mother's antibody. Since the newborn infant does not produce immunoglobulins, any antibody in neonatal blood must have come from the mother. In performing the crossmatch, the mother's serum should be used in the major crossmatch for testing the donor's cells. The baby's serum may contain little or no antibody, and it may be difficult to elute from his cells, but the antibody must necessarily be available in the mother's serum. If the mother's blood is not available, the infant's blood can be used for the crossmatch, but identification of the antibody tends to be less secure. If the mother's blood is used for the crossmatch, a donor can be tested prior to delivery, so that blood can be drawn and administered without delay if the child is severely affected at birth.

Evaluating the Baby

Diagnosis of HDN requires demonstration of an immune hemolytic process. Infants may be anemic for other reasons and may be jaundiced for other reasons. Before the diagnosis can be made, an antibody that is potentially capable of crossing the placenta must be demonstrated in the mother, and its presence in the baby must be documented. The antibody is usually observed coating the baby's red cells (positive direct Coombs test) and sometimes in the baby's serum as well. The infant will also have evidence of massive erythropoietic effort, and some degree of bilirubinemia can usually be demonstrated. The severity of disease can vary tremendously, ranging from the mere presence of a weakly positive direct Coombs test and moderate reticulocytosis to the full-blown state which ends in death or severe retardation.

ABO HEMOLYTIC DISEASE

When immune anti-A or anti-B is the offending antibody, HDN is slightly more difficult to diagnose than when Rh or other antibodies are the cause, and the disease also tends to be milder. Many severe cases of ABO hemolytic disease occur, however, when group O women have children of group A or group B. Although most of the naturally occurring anti-A and anti-B agglutinins are too large to cross the placenta, immune antibodies may, if present in high titer, enter the infant's circulation. The hemolytic process is similar to that caused by Rh antibodies, but frequently the direct Coombs test is only weakly positive.

Various special techniques may be needed to demonstrate the presence of antibody on the infant's cells. The presence of antibody in the serum is not conclusive proof that the infant's cells are being destroyed,[24] but a maternal immune titer of 1:128 or higher is highly suggestive of cell destruction. In a mature infant who becomes jaundiced in the first 24 hours of life, the diagnosis of ABO hemolytic disease should be strongly considered if the mother is group O and the child is of an incompatible group. Investigation should include sensitive modifications of the direct Coombs test on the infant's cells and examination of the mother's serum for high titers of immune antibody. ABO hemolytic disease may occur without any prior immunizing event in the mother, and subsequent children, even those of the same incompatible group, may not be affected.

ANTENATAL DIAGNOSIS

If the hemolytic process is discovered only when the child develops jaundice and anemia, it may be too late to prevent permanent damage. For this reason, the blood of all pregnant women should be screened for antibodies capable of crossing the placenta. Since antibodies other than anti-Rh$_o$(D) can cause HDN, all women—not just Rh negative women—should be examined for irregular antibodies.

Hemolytic disease affects not only the newborn but the fetus in utero. The stillbirth rate in Rh negative women with a demonstrated antibody is 12 per cent,[27,28] rising to 29 per cent in pregnancies after the first-affected child.[18]

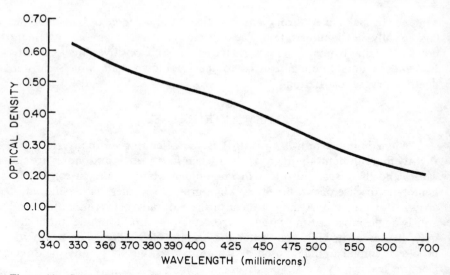

Figure 11. Spectral curve of normal amniotic fluid at term. Compare with Figure 12. (Redrawn, with permission, from Jennings, E. R., in Stefanini, M. [ed.]: Progress in Clinical Pathology. Grune and Stratton, 1966, vol. 1.

Titration

Once a woman develops a potent antibody, her chances of successfully completing the pregnancy are rather poor, and it may be advisable to induce delivery somewhat early. Since prematurity aggravates the problem of HDN, premature delivery should only be undertaken when continuation of the pregnancy appears to endanger the child more than the known risks of prematurity. In the past, the severity of the hemolytic process was inferred from the strength of the maternal antibody. If the antiglobulin titer of a preexisting antibody rose to 1:256 or above in the last months of the pregnancy, the child was considered to be in serious danger,[31] while an unchanging antibody level, or only a slight rise, was suggestive of a less severe process. This practice of frequently titrating the antibody was only moderately successful in predicting the severity of the process.

Amniocentesis

Examination of fluid obtained by amniocentesis appears to offer more accuracy in estimating the severity of the hemolytic process. The observation that severely affected infants were surrounded by deeply stained amniotic fluid led to early, and not very successful, attempts to base prognosis on estimation of amniotic bilirubin levels. More useful has been estimation of total bile pigments by measuring the optical density of amniotic fluid at wave lengths ranging from 700 to 350 mu. When excessive bile pigment is

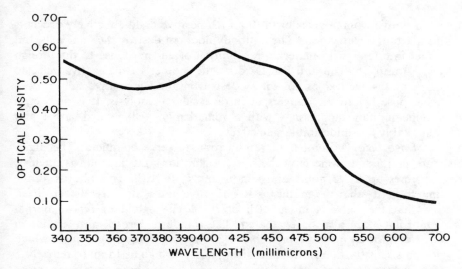

Figure 12. Spectral curve of amniotic fluid, at 31 weeks' gestation, from an infant severely affected by hemolytic disease of the newborn. (Redrawn, with permission, from Jennings, E. R., in Stefanini, M. [ed.]: Progress in Clinical Pathology. Grune and Stratton, 1966, vol. 1.)

present, optical density is increased in the 450 mu area, as compared with the normal curve[14,26] (see Fig. 11 and 12). When meconium or hemoglobin also stains the amniotic fluid, interpretation of the spectral curve is more difficult; in complicated cases, considerable skill and experience are necessary to interpret the data. Nevertheless, examination of amniotic fluid offers by far the most reliable means for antenatal assessment of the severity of the hemolytic process.

PREVENTION

Hemolytic disease of the newborn due to anti-Rh$_o$(D) is now considered a preventable disease. Women already possessing anti-Rh$_o$(D) antibody will continue to have babies at risk, but unsensitized Rh negative women can be protected from developing the antibody. The overwhelming majority of pregnancy-related sensitizations occur at term, during delivery, when fetal Rh positive cells enter the mother's circulation.[5] This transplacental hemorrhage is usually quite small, and cannot be prevented. The infant's Rh$_o$(D) antigen can, however, be prevented from inducing an antibody.

Anti-Rh$_o$(D) Globulin

Purified, standardized anti-Rh$_o$(D) injected within 72 hours after an

Rh negative woman gives birth to an Rh positive child effectively prevents postpartum sensitization.[4] The antibody does not destroy the fetal cells, but rather interferes with maternal recognition of and response to the foreign $Rh_o(D)$ antigen. The anti-$Rh_o(D)$ does the mother's Rh negative cells no harm, and, since it does not act by destroying the Rh positive cells, it does not expose her to the dangers of intravascular hemolysis. It is, in fact, a specific immunosuppressive, with a remarkably well defined target and remarkably few undesirable side effects.

Dose Size. A number of ramifications deserve comment. The maximum permissible time lapse between parturition and injection is unclear, but times up to 72 hours are demonstrably effective. This affords ample time to verify that the mother is Rh negative and is not already sensitized and that the baby is indeed Rh positive. The extent of fetal-maternal hemorrhage can also be evaluated. The standard dose of anti-$Rh_o(D)$ in one very widely used preparation is 300 μg of antibody globulin, which prevents sensitization from immunizing doses as high as 15 ml of red cells.[22] If more than 15 ml of fetal cells have entered the mother's circulation, more antibody should be injected, at the ratio of one vial (300 μg) for each 15 ml of Rh positive cells. Large fetal-maternal bleeds should be suspected if the infant is anemic or hypovolemic, or if delivery has been traumatic. Sensitive anti-$Rh_o(D)$ testing on the mother's blood, comparing a predelivery with postdelivery specimen, is an excellent way to demonstrate that more than the usual number of fetal Rh positive cells are in the mother's circulation.[19]

Abortions. In a few pregnancies fetal-maternal hemorrhage occurs before term, usually late in the third trimester. In these cases, sensitization may already be under way, making postpartum injection ineffective. Unsuspected sensitization may follow abortion, either spontaneous or induced. Rh antigens develop very early in fetal life, so fetal red cells are immunogenic even in the first trimester. Despite the small size of the abortus, fetal cells can enter the mother's blood following many abortions. For this reason, many clinicians prefer routinely to protect Rh negative women with anti-$Rh_o(D)$ following abortions, although the risk of sensitization is probably 2 to 5 per cent.[4,12]

Future Implications

Availability of prophylactic anti-$Rh_o(D)$ should dramatically decrease the incidence of HDN due to that one antibody. It cannot be expected to affect ABO hemolytic disease, which remains common, although rather unpredictable in its occurrence. It cannot be expected to suppress other antigen-antibody systems sometimes implicated in HDN, notably hr'(c) and Kell but sporadically many others. Hemolytic disease of the newborn should become much rarer, but is not likely to disappear entirely; the prudent obstetrician should continue to screen pregnant women for the development of unsuspected antibodies.

GENETIC STUDIES

Blood groups are sometimes used as genetic markers for studies of inheritance, either for anthropologic purposes or for determining paternity. Their inheritance is relatively straightforward, and in most cases the presence of a gene can readily be inferred from simple serologic tests. Nevertheless, the finer points of interpretation require both experience and judgment, and should not be undertaken lightly.

PATERNITY TESTING

Paternity studies are done on the basis of two general rules: 1) Each parent must transmit one gene to the offspring, and 2) a child cannot possess a gene which neither of his parents possesses. These points can be illustrated quite simply as follows. The mating of two group AB individuals cannot produce a group O child, because each parent must pass on either an *A* or a *B*; to be group O, the child has to have two *O* genes. This would exclude both maternity and paternity. A group A individual could have both an *A* gene and an *O* gene, and could transmit the *O* gene, but the group AB parent would still have to pass on either the *A* or the *B*. The mating of a group A with a group A could produce a group O child, because each of the parents could be of the genotype *A/O,* and the child could get one *O* from each parent.

The second rule is most simply illustrated by considering the offspring of two group O individuals. Each of them must have two *O* genes, so the child can receive only the *O* gene and must necessarily be group O. A child of any other ABO group would have to be from an extramarital relationship, for he must have obtained his *A* or *B* gene from a parent.

These rules appear, and are, fairly simple. The problem arises in recognizing which genes control which antigens, and which antigens are identified by which antisera. Paternity studies are ordinarily done on the ABO, Rh, and MN antigens, and in all three systems variant antigens exist which must be recognized and accounted for before statements are made about parental identity.

Serologic tests can never prove that a child *is* the offspring of a given mating, but they may strongly suggest that he could *not* have been conceived by the two individuals involved.

BIBLIOGRAPHY

1. BARKER, L.F., SHULMAN, N.R., MURRAY, R. ET AL.: Transmission of serum hepatitis. J.A.M.A. 211:1509, 1970.
2. BLUMBERG, B.S.: Polymorphisms of the serum proteins and the development of isoprecipitins in transfused patients. Bull. N.Y. Acad. Med. 40:377, 1964.
3. BLUMBERG, B.S., SUTNICK, A.I., LONDON, W.T., AND MILLMAN, I.: Australia antigen and hepatitis: a comprehensive review. Crit. Rev. Clin. Lab. Sci. 2:473, 1971.
4. CLARKE, C.A.: Prevention of Rh isoimmunization. Progr. Med. Genet. 8:169, 1972.
5. COHEN, F., ZUELZER, W.W., GUSTAFSON, D.C., AND EVANS, M.M.: Mechanisms of isoimmunization. I. The transplacental passage of fetal erythrocytes in homospecific pregnancies. Blood 23:621. 1964.
6. COMMITTEE ON STANDARDS: Standards for Blood Banks and Transfusion Services, ed. 6. American Association of Blood Banks, Chicago, 1972.
7. COOMBS, R.R.A., MOURANT, A.E., AND RACE, R.R.: A new test for the detection of weak and "incomplete" Rh agglutinins. Br. J. Exp. Pathol. 26:255, 1945.
8. FUDENBERG, H.H., STIEHM, E.R., FRANKLIN, E.C. ET AL.: Antigenicity of hereditary human gamma-globulin (Gm) factors—biological and chemical aspects. Symp. Quant. Bio. 29:463, 1964.
9. GIBLETT, E.R.: A critique of the theoretical hazard of inter- vs. intraracial transfusion. Transfusion 1:233, 1961.
10. GIBLETT, E.R.: Blood group antibodies causing hemolytic disease of the newborn. Clin. Obstet. Gynecol. 7:1044, 1964.
11. GOCKE, D.J.: A prospective study of posttransfusion hepatitis. J.A.M.A. 219:1165, 1972.
12. GREENWALT, T.J., GAJEWSKI, M., AND McKENNA, J.L.: A new method for preparing buffy-coat poor blood. Transfusion 2:221, 1962.
13. HUMPHREY, J.H. AND WHITE, R.G.: Immunology for Students of Medicine, ed. 3. F.A. Davis Company, Philadelphia, 1970.
14. JENNINGS, E.R.: "Recent advances in diagnosis, treatment and prevention of hemolytic disease of the newborn." In Stefanini, M. (ed.): Progress in Clinical Pathology, Grune & Stratton, Inc., New York, 1966, vol. 1.
15. LANDSTEINER, K., AND WIENER, A.S.: An agglutinable factor in human blood recognizable by immune sera for rhesus blood. Proc. Soc. Exp. Biol. Med. 43:223, 1940.
16. LEVINE, P., CELANO, M.J., WALLACE, J., AND SANGER, R.: A human "D-like" antibody. Nature 198:596, 1963.
17. McELRATH, T.G. AND ASCARI, W.Q.: Prevention of Rh immunization after transfusion with Rh-positive blood. Am. J. Obstet. Gynecol. 110:309, 1971.
18. MOLLISON, P.L.: Blood Transfusion in Clinical Medicine, ed. 4. F.A. Davis Company, Philadelphia, 1967.
19. POLESKY, H.F. AND SEBRING, E.S.: Detection of fetal maternal hemorrhage: An evaluation of serologic tests related to $Rh_o(D)$ immune globulin (human). Transfusion 11:162, 1971.
20. POLLACK, W.: Some physicochemical aspects of hemagglutination. Special Symposium on Recent Advances of Immunohematology in Honor of Philip Levine. Ann. N.Y. Acad. Sci. 127:892, 1965.
21. POLLACK, W., ASCARI, W.Q., CRISPEN, J.F. ET AL.: Studies on Rh prophylaxis. II. Rh immune prophylaxis after transfusion with Rh-positive blood. Transfusion 11:340, 1971.
22. POLLACK, W., ASCARI, W.Q., KOCHESKY, R.J. ET AL.: Studies on Rh prophylaxis. I. Relationship between doses of anti-Rh and size of antigenic stimulus. Transfusion 11:333, 1971.
23. QUEENAN, J.T., KUBARYCH, S.F., SHAH, S., AND HOLLAND, B.: Role of induced abortion in rhesus immunization. Lancet 1:815, 1971.
24. STERN, K.: Clinical value of serologic examinations related to blood groups in pregnant patients. Am. J. Obstet. Gynecol. 75:369, 1958.
25. THOMPSON, E.F., AND WALSH, R.J.: Immunization against the Rh antigen by small amounts of blood. Med. J. Aust. 1:440, 1950.

26. WALKER, W., FAIRWEATHER, D.V.I., AND JONES, P.: Examination of liquor amnii as a method of predicting severity of haemolytic disease of newborn. Br. Med. J. 2:140, 1964.

27. WALKER, W., AND MURRAY, S.: Haemolytic disease of the newborn as a family problem. Br. Med. J. 1:187, 1956.

28. WALKER, W., MURRAY, S., AND RUSSELL, J.K.: Stillbirth due to haemolytic disease of the newborn. J. Obstet. Gynaecol. Br. Commonw. 44:573, 1957.

29. WATKINS, W.: Blood group substances. Science 152:172, 1966.

30. WIENER, A.S.: The Rh-Hr blood types: serology, genetics and nomenclature. Trans. N.Y. Acad. Sci. 13:198, 1951.

31. ZEITLIN, R.A., AND BOORMAN, K.E.: The prognostic value of Coombs and partial absorption titrations in haemolytic disease of the newborn. J. Obstet. Gynaecol. Br. Commonw. 70:798, 1963.

CHAPTER 4

Blood Chemistry

The blood transports a seemingly limitless number of substances, ranging from simple inorganic ions to tremendously complex organic molecules. Most of these substances can be measured fairly precisely by using a variety of techniques which, like the substances involved, range from fairly simple to highly sophisticated. In a book such as this, we can touch only on some of the most frequently measured constituents and comment briefly on problems in measurement and significance of certain abnormalities.

This enormous topic will be approached from several viewpoints. In this chapter the following are considered: glucose; the nitrogen-containing substances in serum, including proteins and the nonprotein elements such as urea, uric acid, ammonia and creatinine; calcium and phosphorus; serum lipids and cholesterol; bilirubin; and a variety of substances of toxicologic importance. In the next chapter (Chap. 5), regulation of acid-base metabolism, fluid balance, and the electrolytes sodium, potassium, chloride, and bicarbonate are discussed. A separate chapter is devoted to serum enzymes of clinical importance (Chap. 6). Certain special topics are discussed in other chapters; thus, iodine metabolism is discussed in the section on the thyroid gland (Chap. 16); measurement of serum iron is considered in the hematology section (Chap. 13); the chapter on inborn metabolic disturbances (Chap. 18) covers certain problems of lipid, copper, uric acid, porphyrin, and carbohydrate metabolism. Measurement of the plasma proteins that participate in blood coagulation is discussed in the chapter on hemostatic mechanisms (Chap. 15). Normal values for a variety of blood constituents are given in Table 9.

GLUCOSE

The principal fuel for all body activities is glucose, a six-carbon sugar

Table 9.   Normal Blood Chemistry Values for Adults

Substance	Serum, Plasma,* or Whole Blood*	Normal Values	Remarks
Acetone	P or S	0-1 mg/100 ml[17]	
Albumin	S	4.3-5.6 Gm/100 ml[29]	
Ammonia	WB	102 ± 23 μg/100 ml[9] (Seligson and Hirahara)[58]	Anticoagulant should not contain ammonium salts. Patient should be fasting.
		45-50 μg/100 ml[9] (Conway)	
Amylase	S or WB	80-150 units[17] (Somogyi)	A unit is 1 mg glucose per 100 ml sample after 30 min incubation.
Ascorbic acid	P	0.8-2.4 mg/100 ml[17]	Patient should be fasting.
Bilirubin	S		
Direct		0.2 mg/100 ml[61]	
Total		1.0 mg/100 ml[61]	
Calcium	S	4.5-5.75 mEq/L[17] 9.0-11.5 mg/100 ml[17]	Serum protein values may affect result.
CO_2	S or P		Heparin.
Combining power		25-33 mM/L[27] 55-75 vol/100 ml[27]	
Content: Arterial		23-31 mM/L[27]	
Venous		25-32 mM/L[27]	
Tension: Arterial		33-48 mm Hg[27]	
Venous		38-53 mm Hg[27]	
Chloride	S	95-106 mEq/L[17]	
Cholesterol	S		
Total		220 ± 50 mg/100 ml[78]	
Esters		163 ± 36 mg/100 ml[78]	
% Esterified		50-70%[61]	
Copper	S	90-150 μg/100 ml[71]	
Creatine	S	0.16-0.4 mg/100 ml[65]	
Creatine phosphokinase	S	0.2-1.42 units [73]	Unit is μ moles creatine liberated/ml serum/hr. Separate and freeze serum immediately.

* See footnote page 106.

Table 9   (Continued)

Substance	Serum, Plasma,* or Whole Blood*	Normal Values	Remarks
Creatinine	S	0.5-1.0 mg/100 ml[65]	
Fatty acids Esterified	S	250-400 mg/100 ml[1] 8-20 mEq/L[17]	
Free		0.35-1.2 mEq/L[17]	
Fibrinogen	P	200-400 mg/100 ml[68]	
Globulin	S	1.3-2.7 Gm/100 ml[29]	
Glucose	WB	90-120 mg/100 ml[17] (Folin-Wu) 65-95 mg/100 ml[27] (Nelson-Somogyi) 60-105 mg/100 ml[14] (Enzymatic) 46-94 mg/100 ml[42] (Ultramicro)	Whole blood diluted in water.
Icterus index	S	2 to 8 units[27]	Compared against 1:10,000 solution of potassium dichromate

Iodine
  Protein-bound
  Butanol-extractable
	S	3.5-8.0 μg/100 ml[16]
		3.2-6.4 μg/100 ml[27]	

Iron	S	56-183 μg/100 ml[21]	
Iron-binding capacity	S	277-379 μg/100 ml[21]	
Lactic acid	S		Patient should be in completely basal state.
Arterial		3.1-7 mg/100 ml[27]	
Venous		5-20 mg/100 ml[27]	
Lactic dehydrogenase	S	200-450 units[27] (Wroblewski and La-Due, modified by Henry, et al.)[28] 40-78 units[28] (Wacker)[70]	Unit is decrease in A of 0.001/min/ml serum. Unit is increase in A of 0.001/min/ml serum.
Lipase	S	0-1.5 units[27]	Unit is ml 0.05 N NaOH needed to neutralize fatty acids in 1 ml serum
Lipids, total	S	450-1000mg/100 ml[27]	Patient should be fasting.

* See footnote page 106.

Table 9 (Continued)

Substance	Serum, Plasma,* or Whole Blood*	Normal Values	Remarks
Magnesium	S	1.4-2.2 mEq/L[4,66] 1.7-2.7 mg/100 ml[4,66]	
Nitrogen (NPN)	WB	25-40 mg/100 ml[5]	Anticoagulant should not contain ammonium salts.
Osmolality	S	281-291 mOsm/kg[26]	
Oxygen Oxygen content	WB		Heparin. Keep sample in ice.
Arterial Venous		15-22 vol/100 ml[17] 11-16 vol/100 ml[17]	
Oxygen saturation	WB		Heparin. Keep sample in ice.
Arterial Venous		98%[27] 55-71%[27]	
pH: Arterial Venous	WB	7.37-7.42[27] 7.34-7.39[27]	
Phosphatase, acid	S	0.5-5[27] (Babson-Read)	Unit is amount of enzyme that liberates 1 mg of α-naphthol/hr.
		0-0.1[27] (Shinowara)	Unit is mg P/hr/100 ml serum.
Phosphatase, alkaline	S	1.5-4.0[27] (Bodansky)	Unit is mg P/hr/100 ml serum.
		3.7-13.1[27] (King-Armstrong)	Unit is mg phenol/30 min/100 ml serum.
		2.2-8.6[27] (Shinowara)	Unit is mg P/hr/100 ml serum.
Phospholipids	S	150-350 mg/100 ml[17]	
Phosphorus, inorganic	S	2.6-4.8 mg/100 ml[13]	Values may rise if serum remains in contact with cells for several hours.
Potassium	S	3.8-5.1 mEq/L[25]	
Proteins (total)	S	6-8 Gm/100 ml[29]	
Electrophoretic fractions Albumin α_1Globulin		52.0-68.0%[29] 2.4-5.3%[29]	

* See footnote page 106.

Table 9   (Continued)

Substance	Serum, Plasma,* or Whole Blood*	Normal Values	Remarks
α_2 Globulin		6.6-13.5%[29]	
β Globulin		8.5-14.5%[29]	
γ Globulin		10.7-21.0%[29]	
A/G ratio		1.5-2.2[29]	
Sodium	S	138-146 mEq/L[17]	
Transaminase			
Glutamic-oxalacetic (SGOT)	S	12-36 units[28]	Unit is change in A of 0.001/min/ml serum.
Glutamic-pyruvic (SGPT)	S	6-53 units[17]	Unit is change in A of 0.001/min/ml serum.
Urea nitrogen (BUN)	S	5-25 mg/100 ml[27]	
Uric acid	S		Separate serum from cells promptly
Males		3.0-7.0 mg/100 ml[8]	
Females		2.0-6.0 mg/100 ml[8]	

* Listed under "Remarks" is information about anticoagulants for specific procedures. If no comment is made, any effective anticoagulant is permissible.

containing, among other side chains, an aldehyde group. Although most of the body's glucose comes from dietary carbohydrates, other sources of this necessary compound are also available. Sugars other than glucose can be utilized either by conversion to glucose within the stomach and intestine prior to absorption or by hepatic transformation of such absorbed sugars as galactose or fructose. The liver can also convert fats and proteins into glucose, pathways that become useful in metabolic emergencies. The liver is the clearinghouse for glucose metabolism; it converts excess glucose to storage forms for later use, and it retrieves the stored material for consumption as needed.

The primary storage form of glucose is glycogen, a complex branched molecule consisting of multiple glucose residues. Excess glucose can be transformed into fat and stored in the body's adipose tissues. Through a complicated series of transformations, products of glucose metabolism can be converted into certain amino acids, but this pathway is not routine for glucose storage. The most efficient retrieval of stored glucose is from glycogen. Utilization of glucose from fat or protein sources results in formation of acidic by-products.

Virtually all cells metabolize glucose, and glucose is continually transported to peripheral sites for utilization. The by-products of metabolism—principally carbon dioxide and water under conditions of optimum energy use—are returned in the venous blood for pulmonary or renal excretion. The regulation of blood glucose concentration is a complex process. Peripheral utilization of glucose depends largely on the presence of adequate supplies of insulin, but the secretions of the adrenal cortex, adrenal medulla, and pituitary and thyroid glands all play a part in regulating glucose mobilization and consumption.

MEASUREMENT

Measuring the blood glucose concentration aids in assessing the body's overall metabolic state, but any single determination must be related to the individual's dynamic physiologic condition. Blood glucose is measured in either the fasting or postprandial state, depending on the type of information desired. Most so-called normal values are for the fasting state.

The importance of glucose in metabolism has been recognized since ancient times, and many tests have been developed for measuring the sugar content of blood and urine. Two principal methods are now in use. One employs the reducing properties of the aldehyde group in glucose, and variations of this method employ different reactions to indicate the reducing effect. The second method employs the enzyme glucose oxidase which oxidizes the sugar and liberates by-products which can then be measured. Although the reducing methods have the advantage of historical precedent and extensive experience, the enzymatic method is more specific. Both methods require adequate control of physical and chemical variables to prevent distortion of the results.

Reducing Methods

The "reducing sugar" tests classically employ copper solutions and measure color change. Two methods are in wide use. For both the reduction methods, and for the glucose oxidase method as well, it is necessary to prepare a protein-free filtrate of the blood sample. For the Folin filtrate, sodium tungstate and sulfuric acid are used, while zinc sulfate and barium or sodium hydroxide are necessary to prepare the Somogyi filtrate. In the Folin filtrate, a proportion of nonglucose reducing substances remains in the filtrate and these saccharoids give falsely high values in nonspecific tests for glucose. The error introduced remains constant, so that valid comparisons can be made against other determinations made with the same method. Confusion arises if the results from different methods must be compared, so it is advisable to know what method is in use.

In the Folin-Wu glucose test, application of heat to a mixture of glucose and alkaline copper sulfate solution results in precipitation of cuprous oxide. Addition of molybdate phosphate solution permits the precipitate to dissolve into a colored solution whose intensity can be measured colorimetrically. In the Somogyi-Nelson determination, the reduced copper acts upon an arsenomolybdate preparation and the color of the resulting complex is measured. In one widely used automated technique, the glucose reduces a copper-containing chelate, producing an intensely colored complex that can readily be measured.

Enzymatic Method

The product measured in the enzymatic reaction is hydrogen peroxide, a by-product of the enzymic conversion of glucose to gluconic acid. The peroxide is measured with a chromogenic indicator in the presence of peroxidase. A number of variables must be controlled with this method, including the temperature, pH, timing, and choice of indicators. Additionally, it is necessary to avoid or remove materials that inhibit enzymic activity. For these reasons, the values reported with the glucose oxidase method may vary from laboratory to laboratory, even though the reaction itself is quite specific.

SIGNIFICANCE OF RESULTS

Normal values for blood glucose are considered to be 80 to 120 mg/100 ml of whole blood for the Folin-Wu method and 65 to 95 mg/100 ml of whole blood for the Somogyi-Nelson method. The values with the glucose oxidase method are approximately the same as for the Somogyi-Nelson method, although Fales[14] suggests 60 to 105 mg/100 ml as a realistic range for normal fasting blood sugar values. The intracellular glucose concentration within red blood cells is lower than the plasma concentration, so serum or plasma glucose levels run approximately 10 per cent higher than those of whole blood.[14]

Elevated Levels

Hyperglycemia is the descriptive term for blood glucose concentrations greater than normal, and hypoglycemia describes lower than normal blood concentrations. Diabetes mellitus is the most frequent cause of marked hyperglycemia, but many other conditions may elevate the glucose level. Disorders of the pituitary gland and certain brain lesions may cause markedly elevated levels, and mildly diabetic levels may accompany Cushing's disease and hyperthyroidism. Any condition in which epinephrine is mobilized will be accompanied by hyperglycemia, usually of relatively mild degree. Examples include acute injury, convulsions, mental stress, and the adrenal tumor pheochromocytoma. Shock and severe hemorrhage cause initial hyperglycemia, but this may be followed by dangerous lowering of the blood glucose level. Acute and chronic infections, eclampsia, and hypertension are often accompanied by mild hyperglycemia, and overweight individuals tend to have high fasting blood sugar levels, possibly indicative of impaired insulin activity. Severe liver disease causes generalized alteration of carbohydrate metabolism, so that a glucose load is removed from the blood less rapidly than normal; but hypoglycemia can also occur since glucose is not adequately mobilized in response to falling blood sugar.

Depressed Levels

Hypoglycemia is characteristic of hyperinsulinism due either to endogenous pancreatic lesions or to exogenous overdosage. Liver disease may cause episodic hypoglycemia, and some of the congenital deficiencies of carbohydrate-regulating enzymes may cause acute and chronic hypoglycemia. Hormonal deficiency of the adrenal, thyroid, or pituitary glands can cause chronically low blood glucose levels, and prolonged poor nutrition from any cause will lower blood sugar levels and deplete glycogen stores so that acute hypoglycemia cannot adequately be compensated.

The dynamics of carbohydrate metabolism are considered briefly in the chapter on endocrine function, and glucose tolerance tests are discussed on page 422.

URINARY GLUCOSE

Glucose levels in the urine often provide valuable clinical information. Glucose is not present in normal urine. Although it passes freely through the glomerular filter, there is virtually complete removal of the sugar from tubular urine, so that none appears in the excreted urine. As long as plasma levels do not exceed 160 to 190 mg/100 ml, the normal kidney can remove all the glucose from the glomerular filtrate. Beyond this renal threshold, complete resorption is no longer possible, and glucose appears in the excreted urine. Some individuals have congenital or acquired tubular defects, so that glucosuria occurs at much lower plasma glucose levels, but these conditions are readily distinguished from diabetes mellitus by demonstration of normal plasma glucose concentration.

Methods for measuring urinary glucose are similar to those for blood glucose, and both the reducing methods and the enzymatic method are currently used. Commercially prepared "instant" tests are available for screening urine sugars, employing either principle.

NITROGENOUS COMPOUNDS

Proteins constitute the bulk of nitrogen-containing compounds in the blood, their concentration per 100 ml being measured in grams, while the remaining nitrogenous constituents are measured in milligrams. Serum proteins and plasma proteins are similar, except that plasma contains fibrinogen, while serum is the fluid portion that remains after fibrinogen has been converted to fibrin. Besides fibrinogen, the principal subdivisions of the protein group are albumin, the α-globulins, and β-globulin, all of which are produced in the liver, and the gamma globulins or immunoglobulins which derive from the lymphocyte-plasma cell system.

Fibrinogen

Fibrinogen is a large complex globulin with no known physiologic function except the formation of fibrin. Fibrin is the end product of blood coagulation, and it also participates in localized inflammatory reactions. Fibrinogen is manufactured by the liver, and plasma concentrations range from 200 to 400 mg per 100 ml, tending to be slightly higher in women than in men. During pregnancy, fibrinogen values may go as high as 600 mg per 100 ml.[64] Elevated fibrinogen levels accompany many systemic or local infections and may occur in multiple myeloma and nephrosis. A sudden decrease in plasma fibrinogen content may occur in episodes of intravascular clotting or disseminated fibrinolysis. These tend to take place when there is disruption or necrosis of tissue, and acquired hypofibrinogenemia may follow obstetrical accidents or extensive surgical procedures, especially those involving the lungs or urinary tract.

SERUM PROTEINS

In healthy individuals, the serum contains between 6.0 and 8.5 grams of protein per 100 ml. Among the many techniques available for measuring proteins, the Kjeldahl method of measuring nitrogen content is usually considered the standard against which other methods are compared. In this method, the nitrogen is converted to ammonium ion which is measured by titration of ammonia into an acid solution of known strength. Total protein weight is calculated by multiplying the nitrogen content by 6.25, a somewhat arbitrary figure derived from the mean nitrogen content of representative human proteins. The Kjeldahl method is reliable and reproducible but requires an investment of time, space, and equipment that makes it unsuitable for multiple routine determinations.

Nonspecific Techniques

Several quick methods are available for measuring total serum proteins when a high degree of accuracy is unnecessary. These include measurement of the specific gravity or of the refractive index of serum. Reliance on these methods depends on the assumption that no qualitatively abnormal proteins are present and that such other serum constituents as glucose, urea, and cholesterol are present in normal concentration.

Biuret Reaction

Perhaps the most common method for measuring proteins utilizes the biuret reaction. A blue compound forms when polypeptides of appropriate configuration combine with copper in an alkaline solution. The simplest nitrogenous compound to give this reaction is biuret, for which the prototype reaction has been named. The intensity of the color is proportional to the concentration of polypeptides. The biuret reaction, suitably modified, is used for automated determination of total protein. The accuracy of the determination is impaired if the protein solution is turbid, a problem often encountered with lipemic sera. High concentrations of bilirubin, bromsulphalein, or other pigments may interfere with the procedure, and hemolysis of the sample will falsely elevate the result by liberating normally intracellular hemoglobin into the serum sample.

Protein Partition. Although the biuret reaction cannot, by itself, distinguish the various proteins in the sample, it can be used for separate quantitation of albumin and globulin. After the total protein concentration has been measured in a serum aliquot, the globulins can be removed from the sample by precipitation with sodium sulfate, with or without sodium sulfite. If the biuret reaction is repeated on the supernatant material, the albumin alone will be measured. The difference between total protein and albumin is reported as the globulin content. Certain cautions must be observed in the salting-out procedure, including adjustment of the salt concentration. If the serum is shaken excessively, some albumin may be denatured and precipitate with the globulin, while incomplete precipitation of globulins causes falsely high albumin values.

An automated technique for measuring albumin specifically puts to use the affinity between albumin and certain charged molecules. The product measured is a colored complex of albumin and an anionic dye, thereby avoiding the problems of salting-out globulins.

Electrophoresis

Electrophoresis provides the most generally satisfactory qualitative separation of serum protein. Since different proteins have different amino acid compositions, the isoelectric point of each protein is unique. Migration in an electric field varies with these physicochemical differences, and migration patterns can be plotted for the different groups of proteins. Although more precise work can be done with moving boundary techniques, electrophoresis on fixed media, such as paper, agar, or acrylamide gel, gives excellent separation into a number of protein components. These protein components can be quantitated either by eluting the proteins from the supporting medium and measuring them directly or by staining the preparation and measuring the relative intensity of each segment. Since the staining method offers only comparative figures, the total serum protein content must be measured if the proportions are to be converted into absolute values. Immunoelectrophoresis, ultracentrifugation, peptide mapping, spectrophotometry, and other methods are available for more precise separation necessary in research contexts.

Albumin. Albumin normally occupies between 52 and 68 per cent of the total protein value[29]; therefore, changes in albumin content affect total protein value more markedly than changes in globulins. The more frequent direction of change is down; the albumin concentration is rarely increased except when there is dehydration and hemoconcentration. Disease of the liver, the site of albumin production, depresses serum albumin levels. This does not follow acute liver damage, because the mean half-disappearance time of albumin is 18 days[62] and even complete cessation of albumin production would take time to become apparent. Chronic liver disease is one of the most common causes of hypoalbuminemia. Since albumin contributes approximately 80 per cent of the serum colloid osmotic pressure,[37] marked hypoalbuminemia may so depress the colloid osmotic pressure that edema and transudation occur. Albumin production declines in such conditions of poor nutrition as advanced malignancy, malabsorption syndromes, starvation, or beriberi. Albumin levels are low in toxemia of pregnancy and in congestive heart failure, in which both impaired production and hypervolemic dilution may play a part. Low levels of albumin may result from excessive protein loss, either through the kidney as in nephrosis or severe nephritis, through the gastrointestinal tract as in protein-losing enteropathies, or through the skin as with extensive burns.

Globulins. The globulins have been divided on the basis of their electrophoretic mobility into α_1, α_2, β_1, and γ fractions. The gamma globulins are the body's antibodies and are subject to considerable variation in disease states. The alpha and beta globulins change significantly in relatively few states and tend as a group to reflect altered liver function.

Low levels of gamma globulins can occur as a congenital abnormality or as an acquired deficiency. In either case, the patient suffers frequent bacterial infections because the normal immunologic defenses are impaired. Diseases that affect lymphocytes and plasma cells, such as lymphoma, myeloma, or macroglobulinemia, may cause deficiencies of functioning antibody gamma globulin even though there may be an increase in nonfunctional, abnormal globulin fractions.

Chronic infections of any kind—bacterial, fungal, or protozoal—produce high levels of gamma globulins. These specific antibodies can often be identified and measured serologically. Nonspecific elevations of gamma globulin occur in all types of chronic liver disease, in many connective tissue disorders, in far-advanced carcinoma, and in lymphomas and leukemias.

High levels of abnormal globulins occur in the so-called gammopathies, diseases of the lymphocytic and plasmacytic system. These abnormal proteins can be identified in a variety of ways, of which the simplest is electrophoresis. Electrophoresis readily demonstrates the existence of circulating abnormal globulins, but immunoelectrophoresis and other immunologic techniques often permit identifying their nature and specificity, if any (see below).

A/G Ratio. The ratio of albumin to globulin (A/G ratio) was considered a useful measurement before the development of accurate protein fractionation. It merely gives the proportion of the two types of protein measured in the salting-out procedure described earlier. Since many diseases affect both albumin and globulin and since the A/G ratio can be affected by changes in either or both, it is an imprecise piece of information at best. Even without the detailed information available from electrophoresis, it is preferable to express albumin and globulin in absolute terms and permit the observer to draw his own conclusions.

Immunoelectrophoresis

Electrophoretic separation of proteins derives from differences in size and electrical charge of different categories of proteins. The resulting bands, although capable of quantitation, tell nothing about their constituent elements. When the separated protein bands are reacted with anti-bodies against known individual proteins or subcategories, more detailed partition develops. Thus haptoglobin and ceruloplasmin, both of which migrate as alpha$_2$ globulins, can be individually demonstrated as separate precipitin arcs with appropriate antiserums.

The selection of antiserum depends upon the number and nature of proteins sought. Antiserums can be raised against classes of immunoglobu-lins (see Chap. 2), against functionally specific proteins, against abnormal protein constituents, or against whole serum or some fraction thereof, which results in a mixture of antibodies. By comparing the patient's results with a normal control or an appropriately quantitated standard, one can observe the number of separate precipitin lines, and roughly quantitate the amount of each constituent. This procedure is also used to demonstrate whether a protein-containing solution has one or several different constitu-ents.

Immunoelectrophoresis is especially useful for documenting suspected deficiencies of specific proteins, such as transferrin, thyroid-binding globu-lin, and so forth, and for investigating qualitatively abnormal globulins. The electrophoretogram provides a starting point by showing the location of abnormality, that is, a tall, narrow peak indicates a quantity of physi-cally homogeneous material moving at a single rate, while a broader hump results from a heterogeneous group of molecules with various rates of migration.

Monoclonal Patterns. The single, well defined peak is usually associ-ated with neoplasms of antibody-producing cells. The unitary nature of the spike (called M-protein or paraprotein) and its light or heavy chain class or both are identified by immunoelectrophoresis. Immunoelectrophoresis also clarifies possibly confusing patterns; for example, it can distinguish a paraprotein from fibrinogen, or from excess lipoproteins, mucoproteins, or glycoproteins arising from carcinomas, or IgG denatured by sample aging or uremia.[30]

The conditions characterized by these electrophoretic spikes are some-times called monoclonal gammopathies, emphasizing that the offspring of a single cell multiply to form the neoplasm. The term gammopathy is mis-leading, however. While approximately 55 per cent of myelomas produce globulins of the IgG class, 22 to 28 per cent produce IgA, and small percentages produce IgM or IgD globulins.[31,79] Lymphomas, lymphocytic leukemia, Waldenstrom's macroglobulinemia, and cold agglutinin disease can also produce paraprotein spikes, while up to 2 per cent of the aging population may have paraproteins (usually IgM) without any associated disease.[3]

BENCE-JONES PROTEIN. Bence-Jones protein, the light chain fragment of myeloma protein, rarely reaches significant levels in the serum, so does not reliably appear on immunoelectrophoresis. Both metabolic high turnover and low molecular weight, which permits escape through the glomerular filter, contribute to the low serum levels of Bence-Jones protein. Half or more of patients with myeloma excrete this microglobulin in their urine. Immunoelectrophoresis of concentrated urine is the best way to document and classify Bence-Jones protein, and may be the best way to diagnose multiple myeloma in the 20 per cent of patients whose only abnormal globulin product is Bence-Jones protein.[30,79]

Polyclonal Patterns. The increased serum globulin pattern that creates a broad, irregularly contoured hump on electrophoresis is sometimes called a polyclonal gammopathy. These multispecific protein patterns reflect the stimulation of many different cells, producing immunoglobulins of different specificities and different physical-chemical characteristics. Even immunization against a single bacterium results in multiple antibodies, since bacteria possess numerous separable antigenic constituents. Antibodies of different immunoglobulin classes or of different binding constants within the same class, may result from a single immunizing event.

Chronic infections with specific agents, such as parasitic infestations, leprosy, lymphogranuloma venereum, and intrauterine syphilis or viral infections, produce a polyclonal pattern with identifiable reactivity. More challenging are the broad, so-called nonspecific hyperglobulinemias associated with chronic liver disease, sarcoidosis, autoimmune diseases, far-advanced carcinomas, and other long-standing necrotizing processes. Although immunoelectrophoresis or immunoglobulin quantitation by radial diffusion may characterize the relative amounts of increased immunoglobulin, it is not presently possible to draw diagnostic conclusions from these patterns.

NONPROTEIN NITROGENOUS COMPOUNDS

The NPN Determination

The nitrogen remaining in the protein-free filtrate can be measured by the Kjeldahl method used for determining the amount of protein nitrogen, using materials and equipment for milligram quantities. In practice, however, this is rarely done. Nonprotein nitrogen (NPN) is usually measured as the derived ammonia, which is quantitated by nesslerization or by reaction with alkaline hypochlorite (Bertholet reaction). Normal values for nonprotein nitrogen are approximately 25 to 40 mg per 100 ml. Approximately 55 per cent of the nonprotein nitrogen comes from urea, the other components being uric acid, creatinine, ammonia, and free amino acids. Since each of these components, including urea, can be determined separately, the value of the NPN determination is somewhat limited. The nonurea constituents change only within a rather narrow range, and specific measurement provides more sensitive information about these variations. Changing urea values affect the NPN most significantly, although uric acid and creatinine values are often altered by conditions that affect urea concentration.

Urea

Urea, the end product of protein metabolism, is produced only in the liver. From its hepatic origin, urea travels through the blood to the kidneys for urinary excretion. Two general methods are used for measuring urea; in both, the results are expressed as milligrams of urea nitrogen, rather than as total urea. In the monoxime method, urea combines with diacetyl monoxime to give a yellow compound which can be measured colorimetrically. In the enzyme method, urease hydrolyzes urea to CO_2 and NH_3, and the resulting ammonia can be measured by nesslerization or the Bertholet reaction. Although the urease method is indirect, in that a metabolite rather than urea itself is measured, it is probably more reliable than the monoxime method, in which the relation between urea concentration and colored product may not be linear. The monoxime method has been adapted, with generally satisfactory results, to automated performance.

The normal value for blood urea nitrogen (BUN) ranges from 5 to 25 mg per 100 ml. Values tend to be slightly higher in males than in females, and persons with unusually high protein intake may have BUN levels at the high end of the scale. There is, however, no significant postprandial change.[28] Urea production rarely declines to any measurable extent, except after loss of 80 to 85 per cent of hepatic function.[61] Low values for urea concentration usually reflect expanded blood volume rather than diminished production.

Uremia. The commonest cause of high BUN values (uremia) is renal disease which may be either acute or chronic. All the inflammatory, degenerative, congenital, traumatic or neoplastic ills that affect the kidney may cause uremia, and the degree of uremia provides a rough index to the severity of the condition. Urinary obstruction at any site can cause uremia. Probably the commonest cause of urinary obstruction is prostatic enlargement, but congenital anomalies, tumors, calculi, pregnancy, or scarring can impair urinary flow. Uremia can also result from conditions not directly related to the kidney or urinary tract. Whenever there is increased protein catabolism, increased urea will be found; if the same problem also decreases renal blood flow or urine production, blood levels of urea will rise.

The list of such conditions includes burns, with subsequent fluid loss; massive hemorrhage into the body cavities or soft tissues; infarction or other accidents to the viscera; pancreatitis; severe diabetic ketoacidosis; and far-advanced carcinoma, with tumor necrosis and cachexia. For all of these extrarenal conditions, appropriate diagnostic and therapeutic measures should be promptly instituted, not because the uremia itself is life-threatening, but because the primary condition is dangerous.

Uric Acid

Uric acid production and excretion are discussed in Chapter 18. Degradation of nucleic acids leads to uric acid formation, and dietary and endogenous purines are the principal sources. Two methods are used to measure blood and urine uric acid. The colorimetric method measures the blue compound formed by the reducing action of uric acid upon alkaline phosphotungstate. This is used in certain automated systems. Large doses of salicylates may interfere with accurate results;[54] this can present difficulties when patients with arthritic disease are evaluated.

A more sensitive, reliable method uses spectrophotometric absorption. Uric acid has a characteristic absorbance peak at 292 mu. The absorbance of the sample is measured before and after treatment with the enzyme uricase, which converts uric acid to allantoin, which does not absorb at this wave length. The concentration of uric acid in the specimen can be calculated from the difference between pretreatment and post-treatment absorbance.

There is some controversy about the normal range of serum uric acid concentration. This is sometimes given as 6.9 to 7.5 mg per 100 ml for men and 5.7 to 6.6 mg per 100 ml for women,[76] but many authorities consider as significantly elevated values above 7.0 mg per 100 ml for men and 6.0 mg per 100 ml for women.[8, 47] Impaired renal function depresses uric acid excretion, and the most frequent cause of high serum levels of uric acid is severe renal disease.

Abnormal Serum Urates. Secondary hyperuricemia is more common than primary hyperuricemia from gout or other metabolic diseases involving purine metabolism. In renal failure, the kidneys cannot excrete nitrogenous wastes, and serum uric acid levels rise, as do the BUN and serum creatinine levels. Temporary depression of urate excretion may also elevate serum urates. This occurs with high circulating levels of lactic acid or ketone bodies, in such conditions as shock, alcoholism, diabetic ketosis, starvation, or certain glycogen storage diseases. Urate excretion is also depressed by thiazide diuretics, and prolonged low doses of aspirin.[53] Certain x-ray contrast media and other drugs may markedly increase uricosuria, causing decreased serum urate level but sometimes producing renal damage from the urates which precipitate out of the supersaturated urine.[51]

A large proportion of patients with gout have relatively impaired urate excretion, but also suffer overproduction. Of primary causes for hyperuricemia, gout is by far the commonest. This condition is considered at greater length in Chapter 18. Whenever nucleic acid turnover is rapid, serum urates rise. In chronic myelogenous leukemia, prolonged hemolytic conditions, and inefficient erythropoiesis, uric acid values are persistently high. Acute elevations, sometimes at dangerously nephrotoxic levels, may follow vigorous cytolytic therapy for leukemia and other neoplasms. Infectious mononucleosis and psoriasis may also produce hyperuricemia, presumably due to impaired renal excretion.

Ammonia

Ammonia, another end product of protein metabolism, is formed from the action of bacteria on the proteins in the intestinal contents. Some ammonia also derives from hydrolysis of glutamine in the kidneys. Ammonia is detoxified in the liver where it is converted to urea. The small quantity of ammonia in the blood is presumably the material in transit from gut and kidneys to the liver. The ammonia in urine does not arise directly from the blood ammonia, but is rather the result of tubular processes for the excretion of H^+ ions as NH_4^+.

Methods for measuring serum ammonia are only moderately accurate. These depend upon liberating ammonia from the sample, and then measuring the quantity liberated by titration or colorimetry. The normal range in whole blood samples is 75 to 200 micrograms (mcg) of ammonia per 100 ml, while values for plasma are somewhat lower, ranging from 56 to 122 mcg per 100 ml.[58] Blood levels vary with dietary intake of protein, and blood should be drawn when the patient is in a fasting condition.

Blood ammonia determinations are used for evaluating the progress of severe liver disease. Since ammonia is removed by the liver, hepatocellular damage may permit blood ammonia levels to rise. In patients with impaired hepatic function, blood ammonia levels can be lowered somewhat by reducing protein intake and by administering antibiotics to reduce the population of intestinal bacteria.

Creatinine

Creatinine is the anhydride of creatine. Creatine exists in skeletal muscle as creatine phosphate, a high-energy compound that functions in reversible energy reactions involving adenosine triphosphate (ATP) and the enzyme creatine phosphokinase. Conversion of creatine to creatinine is nonenzymatic and irreversible. The serum creatinine level reflects total body supplies of creatine and does not vary significantly with exercise or with diet. Individuals with large muscle mass have higher serum creatinine levels than those with less muscle. Normal values for men are slightly higher than those for women, but the overall normal range is between 0.8 and 1.4 mg per 100 ml.

Creatinine is excreted through the kidneys in quantities proportional to the serum content. Creatinine measurements are most useful in evaluating renal function. By comparing serum creatinine concentration with the total quantity excreted within a given time, the *creatinine clearance* can be calculated. This indicates the efficiency with which the kidneys remove creatinine from the blood, and declining renal function leads to declining values for creatinine clearance. As renal function diminishes, serum creatinine rises, but the rise is less acute than the change in BUN. Serum creatinine may be normal in some cases of acute uremia or mild chronic renal disease, but an elevated serum creatinine value indicates severe, long-standing renal impairment.

Creatine. Determination of serum and urine creatine is technically more difficult than determination of creatinine, and it is used principally in evaluating muscle disorders. Normally not more than 0.5 to 0.95 mg per 100 ml of creatine is present in serum. This increases only if degenerative disease of the skeletal muscle releases normally intracellular creatine into the blood. Similarly, creatine is not normally present in urine at levels above 250 mg per day[27] and is present in significant quantities only in degenerative muscle diseases, notably the muscular dystrophies.

CALCIUM AND PHOSPORUS

Calcium and phosphorus are discussed together because the two elements are closely associated physiologically. Most of the body's supplies of both minerals exist in the skeleton, but each element has other physiologic functions as well. Calcium ions affect neuromuscular excitability and cellular and capillary permeability and are necessary for blood coagulation. Phosphorus is essential in the storage and liberation of energy and in the intermediate metabolism of carbohydrates and lipids. Serum inorganic phosphorus levels are measured in terms of the phosphate ions, for ionized free phosphorus does not circulate. The skeleton serves as a storehouse for these elements, and serum values are maintained at the expense of the skeletal minerals.

PHYSIOLOGIC CONSIDERATIONS

Parathyroid hormone promotes excretion and maintains serum calcium levels. Its secretion is regulated by changes in circulating calcium levels. Since serum calcium and phosphorus levels tend to vary reciprocally, parathormone can raise serum calcium levels by promoting urinary phosphate loss. It may also mobilize calcium from bone directly.

Calcium and phosphorus are absorbed from the small intestine, and adequate supplies of vitamin D are necessary for optimum epithelial transport. Calcium absorption is inhibited if the intestinal contents are too alkaline to permit complete solution of the calcium salts. Malabsorption syndromes, steatorrhea and prolonged diarrhea lessen absorption by impairing vitamin D absorption and by removing available calcium through soap linkage with fatty acids.

Both calcium and phosphorus are excreted in the urine, the excretion being regulated by active metabolic processes in the tubular epithelium. When renal damage impairs tubular function, rising serum phosphate levels testify to moderate or severe renal disease. This serum phosphate excess depresses serum calcium values, thus stimulating parathormone production in an attempt to increase phosphate excretion.

MEASUREMENT

Phosphorus

Laboratory measurement of serum phosphate depends upon the reaction of phosphorus with molybdic acid, giving a phosphomolybdate complex. Subsequent reduction of this phosphomolybdate complex produces a blue compound which can be measured colorimetrically and in automated procedures. The reduced compound may reoxidize within a relatively short time, so the procedure requires careful timing. The nature of the reducing agent varies in different methods, and a consistent reducing potential must be maintained if determinations are to be consistently accurate. Serum for phosphate determination should be separated rather promptly from the cells to avoid artefactual alteration as a result of continuing glycolytic activity.

Calcium

Several methods are in use for measuring calcium, but none is completely satisfactory. The flame photometer can be used, but both positive and negative interference can result from the presence of other inorganic ions. The commonest indirect method involves precipitating calcium ions from solution as calcium oxalate, and then measuring the amount of oxalate in the precipitate. In a variation of this method a calcium phos-

Table 10. Summary of Chemical Features of Diseases
with Disturbed Plasma Calcium and Phosphate*

| Disease | Serum | | | Urine | |
	Calcium	Phosphate	Alkaline Phosphatase	Calcium	Phosphate
Hyperparathyroidism	Increased	Decreased	Normal or increased	Increased	Increased
Paget's disease	Normal	Normal	Increased	Normal	Normal
Hypoparathyroidism	Decreased	Increased	Normal	Decreased	Decreased
Renal insufficiency	Decreased	Increased	Normal or increased	Decreased	Decreased
Osteomalacia	Decreased or normal	Decreased	Increased	Decreased	Decreased
Senile osteoporosis	Normal	Normal	Normal	Normal	Normal
Multiple myeloma	Normal to increased	Normal	Normal	Normal to increased	Normal to decreased
Milk-alkali syndrome	Increased	Normal to increased	Normal	Normal to decreased	Normal to decreased
Vitamin D intoxication	Increased	Increased	Normal	Increased	Decreased
Metastatic carcinoma	Normal to increased	Normal	Normal to increased	Increased	Normal
Sarcoidosis	Increased	Normal to increased	Normal to increased	Increased	Decreased
Hyperventilation (alkalosis)	Normal	Normal	Normal	Normal	Normal

* From Bernstein, D.S., and Thorn, G.W., *In* Wintrobe, M.M. et al. (eds.): Harrison's Principles of Internal Medicine, ed. 6. McGraw-Hill Book Company, New York, 1970.

phate precipitate is used, and the phosphate is measured. In still another method, the presence of calcium ions is signalled by the characteristic color assumed by an indicator substance in the presence of dissociated calcium ions. Titration with a chelating agent, which removes ionized calcium from solution, produces a color change when all the free calcium is bound. This method suffers from interference from other metal ions and from colored compounds, such as bilirubin or hemoglobin, in the serum. There is also some difficulty in obtaining sharp end-points. A widely used automated procedure measures the colored complex formed between calcium and an alkaline earth dye. With a fluorescent indicator complex, the end-point can be read fluorometrically. Atomic absorption spectrophotometry is also used for calcium determinations.

Normal values for calcium are given in either milligrams per 100 ml or milliequivalents per liter. These range from 9 to 11 mg per 100 ml, or 4.5 to 5.5 mEq per liter. Conversion is easily done because calcium's molecular weight and valence of 2 permit rapid calculation. Serum phosphorus cannot so easily be converted from milligrams to milliequivalents, because phosphate ions exist at several different valences. The normal range of 2.6

to 4.8 mg per 100 ml is for phosphorus itself, but it must be recalled that the phosphate ion, not free phosphorus, is the biologic form. Serum phosphorus values are higher in children, the normal range for children in the growing years being from 4.5 to 6.5 mg per 100 ml.

A summary of the chemical features of diseases with disturbed plasma calcium and phosphate is given in Table 10.

SIGNIFICANT ALTERATIONS

Hypercalcemia

Hypercalcemia is most conspicuous in hyperparathyroidism which may produce calcium values as high as 18 mg per 100 ml. Hypervitaminosis D also causes high serum calcium. In secondary hyperparathyroidism, parathyroid oversecretion occurs in response to an initially lowered calcium level, so the degree of hypercalcemia is rather mild while the phosphate values are markedly elevated. Hypercalcemia may accompany any condition of bone demineralization, such as multiple myeloma, extensive osseous metastases, or prolonged immobilization leading to bone atrophy. Sarcoidosis occasionally causes hypercalcemia, and high levels of serum calcium can occur in the milk-alkali syndrome. A problem of differential diagnosis may arise here, because peptic ulceration is a moderately common complication of hyperparathyroidism. Thus, the ulcer pain which impels the patient toward overmedication with milk and alkalis may be the presenting symptom of an undiagnosed condition which is the real cause of the hypercalcemia.

Hypocalcemia

Hypocalcemia accompanies hypoparathyroidism, and the various conditions described as pseudohypoparathyroidism and pseudo-pseudohypoparathyroidism. In vitamin D deficiency and vitamin D-resistant rickets, low calcium is the rule, and in steatorrhea and pancreatitis the serum calcium may be low because calcium soaps are formed. In conditions of decreased serum proteins, total serum calcium values will be low, even though the content of ionized calcium may be perfectly normal. Loss of proteins through nephrosis, liver disease, or other diseases removes the binding material for the bound portion of the serum calcium but does not affect the vital physiologic functions served by ionized calcium.

Phosphate Abnormalities

The commonest cause of high serum phosphate levels is renal failure, and values above 8 mg per 100 ml usually indicate severe renal disease. Hypervitaminosis D and hypoparathyroidism may also cause hyperphosphatemia.

Decreased serum phosphate levels characterize hyperparathyroidism and vitamin D deficiency. A variety of renal tubular disorders, such as Fanconi syndrome, vitamin D-resistant rickets, and renal tubular acidosis, cause urinary phosphate wastage with hypophosphatemia. Steatorrhea and the malabsorption syndromes cause hypophosphatemia along with the hypocalcemia, and these are among the few conditions in which calcium and phosphate values are low simultaneously.

LIPIDS

Normal plasma contains a variety of lipid elements, of which the principal groups are free fatty acids, which turn over very rapidly, and provide most of the body's free energy supplies;[18] exogenous triglycerides, which consist of glycerol esterified with fatty acids from dietary intake; endogenous triglycerides, which are manufactured in the liver; cholesterol, an alcohol widely synthesized but esterified and degraded only in the liver; and phospholipids, whose functions in the plasma remain unclear. These lipid elements are insoluble in plasma, an aqueous medium. To be transported, they must interact with proteins which confer polarity and permit dispersion.

LIPID CATEGORIES

Free Fatty Acids

Free fatty acids, which travel complexed to albumin, contribute no more than 25 mg in 350 to 800 mg of total lipids per 100 ml plasma.[57] Although little is present at any one time, up to 25 Gm of fatty acid may pass through the plasma each hour.[18] Measuring the free fatty acids contributes relatively little diagnostic or prognostic information, and is not usually part of clinical lipid evaluations.

Triglyceride

Chylomicrons. Dietary lipids appear in plasma as the triglyceride portion of chylomicrons. These spherical particles are less dense than plasma (average density 0.94) but because they are large (average diameter 5000 Å) they scatter light and, in large quantity, render the serum or plasma turbid. The rate at which chylomicrons are cleared from plasma varies somewhat with the rate of lipid intake. Clearance requires lipoprotein lipase, an enzyme which appears in the blood after heparin stimulation. Chylomicron clearance should be complete approximately six hours after a fat-containing meal.[57] Chylomicrons contain small amounts of cholesterol (10 per cent), phospholipid (7 per cent) and protein (2 per cent). The largest component (81 per cent) is triglyceride. Since these derive directly from ingested lipids, an individual's chylomicron and triglyceride levels vary significantly with his dietary status. Meaningful measurements can be made only under standardized (usually fasting) conditions.

Endogenous Triglycerides. Not all serum triglycerides come directly from dietary lipid. The liver manufactures and exports triglycerides at a level relatively independent of immediate dietary input but reflecting overall dietary composition. If transport is impaired, triglycerides accumulate in the liver cells. Endogenous triglycerides travel mainly in a variety of molecules described as very low density lipoproteins (VLDL). These vary in density from 0.93 to 1.006, and contain between 2 and 15 per cent protein. Triglycerides, virtually all endogenous, constitute about 55 per cent of VLDL while the remaining lipid content includes cholesterol, both free and esterified, and phospholipids.

Cholesterol

Circulating cholesterol derives from endogenous metabolic activity, not directly from dietary intake. The liver is the largest but not the only manufacturer. Only the liver esterifies the sterol with fatty acids, and degrades cholesterol into bile acids for excretion. Approximately 2 Gm of cholesterol are metabolized daily,[12] but half of this appears to follow an enterohepatic cycle of excretion and reabsorption, whose function is unclear. Since dietary intake is only 100 to 500 mg daily,[18] it is clear that circulating cholesterol levels reflect many different factors. Cholesterol is transported largely in the low density (beta) lipoproteins, although some is carried in the high density (alpha) lipoproteins, and a very small amount is found in the pre-beta, or very low density lipoproteins.

Plasma Values. Uncertainty and controversy surround the subject of so-called normal cholesterol values and the significance of deviations from normal. Cholesterol levels rise with age in Western societies. Many consider this an indication of dietary, social, and metabolic pathology rather than a physiologic change that accompanies aging. Frederickson and his colleagues[18] propose a scale of normal values, starting from 120-230 mg per 100 ml in persons below age 20, rising to 160-330 mg per 100 ml in the decade 50 to 59 years. Cholesterol measurement is the oldest, and probably still the most common, test for lipid status, although the role cholesterol plays in overall lipid metabolism is under intensive study.

The Framingham study[34] found serum cholesterol values the best predictor for subsequent coronary artery disease, values above 220 mg per 100 ml in persons below age 50 carrying a two-fold to five-fold risk. For this age group, they classified values between 250 and 350 mg per 100 ml as moderately elevated, but comparable values in healthy older people did not indicate increased risk of late-developing morbidity.

FREE AND ESTERIFIED CHOLESTEROL. Since the liver esterifies cholesterol, the relative amounts of esterified and nonesterified (free) cholesterol may reflect liver function. Normally only 20 to 30 per cent of circulating cholesterol is nonesterified. The amount of free cholesterol rises in biliary obstruction, giving high total cholesterol with reduced esterification. In primary or secondary metabolic hyperlipemias, the total is high, but normal proportions are maintained. Nephrotic syndrome, uncontrolled diabetes mellitus, and hypothyroidism produce secondary hypercholesterolemia of this type. When overall metabolism accelerates, as in hyperthyroidism and acute infections, serum cholesterol falls, as it does in actual starvation or with diets low in fats and total calories. In severe hepatocellular disease, both total and esterified cholesterol levels may drop.

Phospholipids

Phospholipids are complex molecules whose function in plasma is unclear, although their role in membrane metabolism is highly significant. Lecithin and sphyngomyelin are the principal circulating phospholipids; the range in normal serum is approximately 150-375 mg per 100 ml.[57] Phospholipids contribute to both the alpha and beta lipoproteins, primarily the high density alpha molecules. Although phospholipids can be measured independently, separation of the lipoprotein classes provides more valuable information about these molecules and their relation to other serum lipids.

LIPOPROTEIN MEASUREMENT

Electrophoresis

Lipoprotein analysis is most readily done by electrophoresis. At pH 8.6, the chylomicrons remain stationary, and the remaining classes move toward the anode. The alpha lipoproteins move farthest, the beta move least and the pre-beta class falls between alpha and beta. This sequence of chylomicrons at the origin, with beta, pre-beta, and alpha migrating to the anode does not reflect the density of the molecules. Chylomicrons are the least dense, followed in increasing order by the pre-beta (very low density), the beta (low density), and the alpha (high density) lipoproteins. Electrophoresis permits qualitative separation, although beta and pre-beta are sometimes hard to distinguish. The bands are usually characterized only qualitatively by pattern, although the densitometer or elution have been used for quantitation.

Ultracentrifugation

Ultracentrifugation can separate molecules into virtually any number of graded categories. When lipoproteins are studied in the analytical ultracentrifuge at a density of 1.063, the lightest particles float the fastest, and are assigned the highest flotation units (S_f). Thus chylomicrons, which are largely triglycerides and are less dense than 1.000, have the highest S_f value, above 400. The pre-beta group, called very low density lipoproteins because their density is between 0.93 and 1.006, fall between 20 and 400 S_f units. At densities between 1.006 and 1.063, the beta lipoproteins are classed as S_f 0-20. The alpha lipoproteins are more dense than 1.063, hence do not float at all in this system. When abnormal beta or pre-beta migration patterns occur, ultracentrifugation is sometimes helpful. Certain molecules migrate in the beta range, but prove to have a density below 1.006. Practical considerations of cost and availability make ultracentrifugation much less widely used than electrophoresis.

LIPOPROTEIN PATTERNS

Frederickson and Lees[18] have classified the results of lipoprotein electrophoresis into five major abnormal types which can be correlated with clinical hyperlipidemic states. These types refer specifically to electrophoretic patterns, but cholesterol and triglyceride analyses can usefully be related to these categories. Blood for lipid analyses of any kind should be drawn in the fasting state, 12 to 14 hours after food intake. The patient should be in his normal nutritional state without major weight changes or dietary manipulations in the preceding two weeks. Both absolute intake and the relative proportions of carbohydrate and fat will affect circulating lipoprotein levels. The plasma sample, drawn into EDTA, must not be frozen, and should not be exposed to room temperature conditions for prolonged periods.

Problems in Characterization

Table 11 lists the salient features of the five abnormal lipoprotein patterns. Ambiguity most often arises in distinguishing Type III from Type IV or, sometimes, from Type II; and in categorizing Type V, which resembles Type I in many respects and Type IV in other respects. The difficulty in diagnosing Type V hyperlipoproteinemia is reflected in the discrepant incidence figures for this group. Lees and Wilson[38] describe it as "fairly common," while other workers[23,56] consider it uncommon, and Scheig[57] expresses doubt as to "whether this hyperlipoproteinemia actually exists as a separate entity." Critical delineation of Type III requires ultracentrifugation, to demonstrate those abnormal lipoproteins of specific gravity below 1.006 which migrate in a beta pattern.

Type V can be distinguished from Type I by the observation that the turbid or milky serum common to both separates differently after overnight refrigeration. Type I samples develop a top "cream" layer with clear plasma below, while Type V may show some separation, but the lower layer remains cloudy. Type IV and Type V are more difficult to separate.

Clinical Significance

Distinguishing lipoprotein abnormalities has therapeutic significance since diet and drug regimens are different for the different groups. The patterns discussed are generally thought to be familial, although the genetics have not, in all cases, been clearly defined. Type IV and Type V are so intimately related to dietary patterns that both constitutional and exogenous factors are clinically important. Hormonal influences are also involved. In midpregnancy, high density alpha lipoproteins increase. In the third trimester low density and very low density (beta and pre-beta) fractions increase, provoking a Type IV pattern which recedes after delivery. Thyroid hormones increase cholesterol removal from plasma, while hypothyroidism often causes increased cholesterol and beta lipoproteins. Alcohol ingestion, with or without pancreatitis, increases the triglycerides and sometimes the chylomicrons as well. This simulates a Type V pattern, and

Table 11. Types of Familial Hyperlipoproteinemias

Type	Plasma Lipids		Glyceride/ Cholesterol Ratio	Electrophoresis	Other Findings	Incidence
	Triglycerides	Cholesterol				
I	↑↑↑	↑	>8	Prominent chylomicron band Other bands decreased	Abdominal crises, pancreatitis Eruptive xanthomas Glucose tolerance normal Postheparin lipolytic activity low Turbid or milky serum, layers on standing	Rare Very early onset
II	±	↑↑↑	<1	Prominent, clearly defined beta band Other bands normal	Severe, early atherosclerosis, especially coronary Tendinous and tuberous xanthomas Glucose tolerance normal Postheparin lipolytic activity normal Clear serum	Common Early onset
III	↑↑ (variable)	↑ (variable)	<2	Broad beta band, indistinctly defined Other bands normal	Accelerated atherosclerotic disease, especially peripheral Palmar xanthomas Glucose tolerance abnormal Postheparin lipolytic activity normal Turbid serum High serum uric acid	Uncommon Variable age at discovery

Table 11 (Continued)

Type	Plasma Lipids Triglycerides	Cholesterol	Glyceride/ Cholesterol Ratio	Electrophoresis	Other Findings	Incidence
IV	↑↑ (varies with diet)	↑	1-5	Pre-beta band increased Other bands decreased	Coronary artery disease prominent Xanthomas uncommon Glucose tolerance abnormal Postheparin lipolytic activity may be low, if triglycerides especially high Turbid serum Carbohydrates produce triglyceride increase	Most common type Usually identified in middle life
V	↑↑	↑	>5	Chylomicron band present Pre-beta band increased	Abdominal crises Eruptive xanthomas Obesity usual Glucose tolerance abnormal Postheparin lipolytic activity normal or slightly low Carbohydrate or fat intake alters pattern Serum turbid or milky, layers on standing, but lower layer remains turbid	Unclear Onset usually in early adulthood

many Type V patients are heavy drinkers. Patients with nephrotic syndrome have high serum levels of beta and pre-beta lipoproteins, and may also have impaired lipoprotein lipase activity.

LIPOPROTEIN LIPASE ACTIVITY

Lipoprotein lipase clears triglycerides from circulating plasma. Its particular target is dietary triglycerides in the chylomicrons. It differs from pancreatic lipase in its sites of production and storage, its site of action, and its diagnostic significance. Pancreatic lipase is found in serum only following damage to its parent organ, but serum lipoprotein lipase activity occurs in normal and many hyperlipidemic individuals following heparin injection. This activity, called postheparin lipolytic activity, or clearing factor, is deficient in patients with Type I hyperlipidemia, and may be reduced in nephrotic syndrome, hypothyroidism, in severe alcoholism, and following prolonged low fat intake.

BILIRUBIN

Bilirubin is the predominant pigment of human bile and gives it the characteristic golden yellow color. Bilirubin is formed from hemoglobin of destroyed erythrocytes by the reticuloendothelial system, including the Kupffer cells of the liver. It is, therefore, found normally at a level of about 0.7 mg per 100 ml *en route* to the liver for excretion. The polygonal cells of the liver have nothing to do with the production of this pigment, but they do withdraw it from the blood and excrete it in the bile. In cases of hemorrhage into connective tissue and serous cavities, hemoglobin is converted directly into bilirubin. Following such hemorrhage, hyperbilirubinemia may develop.

THE LIVER

It should be recognized that there is a difference between the bilirubin before (prehepatic) and after (posthepatic) it has passed through the liver cells. Bilirubin that has passed through the polygonal cells of the liver is more dialyzable, more oxidizable, more readily absorbed by precipitated protein, and is not soluble in chloroform. Within the liver, bilirubin is enzymatically conjugated with glucuronic acid, and the characteristic posthepatic form of bilirubin is actually bilirubin diglucuronide. Because of its ability to cross membranes, only posthepatic bilirubin appears in the urine. Newborn infants, whose livers have inadequate enzyme levels, are

Table 12.   The Two Types of Bilirubin

Type of Bilirubin	Synonyms	Characteristics
Prehepatic	Unconjugated Free Indirect-reacting	Does not cross glomerular filter Harmful to neonatal nervous system Formed in reticuloendothelial system (peripheral) Requires organic solvent for diazo reaction
Posthepatic	Conjugated Glucuronide Direct-reacting	Freely crosses glomerular filter Formed by enzymatic activity, in liver Gives diazo reaction in aqueous medium

poorly equipped to convert bilirubin to the glucuronide, so that most of the circulating bilirubin is of the prehepatic type in hemolytic disease of the newborn.

The Diazo Reaction

Prehepatic and posthepatic forms of bilirubin are distinguished by the different manner in which they react with diazo reagents. In the van den Bergh reaction, sulfanilic acid and bilirubin—in the presence of nitrous acid—undergo a diazo reaction to form pink azobilirubin, which can be measured colorimetrically. Posthepatic bilirubin, the glucuronide, participates in this reaction in an aqueous medium, while the prehepatic, unconjugated form reacts only after addition of methyl alcohol. This procedural necessity has produced another set of terms to describe the different forms of bilirubin. Since the posthepatic form reacts promptly when the reagents are added, it is called direct-acting bilirubin; the prehepatic form, which requires methyl alcohol as an additional reagent, is called the indirect form. In Table 12 certain features of the two types of bilirubin are listed. Normal total serum bilirubin ranges between 1.0 and 1.5 mg per 100 ml, varying somewhat from laboratory to laboratory. Of this, no more than 0.3 to 0.5 mg is ordinarily in the posthepatic form.

DIFFERENTIAL DIAGNOSIS

The separation of bilirubin into prehepatic and posthepatic forms appears to offer a splendid means of differentiating the various etiologies of jaundice. Jaundice simply refers to the yellow coloration imparted by increased circulating bilirubin. In theory, it would appear that an increase in posthepatic bilirubin must derive from obstruction of the biliary tract, through which conjugated bilirubin must pass on its way from the liver into the intestinal lumen. Conversely, an increase in prehepatic bilirubin implies hepatic inability to keep up with the input of newly formed bilirubin, due either to hepatic insufficiency or to the presence of vast quantities of bilirubin, as may occur in severe hemolytic processes.

In clinical situations, the laboratory findings are seldom clear-cut. Hemolysis does, indeed, produce a pure increase in prehepatic bilirubin, but there is usually little difficulty in diagnosing hemolytic anemia on the basis of hematologic findings. Disease of the hepatobiliary tract is almost always complex so that, for example, hepatitis may cause hepatocellular insufficiency and increased levels of prehepatic bilirubin, but the posthepatic form is also increased owing to increased permeability of the inflamed biliary radicles. Although pure, acute obstruction of the biliary tract causes increased posthepatic bilirubin, persistence of the obstruction for any length of time causes secondary hepatocellular damage with a consequent increase in prehepatic bilirubin.

Prehepatic Bilirubin

Elevated levels of prehepatic bilirubin occur in autoimmune or transfusion-induced hemolysis and in hemolytic processes due to sickle cell disease, pernicious anemia, various other intrinsic red cell defects, malaria, and septicemia. Hemorrhage into the body cavities or soft tissues is followed by a bilirubin rise within 4 to 6 hours. In hemolytic disease of the newborn, levels of indirect bilirubin may rise to levels above 20 mg per 100 ml within a few hours, owing to the biochemical immaturity of the infant's liver.

Posthepatic Bilirubin

Posthepatic bilirubin is increased in obstructive diseases of the biliary system due to calculi, tumors, extrinsic pressure, or intrahepatic abnormalities. Toxic, infectious, or autoimmune hepatitis results in increase of both fractions, and cirrhosis produces both hepatocellular and biliary tract damage.

ICTERUS INDEX

The icterus index is an approximate measure of the degree of jaundice and does not measure bilirubin as such. The serum is compared against standardized solutions of potassium dichromate, a golden yellow compound, and the comparative results are expressed in arbitrary units. The icterus index of normal serum, which has a yellowish tinge, ranges from 2 to 8 units, and clinical jaundice is usually evident at approximately 15 units. Rough quantitation is possible, using a conversion factor of 10 index units to equal one milligram of bilirubin. This does not, of course, distinguish between prehepatic and posthepatic forms of bilirubin. The serum must be clear, unhemolyzed, without undue lipemia, and free of other pigments (usually carotene is the only offender).

TOXICOLOGY

Complete discussions of the clinical, legal, and biochemical implications of toxicology are available in specialized monographs. In this chapter, we can appropriately address only a few lines to the commoner types of poisoning encountered in clinical practice, especially those for which adequate diagnosis and treatment are available in a general hospital.

ARSENIC

Arsenic intoxication may be acute or chronic and may occur either accidentally or with suicidal or homicidal intent. Accidental chronic exposure may occur in industrial processes involving metals, paints, dyes, cosmetics, and insecticides. The most common arsenic-containing preparations are household and agricultural insecticides, but an appreciable amount of arsenic is present in some veterinary medications and in antiprotozoal medications. Acute arsenic poisoning can follow ingestion of large doses of these preparations while prolonged exposure to small doses can cause chronic intoxication.

In acute poisoning, a dose of 100 mg of arsenic may be fatal, leading to gastrointestinal irritation, dehydration, electrolyte imbalance, hypoxia, and convulsions. Chronic toxicity is characterized by nonspecific malaise and gastrointestinal disorders, various dermatologic abnormalities, inflammatory reactions of the respiratory tract, progressive liver damage, peripheral nerve damage, and encephalopathy.

If arsenic poisoning is suspected, a screening test for heavy metals can readily be performed on gastric contents, urine, blood, or preparations from hair or nails. In this test, a strip of copper or twist of copper wire is placed in the sample, and hydrochloric acid is added to achieve approximately 5 to 10 per cent acidity. If heavy metals are present, characteristic deposits form on the copper surface after an hour of gentle heating. Arsenic coats the copper with a dull black deposit; mercury produces a shiny silvery coat; bismuth, a shiny black deposit; and antimony, a dark purple sheen. More detailed procedures are available for complete identification and quantitation, but these should be done in approved toxicology laboratories because the results often have legal implications.

BARBITURATES

This group of compounds depresses the central nervous system and the activity of nerves and muscles at all sites. A variety of preparations exists, differing in the duration of their activity. The physiologic effects of any barbiturate vary with the route of administration, the degree of individual tolerance, and the presence or absence of modifying compounds. The combination of alcohol and barbiturates greatly potentiates the depressive effect of each.

According to the dose and nature of the drug, barbiturate intoxications produce nervous system depression, respiratory depression, bradycardia, and circulatory collapse. Clinical staging has been attempted by judging the presence of various reflex responses. Shock, profound respiratory depression, and absence of deep reflexes constitute the most severe intoxication. During therapy, tubular damage from renal ischemia may complicate recovery, and prolonged respiratory depression accounts for serious morbidity.

Diagnostic Problems

Diagnosis of barbiturate intoxication may be difficult since a variety of conditions can produce coma, and more than one drug may be involved in accidental or intentional overdosage. Even when barbiturates are known to be involved, prognosis is difficult to estimate because serum levels may not accurately reflect the overall physiologic condition. As a general rule, higher serum levels can be tolerated from long-acting barbiturates, while lower doses of short-acting drugs carry more immediate risk. One scale of potentially lethal serum concentrations starts with 3 mg per 100 ml for very short-acting preparations and goes up to 10 mg per 100 ml for the longest-acting preparations such as phenobarbital.[60] Although the dose and other contributing factors may be unknown, clinical course and the changing blood levels over the initial treatment phases may help in prognosis. Opinions vary as to the efficacy of analeptics in treating severe barbiturism. Hemodialysis, when readily available, can be extremely helpful. The most important problems in all patients are respiratory support and the avoidance or correction of shock and hemoconcentration.[25,41,59]

A useful screening test gives a colored mercury diphenyl-carbazone complex when any of the common barbiturates, the hydantoins, or glutethimide (Doriden) is present. Although a positive result does not identify the specific offender, a negative result eliminates a large group of potential intoxicants.[46]

The barbiturates are soluble in organic solvents, and methods of determination depend on extraction from blood or urine with chloroform or acid-ether. Quick qualitative identification of barbiturates in urine can be done if color develops when cobalt acetate and isopropyl amine are added to a concentrated acid-ether extract of urine. Intermediate- and short-acting preparations produce a blue-violet compound on addition of cobalt acetate alone, while phenobarbital requires addition of isopropyl alcohol as well. Quantitative methods involve measuring ultraviolet absorption, and paper chromatography can be used for accurate identification.

BROMIDE

Bromide is a central nervous system depressant which formerly enjoyed widespread medical endorsement but is now found largely in patent medicine preparations and nerve tonics. The gastrointestinal irritant effect usually foils attempts at massive acute ingestion, but chronic bromide intoxication is by no means uncommon, especially in individuals given to self-medication. Symptoms are nonspecific and include emotional lability, impaired intellectual function, motor incoordination, and nodular or acneform dermatitis. Anorexia, constipation, and weight loss also occur with chronic bromide ingestion, and a variety of organic and psychic illnesses may be diagnosed in patients with any or all of the above symptoms of bromism. Psychic disturbances are fairly common in the population that ingests large quantities of bromide nostrums, so the diagnostic problems may become rather complicated.

Bromide excretion occurs through the renal pathways for chloride excretion. The plasma half-life of a moderate dose of bromide is 12 days.[63] Treatment is directed at accelerating urinary excretion primarily by administering mercurial diuretics and copious amounts of chloride ion.

Serum bromide levels above 90 mg per 100 ml tend to cause toxic symptoms, but there is considerable variation in individual effect. When gold chloride is added to a protein-free filtrate of serum containing bromide, a yellow-orange color results and can be measured colorimetrically. One qualitative method involves silver nitrate precipitation to silver bromide. In another qualitative technique, a mixture of serum and chlorine water causes yellow discoloration of added chloroform if bromides are present; in this procedure, a purple discoloration occurs in the presence of iodides.

CARBON MONOXIDE

Carbon monoxide is toxic because it combines with hemoglobin to produce carboxyhemoglobin, a physiologically inert compound that damages the victim by reducing the quantity of hemoglobin available for oxygen transport. Because injury occurs from hypoxia, carbon monoxide is especially dangerous to those whose oxygen needs are high or whose oxygen transport system is precarious. Thus, children with their high metabolic rate, anemic patients with a low hemoglobin mass, and patients with cardiorespiratory disease are particularly susceptible to carbon monoxide toxicity.

Carbon monoxide, a product of incomplete combustion of carbon-containing compounds, occurs in automobile exhausts, illuminating gas, and the fumes from improperly functioning furnaces. Both accidental and suicidal intoxication occur, and the principal early symptoms are headache and dizziness. Continuing exposure causes increasing quantities of carboxyhemoglobin to replace oxyhemoglobin until carboxyhemoglobin levels of 60 to 80 per cent lead to coma and death.[35] Treatment is directed at displacing carbon monoxide from the hemoglobin and is best done by administering high concentrations of oxygen.

Carbon monoxide poisoning can usually be diagnosed from the situation in which the patient is found, although unsuspected chronic intoxication may result from repeated exposure to the fumes of a poorly functioning heating unit. The blood has a characteristic bright cherry-red appearance, and in individuals who have died following carbon monoxide poisoning, the mucous membranes and vascular endothelium may be bright red. Several quick qualitative tests are available for identification of carboxyhemoglobin. When 20 per cent sodium hydroxide solution is added to a drop of blood diluted in 10 to 15 ml of water, normal blood turns straw yellow immediately, while blood with more than 20 per cent carboxyhemoglobin remains pink for several seconds before changing color. A normal control should be run simultaneously. Another method involves evaporating one milliliter of blood to dryness. At carboxyhemoglobin concentrations of 40 per cent or above, the residue is brick red, while normal blood produces a brownish black deposit. Quantitative methods are available using the reduction of palladium chloride, while the most accurate method is gas chromatography. Fatal concentrations range between 40 and 80 per cent, while values as high as 5 per cent may occur in otherwise normal individuals who are heavy smokers.[35]

ALCOHOL

Ethyl alcohol becomes a subject of laboratory concern in cases of coma of unknown etiology, or when the amount of alcohol present must be quantified, usually for legal purposes. Qualitative tests for alcohol employ the reducing property common to ethyl alcohol, methyl alcohol, formaldehyde, paraldehyde, acetaldehyde, and acetone. Rapid diffusion techniques and more quantitative distillation techniques use potassium dichromate as the indicator substance. These are not specific for ethanol, but most often clinical circumstances indicate that ethyl alcohol is the reducing substance present.

Etiologic Agents of Coma

In cases of coma of unknown etiology, it may be necessary to discriminate among these substances. Gas-liquid chromatography is probably the procedure of choice. Specific chemical tests are available when appropriate indications warrant individual testing. Acetone can be identified in blood or urine with sodium nitroprusside. Paraldehyde has a characteristic odor, and also imparts reducing properties to the urine. Formaldehyde is not usually a clinical problem. The screening and quantitative procedures for methyl alcohol actually measure its oxidation product, formaldehyde. This is produced by preliminary oxidation of the sample, but if the specimen has been taken at autopsy, formalin contamination may present a problem. Both heparin and EDTA produce false positives,[35] so other anticoagulants should be employed.

Ethyl Alcohol

Legal considerations often surround tests to quantify ethyl alcohol. Most jurisdictions consider blood ethanol levels of 150 mg per 100 ml (0.15 Gm per cent) as prima facie evidence of being "under the influence," but levels between 50 and 150 mg per 100 ml exert unmistakable effects on behavior, especially on driving. The blood alcohol levels associated with fatal ethanol intoxication vary over a remarkably wide range depending upon the individual's prior condition, other drugs present, elapsed time after ingestion, speed of absorption, and so forth. Alcohol potentiates the depressant effects of innumerable other substances, so that low blood alcohol levels should not lull the practitioner into a sense of security. Barbiturates, antihistamines, anticonvulsants, morphine derivatives, and tranquilizers are frequently found in association with alcohol, and should be considered in cases of accidental or, especially, suicidal poisoning.

LEAD

Lead intoxication is usually chronic and unintentional. Lead fumes may be inhaled during repeated exposure to paints, acetylene torches, or combustion products from burning battery casings. Oral ingestion is most common in children who consume lead-containing paint from flaking surfaces or from toys and furniture, and in persons who drink whiskey that has been distilled through lead-contaminated equipment. Toxic blood levels are considered to be above 0.10 mg per 100 ml, although symptoms may occur at lower levels. Urinary lead excretion in concentrations higher than 0.08 mg per liter is suggestive of excessive lead exposure, while values above 0.15 mg per liter usually indicate toxicity. Accurate measurement of lead levels in blood and urine requires meticulous technique and scrupulously clean equipment. In cases of suspected lead poisoning, other laboratory determinations are usually done first.

Lead poisoning should be suspected in any anemic child with a history of eating dirt or other nonfood materials or of exposure to battery fumes. Industrial workers in high risk occupations should be under periodic surveillance. A mild, normochromic, hemolytic anemia is usually found in chronic lead poisoning, and among the early signs are increased urinary levels of delta-amino levulinic acid and coproporphyrin III. Since these compounds can be measured more easily than urinary lead, they constitute effective screening procedures for group or individual studies. In children, severe lead intoxication may cause encephalopathy characterized by clumsiness, irritability, and progressive neuromuscular excitement. Lead encephalopathy is uncommon in adults who more often suffer anorexia, muscle pains, and constipation. Severe involvement may cause lead colic. Long-continued exposure, especially in children, may result in deposition of lead compounds at the base of the teeth and in bones, but the so-called lead line does not always occur.

PHENOTHIAZINES

Severe phenothiazine intoxication, as an isolated phenomenon, is relatively rare. The drugs may cause dermatologic reactions, hypotension, extrapyramidal motor disorders, or jaundice in susceptible patients, but these problems usually constitute side effects of therapeutic administration. The phenothiazines become important in toxicology because they are widely distributed, readily available, and are frequently included in a group of agents taken with suicidal intent. Proprietary drugs in this group include Sparine (promazine), Thorazine (chlorpromazine), Compazine (prochlorperazine), and Phenergan (promethazine hydrochloride), among others. Fatalities due to the phenothiazines alone are exceedingly rare, but this group of drugs potentiates the depressant effects of alcohol, barbiturates, morphine, and meperidine, any or all of which may be used in suicide attempts.

The presence of phenothiazines can best be demonstrated in urine or on tissue samples. The blood level tends to be low, since the material is bound very rapidly in tissue and is slowly excreted in feces and urine. Phenothiazine metabolites may persist in the body and sometimes in the urine for many months following discontinuance of a therapeutic regimen.[33] The simplest urine test for phenothiazines is addition of 6 drops of sulfuric acid and 1 drop of 10 per cent ferric chloride to 1 ml of urine. If phenothiazines are present, a lilac color develops. The simultaneous presence of salicylates does not interfere with this test. Quantitative tests can be done on tissue or urine by measuring ultraviolet absorbance after adding sulfuric acid to a sodium hydroxide-ether extract of the sample. The identity of the particular phenothiazine compound does not affect the results.

SALICYLATES

Salicylate intoxication is a common medical problem in both pediatric and adult age groups, accounting for as many as one quarter of all accidental intoxications.[46] In children, toxicity may occur through over-zealous therapy or from accidental ingestion by the inquisitive child. In adults, aspirin is often used in suicide attempts, and remarkably large doses of salicylates may be taken by enthusiastic self-medicators. Nonfatal ingestion of 130 Gm of aspirin by an adult has been reported, but adult fatalities occur at doses as low as 10 Gm, or 30 to 40 regular-sized tablets.[75] Fatalities more often occur in children, especially if preexisting fever or infection aggravates the metabolic effects of the drug.

The problems of acute salicylate toxicity arise chiefly from acid-base disturbances. Initial respiratory alkalosis occurs from direct stimulation of the respiratory center. To maintain the blood pH, pulmonary loss of carbon dioxide is compensated by renal excretion of bicarbonate, and the result is carbon dioxide deficit accompanied by loss of sodium and potassium in the urine. A later effect of salicylism is metabolic acidosis from organic acids and salicylic acid derivatives, resulting in still further drain on the body's buffering capacity. Although the effects on pH may counterbalance each other, the effect on the buffer mechanism is cumulative. Renal function may be impaired by dehydration, bicarbonate alterations, and severe potassium depletion, and depressed renal function further complicates the metabolic derangements.

Mild degrees of salicylate intoxication cause headache, audial and visual disturbances, dizziness, hyperventilation, and gastrointestinal irritation. Although salicylates affect the concentration of several clotting factors, overt bleeding is a rare complication of mild or moderate intoxication. Purpuric manifestations may accompany fatal salicylism.

The therapy of salicylism is too complicated to be detailed here.

Salicylates are excreted through the kidney, so that toxic renal damage may complicate efforts to reduce blood salicylate level. Exchange transfusion and hemodialysis have been used as life-saving measures when salicylate levels are extremely high.

Initial Blood Level

The blood salicylate level correlates fairly closely with the severity of symptoms and prognosis in children, provided that correction is made for the time elapsed after ingestion. Thus, a moderate elevation persisting many hours after ingestion may carry a graver prognosis than a higher figure occurring a short time after the drug was taken. The prognosis should be based on calculated initial blood level rather than on the actual level at the time of examination. Done[10,11] gives formulas and a nomogram for calculating initial blood levels and offers the following prognostic data, based on calculated initial serum concentration: Up to 50 mg per 100 ml tends to cause no ill effects; 50 to 80 mg per 100 ml causes mild symptoms; moderate intoxication follows levels of 80 to 100 mg per 100 ml; and severe toxicity occurs with levels between 110 and 160 mg per 100 ml. An initial salicylate level above 160 mg per 100 ml almost always carries a fatal outcome. If the blood level is measured within six hours of acute ingestion, the actual determination can be used as the initial level. The metabolism and excretion of salicylates occurs at a constant rate or may slow as the size of the ingested dose increases.[77] Induced diuresis may speed excretion, but in very severe cases, dialysis has proved useful.[11,41]

Measurement

The ferric chloride test on urine is a quick means for demonstrating the presence of salicylates, but positive reactions occur after doses as small as 5 grains (300 mg, or one adult-size tablet).[74] The quantity can be very roughly guessed from the intensity of purple color resulting when 1 ml of 10 per cent ferric chloride is added to 3 ml of urine. This screening test has its greatest value in the differential diagnosis of coma due to unknown causes. Both glucose and salicylates appear as reducing substances in the urine, and it is often essential to distinguish between diabetes and salicylate intoxication as the cause of acidosis and coma. The urine should be gently heated to drive off acetone bodies, which tend to accompany both conditions and which produce a positive ferric chloride test. More accurate measurement is done on blood samples, according to a variety of colorimetric and spectrophotometric techniques.

BIBLIOGRAPHY

1. ANNINO, J.S.: Clinical Chemistry, Principles and Procedures, ed. 3. Little, Brown & Company, Boston, 1964.
2. ANNINO, J.S.: Normal values for serum glutamic oxalacetic transaminase and lactic dehydrogenase activities. Am. J. Clin. Pathol. 46:397, 1966.
3. AXELSSON, U., BACHMANN, R., AND HALLEN, J.: Frequency of pathological proteins (M-components) in 6,995 sera from an adult population. Acta Med. Scand. 179:235, 1967.
4. BASINSKI, D.H.: "Magnesium (titan yellow)," *In* Meites, S. (ed.): Standard Methods of Clinical Chemistry. Academic Press, New York, 1965, vol. 5.
5. BEACH, E.F.: "Non-protein nitrogen," *In* Seligson, D. (ed.): Standard Methods of Clinical Chemistry. Academic Press, New York, 1958, vol. 2.
6. BOWERS, G.N.: "Lactic dehydrogenase," *In* Seligson, D. (ed.): Standard Methods of Clinical Chemistry. Academic Press, New York, 1963, vol. 4.
7. BRANDSTEIN, M., AND CASTELLANO, A.: A simple method for determination of total lipids in serum. J. Lab. Clin. Med. 57:300, 1961.
8. CARAWAY, W.T.: "Uric acid," *In* Seligson, D. (ed.): Standard Methods of Clinical Chemistry. Academic Press, New York, 1963, vol. 4.
9. CONN, H.O.: "Blood ammonia," *In* Meites, S. (ed.): Standard Methods of Clinical Chemistry. Academic Press, New York, 1965, vol. 5.
10. DONE, A.K.: Salicylate intoxication. Significance of measurements of salicylate in blood in cases of acute ingestion. Pediatrics 26:800, 1960.
11. DONE, A.K.: Treatment of salicylate poisoning: review of personal and published experiences. Clin. Toxicol. 1:451, 1968.
12. DRYER, R.L.: "The lipids," *In* Tietz, N.W. (ed.): Fundamentals of Clinical Chemistry. W. B. Saunders Company, Philadelphia, 1970.
13. DRYER, R.L., AND ROUTH, J.I.: "Determination of serum inorganic phosphorus," *In* Seligson, D. (ed.): Standard Methods of Clinical Chemistry. Academic Press, New York, 1963, vol. 4.
14. FALES, F.W.: "Glucose (enzymatic)," *In* Seligson, D.(ed.): Standard Methods of Clinical Chemistry. Academic Press, New York, 1963, vol. 4.
15. FOSS, D.P.: "Determination of protein-bound iodine in serum," *In* Seligson, D. (ed.): Standard Methods of Clinical Chemistry. Academic Press, New York, 1963, vol. 4.
16. FOSS, D.P., HANKES, L.V., AND VAN SLYKE, D.D.: A study of the alkaline ashing method for determination of protein-bound iodine in serum. Clin. Chim. Acta 5:301, 1960.
17. FRANKEL, S., REITMAN, S., AND SONNENWIRTH, A.C. (EDS.): Gradwohl's Clinical Laboratory Methods and Diagnosis, ed. 7. The C.V. Mosby Company, St. Louis, 1970.
18. FREDERICKSON, D.S., LEVY, R.I., AND LEES, R.S.: Fat transport in lipoproteins—an integrated approach to mechanisms and disorders. N.Engl.J.Med. 276:34, 1967.
19. FREIMUTH, H.C.: Toxicology for the general hospital laboratory. Hosp. Progr. 47:90, 1966.
20. GAMBINO, S.R.: "pH and P_{CO_2}," *In* Meites, S. (ed.): Standard Methods of Clinical Chemistry. Academic Press, New York, 1965, vol. 5.
21. GIOVANNIELLO, T.J., AND PETERS, T., JR.: "Serum iron and serum iron-binding capacity," *In* Seligson, D. (ed.): Standard Methods of Clinical Chemistry. Academic Press, New York, 1963, vol. 4.
22. GRAY, C.H.: Clinical Chemical Pathology, ed. 5. The Williams & Wilkins Co., Baltimore, 1968.
23. HARLAN, W.R.: A nomogram for determining types of hyperlipidemia. Arch. Intern. Med. 124:64, 1969.
24. HARRIS, R.C.: "Peak levels of serum bilirubin in normal premature infants," *In* Sara-Kortsak, A. (ed.): Kernicterus. University of Toronto Press, Toronto, Ontario, 1961.
25. HENDERSON, L.W., AND MERRILL, J.P.: Treatment of barbiturate intoxication, with a report of recent experience at Peter Bent Brigham Hospital. Ann. Intern. Med. 64:876, 1966.

26. HENDRY, E.B.: Osmolarity of human serum and of chemical solutions of biologic importance. Clin. Chem. 7:156, 1961.
27. HENRY, R.J.: Clinical Chemistry: Principles and Technics. Harper & Row, New York, 1964.
28. HENRY, R.J., CHIAMORI, N., GOLUB, O.J., AND BERKMAN, S.: Revised spectrophotometric methods for the determination of glutamic-oxalacetic transaminase, glutamic-pyruvic transaminase, and lactic acid dehydrogenase. Am. J. Clin. Pathol. 34:381, 1960.
29. HENRY, R.J., GOLUB, O.J., AND SOBEL, C.: Some of the variables involved in the fractionation of serum proteins by paper electrophoresis. Clin. Chem. 3:49, 1957.
30. HOBBS, J.R.: Disturbances of the immunoglobulins. Sci. Basis Med. Annu. Rev. 106, 1966.
31. HOBBS, J.R.: Immunoglobulins in clinical chemistry. Adv. Clin. Chem. 14:219, 1971.
32. HSIEH, K.M., AND BLUMENTHAL, H.T.: Serum lactic dehydrogenase levels in various disease states. Proc. Soc. Exp. Biol. Med. 91:626, 1956.
33. JARVIK, M.E.: "Drugs used in the treatment of psychiatric disorders," In Goodman, L.S., and Gilman, A. (eds.): The Pharmacologic Basis of Therapeutics, ed. 4. The Macmillan Company, New York, 1970.
34. KANNEL, W.B., CASTELLI, W.P., GORDON, T., AND MCNAMARA, P.M.: Serum cholesterol, lipoproteins, and the risk of coronary heart disease. The Framingham study. Ann. Intern. Med. 74:1, 1971.
35. KAYE, S.: Handbook of Emergency Toxicology, ed. 3. Charles C Thomas, Springfield, Ill., 1970.
36. KESSLER, G.: "An automated system of analysis." In Frankel, S., Reitman, S., and Sonnenwirth, A.C. (eds.): Gradwohl's Clinical Laboratory Methods and Diagnosis, ed. 7. The C.V. Mosby Company, St. Louis, 1970.
37. KORNGOLD, L.: "Plasma proteins: methods of study and changes in disease," In Stefanini, M. (ed.): Progress in Clinical Pathology. Grune & Stratton, New York, 1966, vol. 1.
38. LEES, R.S., AND WILSON, D.E.: The treatment of hyperlipidemia. N.Engl.J. Med. 284:186, 1971.
39. MACDONALD, R.P.: "Bilirubin (modified Malloy and Evelyn)," In Meites, S. (ed.): Standard Methods of Clinical Chemistry. Academic Press, New York, 1965, vol. 5.
40. MACDONALD, R.P.: "Salicylate," In Meites, S. (ed.): Standard Methods of Clinical Chemistry. Academic Press, New York, 1965, vol. 5.
41. MANN, J.B. AND SANDBERG, D.H.: Therapy of sedative overdosage. Pediatr. Clin. North Am. 17:617, 1970.
42. MEITES, S.: "Ultramicroglucose (enzymatic)," In Meites, S. (ed.): Standard Methods of Clinical Chemistry. Academic Press, New York, 1965, vol. 5.
43. MEITES, S., AND BOHMAN, N.: Evaluation of an ultramicro method for glucose determination. Am. J. Med. Technol. 29:327, 1963.
44. MIDDLETON, J.E., AND GRIFFITH, W.J.: Rapid colorimetric micromethod for estimating glucose in blood and C.S.F. using glucose oxidase. Br. Med. J. 2:1525, 1957.
45. MIKKELSEN, W.M., DODGE, H.J., AND VALKENBURG, H.: The distribution of serum uric acid values in a population unselected as to gout or hyperuricemia; Tecumseh, Michigan, 1959-60. Am. J. Med. 39:242, 1965.
46. NOBEL, S.: "Toxicology in a general hospital," In MacDonald, R.P. (ed.): Standard Methods of Clinical Chemistry. Academic Press, New York, 1970, vol. 6.
47. PAULUS, H.E., COUTTS, A., CALABRO, J.J. AND KLINENBERG, J.R.: Clinical significance of hyperuricemia in routinely screened hospitalized men. J.A.M.A. 211:277, 1970.
48. PETERMAN, M.L.: Plasma protein abnormalities in cancer. Med. Clin. North Am. 45:537, 1961.
49. PETERS, T., JR.: Serum albumin. Adv. Clin. Chem. 13:37, 1970.
50. PILEGGI, V.J., LEE, N.D., GOLUB, O.J., AND HENRY, R.J.: Determination of iodine compounds in serum. I. Serum thyroxine in the presence of some iodine contaminants. J. Clin. Endocrinol. Metab. 21:1272, 1961.
51. POSTLETHWAITE, A.E., BARTEL, A.G., AND KELLEY, W.N.: Hyperuricemia due to ethambutol. N. Engl. J. Med. 286:761, 1972.
52. PRUZANSKI, W., AND OGRYZLO, M.A.: Abnormal proteinuria in malignant diseases. Adv. Clin. Chem. 13:335, 1970.
53. RASTEGAR, A., AND THEIR, S.O.: The physiologic approach to hyperuricemia. N. Engl. J. Med. 286:470, 1972.

54. REMP, D.G.: "Uric acid (uricase)," *In* MacDonald, R.P. (ed.): Standard Methods of Clinical Chemistry. Academic Press, New York, 1970, vol. 6.
55. RICE, E.W., FLETCHER, D.C., AND STUMPF, A.: "Lead in blood and urine," *In* Meites, S. (ed.): Standard Methods of Clinical Chemistry. Academic Press, New York, 1965, vol. 5.
56. SCHATZ, I.J.: Classification of primary hyperlipidemia. J.A.M.A. 210:701, 1969.
57. SCHEIG, R.: "Diseases of lipid metabolism," *In* Bondy, P.K. (ed.): Duncan's Diseases of Metabolism, ed. 6. W.B. Saunders Company, Philadelphia, 1969.
58. SELIGSON, D., AND HIRAHARA, K.: The measurement of ammonia in whole blood, erythrocytes, and plasma. J. Lab. Clin. Med. 49:962, 1957.
59. SETTER, J.G., MAHER, J.F., AND SCHREINER, G.E.: Barbiturate intoxication: evaluation of therapy including dialysis in a large series selectively referred because of severity. Arch. Intern. Med. 117:224, 1966.
60. SHARPLESS, S.K.: "Hypnotics and sedatives, I. The Barbiturates," *In* Goodman, L.S., and Gilman, A. (eds.): The Pharmacologic Basis of Therapeutics, ed. 4. The Macmillan Company, New York, 1970.
61. SHERLOCK, S.: Diseases of the Liver and Biliary System, ed. 4. F.A. Davis Company, Philadelphia, 1968.
62. SOOTHILL, J.F.: Quantitative disturbance of plasma proteins in disease. Sci. Basis Med. Annu. Rev. 1967.
63. SÖREMARK, R.: The biologic half-life of bromide ions in human blood. Acta Physiol. Scand. 50:119, 1960.
64. TALBERT, L.M., AND LANGDELL, R.D.: Normal values of certain factors in the blood clotting mechanism in pregnancy. Am. J. Obstet. Gynecol. 90:44, 1964.
65. TAUSSKY, H.H.: "Creatine and creatinine in urine and serum," *In* Seligson, D. (ed.): Standard Methods of Clinical Chemistry. Academic Press, New York, 1961, vol. 3.
66. THIERS, R.E.: "Magnesium (fluorometric)," *In* Meites, S. (ed.): Standard Methods of Clinical Chemistry. Academic Press, New York, 1965, vol. 5.
67. TIETZ, N.W.: "Electrolytes," *In* Tietz, N.W. (ed.): Fundamentals of Clinical Chemistry. W. B. Saunders Company, Philadelphia, 1970.
68. TOCANTINS, L.M., AND KAZAL, L.A.: Blood Coagulation, Hemorrhage and Thrombosis. Grune & Stratton, New York, 1964.
69. VALBERG, L. S., CORBETT, W.E.N., McCORRISTON, J.R., AND PARKER, J.O.: Excessive loss of plasma protein into the gastrointestinal tract associated with myocardial disease. Am. J. Med. 39:668, 1965.
70. WACKER, W.E.C., ULMER, D.D., AND VALLEE, B.L.: Metalloenzymes and myocardial infarction. II. Malic and lactic dehydrogenase activities and zinc concentrations in serum. N. Engl. J. Med. 255:449, 1956.
71. WALSHE, J.M.: "Wilson's disease, a review," *In* Peisach, J., Aisen, P., and Blumberg, W.E. (eds.): The Biochemistry of Copper. Academic Press, New York, 1966.
72. WATSON, D.: "Albumin and 'total globulin' fractions of blood," *In* Sobotka, H., and Stewart, C.P. (eds.): Advances in Clinical Chemistry. Academic Press, New York, 1965, vol. 8.
73. WILKINSON, J.H.: An Introduction to Diagnostic Enzymology. Williams & Wilkins Co., Baltimore, 1962.
74. WILLIAMS, L.A.: "Toxicology," *In* Frankel, S., Reitman, S., and Sonnenwirth, A.C. (eds.): Gradwohl's Clinical Laboratory Methods and Diagnosis, ed. 7. C.V. Mosby Company, St. Louis, 1970.
75. WOODBURY, D.M.: "Analgesics-antipyretics, anti-inflammatory agents, and inhibitors of uric acid synthesis," *In* Goodman, L.S., and Gilman, A. (eds.): The Pharmacologic Basis of Therapeutics, ed. 4. The Macmillan Company, New York, 1970.
76. WYNGAARDEN, J.B., AND KELLEY, W.N.: "Gout," *In* Stanbury, J.B., Wyngaarden, J.B., and Frederickson, D.S. (eds.): The Metabolic Basis of Inherited Disease, ed. 3. McGraw-Hill Book Company, New York, 1972.
77. YAFFE, S.J., SJÖQVIST, F., AND ALVAN, G.: Pharmacologic principles in the management of accidental poisoning. Pediatr. Clin. North Am. 17:495, 1970.
78. ZAK, B.: "Total and free cholesterol," *In* Meites, S. (ed.): Standard Methods of Clinical Chemistry. Academic Press, New York, 1965, vol. 5.
79. ZAWADSKI, Z.A., AND EDWARDS, R.V.: M-components in immunoproliferative disorders. Am. J. Clin. Path. 48:418, 1967.
80. ZIMMER, J.G., AND DEMIS, D.J.: Associations between gout, psoriasis, and sarcoidosis. Ann. Intern. Med. 64:786, 1966.

CHAPTER 5

Acid-Base and Electrolyte Regulation

ACID-BASE REGULATION

The pH of normal circulating blood ranges from 7.38 to 7.44, while the limits compatible with life are approximately 6.8 to 7.8. The pH is the negative logarithm of the hydrogen ion concentration, a term used because the number of decimal places involved can become cumbersome; i.e., a concentration of 0.000001 hydrogen ions per liter is more effectively expressed as pH 5.0. The pH is a concept rather than a concentration. It is, of course, dependent upon the number of free hydrogen ions in a solution; the larger the number of hydrogen ions, the smaller the pH value. In the blood, free hydrogen ions are present in very small numbers. Complete neutrality is expressed by pH 7.0. The blood contains between 36 and 44 nanoequivalents of free hydrogen ions per liter, at the normal pH range of 7.36 to 7.44.[14] The pH range compatible with life is much greater, approximately 6.9 to 7.8. This rather narrow numerical spread in pH units corresponds to H^+ concentrations between 16 and 110 nanoequivalents per liter.[10]

FUNDAMENTAL CONCEPTS

Acids and Bases

An *acid* is any substance capable of liberating a hydrogen ion into the solution; a *base* is any substance that can accept a hydrogen ion from the solution. The ability of a compound to donate or to accept a hydrogen ion depends, among other things, on the pH of the medium. Compounds that are commonly called "acids" must be considered as pairs of an acid and a base. A hypothetical acid, HAc, consists of the ions H^+ and Ac^-. The compound acid, when it dissociates, donates an H^+ ion into the medium; the Ac^- ion, in its dissociated state, is a base because it can combine with (accept) a hydrogen ion.

Some compounds that are not, in common parlance, "acids" are in fact hydrogen ion donors under appropriate circumstances. For example, both NH_4^+ and $HPO_4^=$ can liberate a hydrogen ion into a medium relatively low in hydrogen ions. If the medium contains a large number of hydrogen ions, $HPO_4^=$ can act as a base, accepting a hydrogen ion to become $H_2PO_4^-$. The number of anions and cations in a solution must always be equal; therefore, none of the ions just mentioned could exist in a solution without a balancing ion. Some combinations of anion and cation dissociate freely, and each ion floats separately in the medium. Other combinations remain more closely tied to one another. The tendency of a compound to dissociate is described by the terms weak and strong.

Strong and Weak Acids

A *strong acid* is one which dissociates to liberate its H^+ under a wide range of conditions, even into mediums with an already high hydrogen ion concentration. A *weak acid* is one which dissociates poorly; that is, relatively few free ions enter the medium, and the positive ion and negative ion remain closely associated with each other. To form the salt of an acid, the hydrogen ion is replaced by a cation which does not affect the pH of the medium. If we replace the H^+ by Na^+ in the acid HAc, we then have two electrically balanced ions, Na^+ and Ac^-. Although the Na^+ ion does not alter the pH, the Ac^- ion remains capable of combining with (accepting) an H^+ ion.

If the acid HAc is a weak acid, it will dissociate into H^+ and Ac^- only if very few H^+ ions are present in the medium; that is, it dissociates at a relatively high pH. The salt NaAc dissociates much more freely, and the Ac^- floats free and is capable of combining with any H^+ ions that might be available. The resultant compound HAc is, as we have said, a weak acid; as long as the medium is moderately acidic, it does not dissociate its H^+ back into the medium. The result of adding the salt of a weak acid to a moderately acid medium is that dissociated hydrogen ions combine with the anions to form undissociated weak acid, and the medium becomes less acid. This is shown in the following equations:

NaAc $\rightleftarrows$ Na^+ + Ac^- (the salt of a weak acid)
HCl $\rightleftarrows$ H^+ + Cl^- (a strong acid, freely dissociated)
Na^+ + Ac^- added to H^+ + Cl^- gives HAc + Na^+ + Cl^-

Buffer Solutions

A solution that contains a weak acid together with the salt of that weak acid is called a buffer solution, meaning that it is capable of assimilating (buffering) added H^+ or OH^- ions with relatively little change in pH. This is true because the ionization of the weak acid varies with the number of H^+ ions in the solution. If additional H^+ ions enter the solution, the Ac^- ion from the dissociated salt combines with the H^+ ion to form the poorly dissociated acid. If OH^- ions are added, the medium becomes much less acidic, and the weak acid dissociates to provide H^+ ions which neutralize the added OH^-. These situations are shown in the following equations, in which strong acid or strong base is added to a buffer solution of the weak acid HAc and its salt NaAc:

$$H^+ \text{ and } Cl^- \text{ added to } HAc + Na^+ + Ac^- = 2HAc + Na^+ + Cl^-$$
$$Na^+ \text{ and } OH^- \text{ added to } HAc + Na^+ + Ac^- = H_2O + 2Na^+ + 2Ac^-$$

In both cases, the pH remains unchanged. Obviously, if more H^+ or OH^- were added, the pH would change when the weak acid or its salt was exhausted. The ideal buffer pair consists of equal quantities of salt (base) and acid, so that dissociation or recombination can occur in either direction without exhausting the supply of either base or acid.

The Henderson-Hasselbalch Equation

The buffering capacity of a salt-acid pair depends upon the number of hydrogen ions already present (i.e., the pH of the solution) and the physical property of the acid (i.e., its inherent tendency to dissociate). These relationships are illustrated in the Henderson-Hasselbalch equation:

$$pH = pK + \log \frac{[A^-]}{[HA]}$$

It is not necessary, for our purpose, to show how this equation is derived. The terms used are as follows: pH is the hydrogen ion concentration in the solution at the time under consideration; pK is a constant specific for each base-acid combination, designating that pH at which the compound is half dissociated and half undissociated; the proportion $\frac{[A^-]}{[HA]}$ refers to the actual concentrations of base (dissociated anion capable of uniting with an H^+ ion) and acid (undissociated form in which the H^+ ions do not affect the pH) in the solution at the time under consideration.

In simple nonmathematical terms, the Henderson-Hasselbalch equation tells us that the pH of an acid-containing medium is proportional to the existing concentration of dissociated salt and combined acid. Different acids have different buffering capacity depending upon their pK (i.e., the pH at which half the acid is undissociated) and upon the pH at which they are required to act. Even the best of buffer pairs can accept only a limited challenge of H^+ or OH^-. Once the acid or the salt has been consumed in the buffering process, additional H^+ or OH^- changes the pH unhindered.

BLOOD pH

The pH of the blood critically affects the health of the organism; the body must continually protect itself against drastic pH changes. Most metabolic reactions produce acid end products. Vast quantities of carbon dioxide are produced as energy is generated and consumed; CO_2, in hydrated form, is the acid H_2CO_3. However, CO_2 is volatile and can readily be excreted through the lungs once it arrives there from the site of production. In conditions of normal respiratory function, CO_2 is transported and rapidly excreted without affecting the blood pH. Certain nonvolatile acids are also produced; these originate from sulfur- and phosphate-containing compounds and from various incomplete combustion reactions. The nonvolatile acids are normally excreted through the kidneys. Both CO_2 and the nonvolatile acids must be neutralized at the site of production and transported through the blood to the site of excretion.

Physiologic Buffers

There are in the circulating blood many buffer compounds that prevent local acid accumulation and permit the transportation of acids through the body. Some available buffer pairs derive from amino acids of the serum proteins, from the phosphate compounds in plasma and red cells, and from the amino acids of intracellular hemoglobin. The most significant of the blood buffers, however, is the bicarbonate—carbonic acid pair. Carbonic acid is weakly dissociated, and large quantities of bicarbonate exist in the plasma. The bicarbonate—carbonic acid system has its pK, hence optimal buffering capacity, at pH of 6.1, far below the pH of normal blood. In addition, the proportion of bicarbonate to carbonic acid is 20:1, far removed from the optimal buffering ratio of 1:1. At first glance, this seems an unpromising combination. The peculiarities of physiology are such, however, that the bicarbonate buffer system is remarkably effective and the other buffer systems mentioned play a much smaller part in pH regulation.

The Bicarbonate System. As we pointed out earlier, a buffer pair (i.e., the base and the acid form) loses its buffering capacity if either member is totally consumed. In the body, several mechanisms combine to maintain the normal 20:1 proportion between bicarbonate and carbonic acid, thus to maintain the blood at its normal pH. For convenience, let us restate the Henderson-Hasselbalch equation, using the actual compounds involved:

$$pH = pK + \log \frac{[HCO_3^-]}{[H_2CO_3]}$$

The denominator is kept low by continuous excretion of CO_2, so H_2CO_3 accumulation is prevented. The numerator, or bicarbonate portion, can be increased or decreased as necessary through renal excretion mediated by carbonic anhydrase activity. If anything happens to increase the bicarbonate or decrease the CO_2 concentration, the blood pH will rise, and anything that increases the CO_2 concentration or diminishes the bicarbonate will lower the pH. In metabolic balance, however, acids are produced, neutralized, and excreted, and the buffer pair remains constant.

LABORATORY MEASUREMENT

A variety of derangements can alter the normal condition, and when this occurs, it is necessary to measure the changes in pH and buffering capacity. Blood pH can be measured directly, and under certain conditions this determination is invaluable. If pH change occurs, the body has sustained serious metabolic derangement. The blood pH portrays the end result of the buffering process; measurement of the buffer components provides dynamic information about ongoing processes of compensation. The ratio between bicarbonate and carbonic acid, as stated in the Henderson-Hasselbalch equation, determines the blood pH. Thus, measurement of any two variables permits calculation of the third variable.

pH Determination

Since changes as slight as 0.01 pH units may have considerable physiologic significance, pH determinations must be highly accurate if they are to be used at all. Titrimetric methods, although potentially extremely accurate, are difficult and time-consuming. Electrometric pH measurement is now used almost exclusively in clinical situations. Electrometric methods measure the potential generated across a glass membrane separating two solutions of unequal hydrogen ion concentrations. The sample to be measured is placed on one side of the membrane, and a standard solution of known hydrogen ion concentration is on the other.

Suitable Blood Sample. For pH determinations, either whole blood or plasma can be used; arterial, venous, or capillary blood may be suitable. Venous blood has a pH approximately 0.03 pH units below arterial blood,[5] owing to accumulation of metabolic acids; if venous blood is used, it should be "arterialized" by warming the site for 15 minutes before venepuncture. To avoid accumulating additional acids, the patient should maintain a relaxed state and not "pump" his fist. A tourniquet, if required, should exert pressure no greater than the mean arterial blood pressure and should remain in place as blood is withdrawn.

Artefacts. Many artefacts can affect the pH of the sample. Ideally, the blood should be maintained anaerobically, and the test should be started within five minutes. As time passes, glycolytic activity produces acid metabolites that lower the pH; storage at room temperature accelerates the fall. If the test cannot be done immediately, the sample can safely be kept, anaerobically and in ice, for up to two hours. In bloods with high white counts, glycolysis is increased and the pH drops more rapidly. Sodium fluoride, sometimes used to inhibit glycolysis, introduces artefacts in either direction if the concentration is not rigidly standardized.

WHOLE BLOOD VS. PLASMA. Temperature change also affects the pH by altering protein ionization. Since red cells contain more protein than plasma, whole blood pH is more temperature sensitive than plasma pH. The measured pH of whole blood is 0.01 units lower than that of plasma, partly because the red cells accumulate at the reference electrode.[5] The pH of whole blood may be unpredictably altered by the carbonic anhydrase activity of the red cells; therefore, if time must elapse between collection and determination, plasma is probably more reliable. The anticoagulant should always be heparin, since oxalate tends to raise the pH, and citrate and EDTA tend to lower it.[5]

Results. Two sets of terms are used to describe the physiologic conditions in which pH change occurs; acidosis and alkalosis; and acidemia and alkalemia. Those who advocate using the latter terms suggest that *acidosis* and *alkalosis* describe pathologic conditions in which buffering action is necessary to prevent pH change, while the terms *acidemia* and *alkalemia* make it clear that actual pH change has occurred. This usage distinguishes between uncompensated conditions in which the pH does change, and compensated conditions in which the pH is preserved but at the expense of buffer constituents.

Measuring the Buffer Pair

The proportion of free bicarbonate to carbonic acid determines the

blood pH, the critical proportion being $\dfrac{[HCO_3^-]}{[H_2CO_3]}$

Both numerator and denominator contain measurable carbon dioxide. At pH of 7.4, the proportion is 20:1, and the dominant carbon dioxide-containing compound is bicarbonate. The denominator, written as H_2CO_3, consists partly of undissociated carbonic acid but mostly of physically dissolved carbon dioxide. The volume of dissolved CO_2 is directly proportional to the partial pressure of carbon dioxide in the alveolar air.

If the concentration of buffer compounds is measured as total CO_2 content, both numerator and denominator are included in one figure without partition. If the partial pressure of carbon dioxide (Pco_2) is determined also, the proportion can be fully defined. In most cases, especially when the history is clear-cut, CO_2 content alone can indicate the extent of the metabolic derangement. In more complex situations, when more than one mechanism may be operative, the fullest information possible must be obtained.

COLLECTING THE SAMPLE. For all types of test, there is the problem of maintaining the blood sample in the same condition as when the blood was drawn. Since carbon dioxide enters and leaves the blood freely and since the partial pressure of atmospheric carbon dioxide is far lower than in alveolar air, significant CO_2 tends to escape from the blood sample if the sample is freely exposed to the atmosphere. Collection of the blood under mineral oil in a test tube is not entirely satisfactory for preventing loss of CO_2. In addition to the difficulty of handling the oil without spilling, carbon dioxide can diffuse into the overlying oil. It is preferable to seal the blood in the syringe used for venepuncture or to collect the blood in a vacuum tube which contains heparin, taking care to fill the tube to capacity.[6]

Carbon Dioxide Combining Power. The earliest meaningful test of buffer capacity was determination of the carbon dioxide combining power. In this test, the problem of CO_2 escape was avoided by arbitrarily equilibrating the sample with an atmosphere having a Pco_2 of 40 mm Hg, the normal Pco_2 of alveolar air. Using his own alveolar air, the technician restored the dissolved CO_2 to a uniform, arbitrary value which was then subtracted from the final figure. The remaining volume of CO_2 came from the bicarbonate in the sample, so that the test effectively measured only the numerator. Since the numerator is always much larger than the denominator, and since changes in bicarbonate alone often indicate the severity of the problem, this test has proved clinically useful. It does not, however, measure subtle changes arising from alterations in the denominator.

The CO_2 combining power is reported in milliequivalents per liter (mEq/L), representing the $HCO_3{}^-$. Normal values are 26 to 29 mEq/L. Earlier workers expressed their findings as volumes (milliliters) per 100 ml of serum, and the normal range was 55 to 65 volumes per cent (vol per cent). To convert from one set of units to the other, volumes per cent is multiplied by 0.45 to give milliequivalents per liter.

Carbon Dioxide Content. Total carbon dioxide content measures both elements of the proportion and permits somewhat more accurate assessment of clinical problems. If carbon dioxide content is to be measured, blood must be drawn anaerobically, separated promptly, and stored anaerobically until the test is run. Arterialized venous blood, freely flowing capillary blood, or arterial blood are all suitable for tests of CO_2 content. The quantity of CO_2 is expressed as millimoles per liter. Since H_2CO_3 dissociates into univalent ions, the value in millimoles can be expressed directly as milliequivalents. The normal range for CO_2 content is 25 to 32 mEq/L. The CO_2 content gives the total of the numerator and denominator but does not assign values to either. These values can be calculated or derived from a nomogram if the pH and total CO_2 are known.

The Pco_2.

MEASURED IN ALVEOLAR AIR. The denominator in the Henderson-Hasselbalch equation can be evaluated directly by measuring dissolved CO_2, since little of the H_2CO_3 is present as undissociated carbonic acid. Dissolved CO_2 is proportional to partial pressure of CO_2 in the alveolar air, which is the gaseous atmosphere at equilibrium with the blood. If the Pco_2 of alveolar air can be measured directly, this value, in mm Hg, is used to represent the Pco_2 of arterial blood. Collection of alveolar air requires the patient's active participation, and is often most difficult in the very patients for whom the determination is most important.

MEASURED BY ELECTRODE. Recent advances in electrometry permit Pco_2 to be measured directly, using an electrode analogous to that used for pH determination. In laboratories where this equipment is available, blood Pco_2 can be measured accurately, with little delay, on very small samples of blood.

THE ASTRUP TECHNIQUE. This technique employs both measurement and calculation. The pH of the patient's blood is first determined directly. Two aliquots of blood are then equilibrated with carbon dioxide, one with 2 per cent carbon dioxide and the other with 6 per cent carbon dioxide. The pH of these two samples is determined after full equilibration has occurred. With this information, both the Pco_2 and pH of two blood samples are known, so that a graph can be constructed to express the relationship of pH and P_{CO_2}. By locating the pH of the original sample on this line, one can calculate from the graph what the native P_{CO_2} must have been to give the original pH.

Other Approaches in Laboratory Measurement

There is considerable debate about the best ways of obtaining and using data to evaluate acid-base status. Various special techniques and terminologies[3,14,15] are used in various laboratories. Chief among these are the concepts of buffer base, standard bicarbonate, and base excess. Consideration of the relative merit of these approaches is beyond the scope of the discussion here.

EFFECT OF ELECTROLYTES

Changes in such serum electrolytes as Na^+, K^+, Ca^{++}, Cl^-, and others do not themselves affect the pH, but the electrolyte changes reflect physiologic derangements which may also affect acid-base balance. Renal excretory pathways are such that, in normal conditions, either Na^+ or K^+ is the primary urinary cation. If a sodium ion is reabsorbed from tubular urine, then a potassium ion is excreted in its place; the reverse occurs if potassium is reabsorbed. Hydrogen ions, either H^+ or NH_4^+, compete with K^+ in this exchange. In conditions of H^+ excess or K^+ deficit, hydrogen ions are excreted to replace Na^+.

Unmeasured Anions

Sodium is the principal cation of blood and has a normal concentration of 132 to 142 mEq/L. Potassium, the other significant cation, varies over a very narrow range even in disease, but contributes, normally, 4 or 5 mEq/L to the cationic total. Chloride is the principal anion, ranging normally from 98 to 106 mEq/L. The carbon dioxide content, which includes bicarbonate, dissolved carbon dioxide, and carbonic acid, contributes 25 to 32 mEq/L. The carbon dioxide anions added to the chloride anions normally total 6 to 12 mEq/L less than the number of potassium and sodium cations. This difference of 6 to 12 anionic milliequivalents, sometimes called the unmeasured anions, derives from nonvolatile acids such as phosphates, sulfates, proteinates, and miscellaneous organic acids. This figure—the difference between sodium plus potassium concentration and the sum figure of chloride concentration and CO_2 content—can vary with changes in any one of the determinants. Used in conjunction with the pH and the CO_2 combining power, the figure may indicate that the acid-base change is probably due to retention of nonvolatile acids, to bicarbonate loss, or to chloride retention.[12] Retained nonvolatile acids often derive from ingested agents such as salicylates or methyl alcohol, or may represent accumulation of endogenous products, notably lactic acid or ketone bodies. The term *anion gap* is sometimes used to describe such increase in unmeasured anions.

The Principal Buffer System

The bicarbonate-carbonic acid buffer system is peculiarly effective because the carbonic acid level can be rapidly altered by pulmonary CO_2 excretion, and the bicarbonate concentration is regulated in the kidney by excretion, reabsorption, and regeneration of the ion. Pulmonary compensation occurs very rapidly, but renal changes require several hours. The kidney also excretes nonvolatile acids by excreting the anion as the salt and disposing of the hydrogen ion. An excess acid load cannot simply be excreted as the hydrogen ion H^+ and the anion Ac^-, for this would lower the urinary pH beyond physiologic tolerance. Instead the Ac^- is excreted with Na^+, K^+, or other cations. Excess H^+ can be converted to NH_4^+ for excretion or may remain in the blood where it must be buffered.

When acid production or retention produces a hydrogen ion load, the body can neutralize the H^+ by conversion of HCO_3^- to H_2CO_3. This produces an increase in blood carbon dioxide, thus stimulating respiratory activity so that the carbon dioxide is blown off and the acid causes no physiologic damage. When the body's supply of HCO_3^- is depleted, this buffering activity must stop, and hydrogen ion accumulates. The ultimate solution, of course, is to reverse whatever process caused the build-up of acids. To consider all the complexities of acid-base and electrolyte interaction and appropriate therapeutic measures is beyond the scope of this discussion. We can, however, consider the main categories of acid-base disturbance, their usual etiologies, and associated laboratory findings.

DISORDERS OF ACID-BASE REGULATION

Let us, at this point, restate the Henderson-Hasselbalch equation, which describes the relationship between pH and the concentration of the buffer compounds:

$$pH = pK + \log \frac{[HCO_3^-]}{[H_2CO_3]}$$

In subsequent paragraphs, the bicarbonate concentration will sometimes be

Table 13.   Carbon Dioxide Changes and pH Change

	Direction of pH Change	Direction of Change of CO_2 Content
Metabolic acidosis	↓	↓
Respiratory acidosis	↓	↑
Metabolic alkalosis	↑	↑
Respiratory alkalosis	↑	↓

referred to as the numerator, and the P_{CO_2} (or transported CO_2) is referred to as the denominator; both these terms refer to the Henderson—Hasselbalch equation. At the normal pH of 7.4, the normal ratio between numerator and denominator is 20:1.

A pH rise is termed alkalosis or alkalemia. This can result from respiratory CO_2 loss (decrease in the denominator) or from a metabolically induced increase in bicarbonate (increase in the numerator). Acidosis or acidemia is a decrease in pH, which can have either a respiratory origin as carbon dioxide retention or metabolic origin as loss of bicarbonate. Bicarbonate is lost when nonvolatile acids increase, since the bicarbonate must become H_2CO_3 to buffer the excess hydrogen ion, and the resulting carbon dioxide is lost to the body through respiratory excretion. The direction of pH change cannot be inferred simply from determination of bicarbonate content, as can be seen in Table 13.

METABOLIC ACIDOSIS

Diabetic Ketoacidosis

The most dramatic example of metabolic acidosis is diabetic ketoacidosis, in which incomplete combustion of proteins and fatty acids produces nonvolatile ketoacids. These acids must be excreted in the urine along with some of the body's cations, and they must be buffered in the blood by conversion of bicarbonate into carbonic acid. The body, in trying to maintain the proportion of bicarbonate to carbonic acid at 20:1, continually decreases the denominator by respiratory excretion of CO_2 as the numerator decreases. The result is tremendous loss of total CO_2 and a reduction in buffering capacity. Massive excretion of glucose and ketoacids leads to dehydration by osmotic diuresis. The osmotic diuresis impairs renal concentrating mechanisms, leading to still further water loss. Hyperventilation accentuates dehydration, by insensible water loss. With dehydration, body temperature rises, and the resulting hypermetabolism induces further incomplete combustion and ketoacid production. To balance the excretion of ketoacid anions, massive cation loss occurs in the urine, leading to Na^+ and K^+ depletion.

The Potassium Problem. Another mechanism for stabilizing blood pH is the exchange of serum hydrogen ions for intracellular potassium ions. When hydrogen ions disappear into the cells, the blood pH is partially protected, but the intracellular pH suffers. Furthermore, potassium ions which enter the blood from their previous intracellular location rapidly leave the body as urinary cations, so that whole-body stores of potassium are seriously depleted. The serum potassium concentration at any given moment may be normal or low but does not reflect the whole-body state.

Laboratory Findings. Typical laboratory findings in diabetic ketoacidosis include marked reduction in total CO_2 and significant fall in P_{CO_2}; pH drop proportional to the severity of the condition; decreased serum sodium, with a variable level of serum potassium; marked increase in unmeasured anions and relatively small change in chlorides; and, of course, tremendously elevated blood glucose levels.

Acidosis of Renal Disease

Another relatively common cause of metabolic acidosis is severe renal disease, which ordinarily produces a chronic condition rather than a sudden, dramatic episode. Overall metabolism produces approximately 50 to 75 mEq of hydrogen ion daily, an amount which, if retained, depresses the bicarbonate buffer by approximately 3 or 4 mEq/L in a 70 kg individual.[10] This acidosis may develop rapidly in acute renal failure, but more often the hydrogen ion excretion is partially effective and other defects combine to produce a series of problems. As the kidney loses its ability to excrete nonvolatile acids, carbonic anhydrase activity also diminishes, so that bicarbonate reabsorption and regeneration are severely impaired. The combination of nonvolatile acids and decreased bicarbonate is similar in general outlines to diabetic acidosis. In the chronic state, CO_2 content persists at a low level. Because there is no acute rise in denominator to precipitate hyperventilation, the P_{CO_2} is less depressed than in diabetic ketoacidosis. Cation loss is not significant, and as the renal disease worsens, hyperkalemia may occur. The blood glucose is normal, but there is an increase in unmeasured anions, and there are high levels of BUN and creatinine.

Intoxications

Acidosis with increased unmeasured anions occurs with certain intoxications, notably from salicylates, methanol, and paraldehyde. Salicylism is an especially complex problem (see p. 139), since there are elements which dispose toward both respiratory alkalosis and metabolic acidosis.

Lactic Acidosis

A very pronounced acidosis, accompanied by increased serum osmolality and disproportionately large anion gap, occurs in lactic acidosis. Lactic acid, a terminal product of glycolysis, may accumulate whenever anaerobic glycolysis is accelerated, but ordinarily levels recede to normal when the metabolic stress subsides. Uncontrolled lactic acid production or retention or both occur as a severe, unpredictable, and frequently fatal complication of a diverse group of diseases. Individuals with diabetes mellitus,[1] with ketotic or nonketotic[14] coma, may develop this complication, but severe diseases of kidney, liver, heart, blood vessels, and the hematologic system have all been implicated,[9,13,16] and the condition assumes a critical identity apart from the underlying disease. Besides the acidosis, pronounced hyperosmolality, and an anion gap not satisfactorily explained by elevated lactate levels alone, the patient has increased serum levels of lactate dehydrogenase and glutamic-oxalacetic transaminase, and often increased inorganic phosphate levels as well.[16]

Primary Bicarbonate Alteration

Acidosis without increased unmeasured anions occurs when large amounts of bicarbonate are lost, typically from prolonged or severe diarrhea. Distal to the entrance of the alkaline pancreatic juice, intestinal contents contain large amounts of bicarbonate. Excessive fecal excretion seriously depletes this anion. Renal disease, in which bicarbonate reabsorption and regeneration are impaired, may cause a similar situation. This type of renal tubular acidosis results from hereditary or acquired tubular defects or from massive ingestion of a carbonic anhydrase inhibitor or ammonium chloride (see p. 231).

Significant findings in such cases include increased serum chlorides, which rise to compensate the anion deficit caused by bicarbonate loss. Serum sodium and potassium are variably diminished, and total CO_2 content is usually only moderately reduced. If compensatory mechanisms are adequate the pH change is relatively slight, but if the diarrheal process is catastrophic, as it may be in small children or in any patient with certain bacterial infections, rapid and severe acidosis may occur.

RESPIRATORY ALKALOSIS

As in metabolic acidosis, CO_2 content diminishes in respiratory alkalosis. The primary defect is increased pulmonary loss of carbon dioxide, which decreases the denominator of the Henderson-Hasselbalch equation and disposes toward pH rise. To prevent this pH change, the body increases bicarbonate excretion and lowers the numerator to maintain the proportion. The net result is depletion of both bicarbonate and carbonic acid, with ultimate loss of buffering capacity and rise in pH. Respiratory alkalosis is more often acute than chronic, and the most usual cause is psychogenic hyperventilation. Salicylate intoxication, early in the disease, causes respiratory alkalosis by directly stimulating the respiratory center. Later, metabolic acidosis supervenes, intensifying the loss of total CO_2 even though the direction of pH change is reversed. Any condition of high body temperature or hypermetabolism, such as severe febrile illness or thyrotoxicosis, may cause CO_2 loss through increased respiration. Chronic states of hyperventilation are rare, but occur in certain central nervous system lesions.

Laboratory Findings

In chronic conditions, urinary bicarbonate excretion increases, and excretion of this anion requires the balancing presence of such cations as sodium, potassium, or calcium. Serum chloride rises as bicarbonate levels fall, and serum sodium and potassium values are low. In acute episodes, the only abnormal laboratory findings may be low P_{CO_2} and high pH, since compensatory bicarbonate change requires several hours. Fairly common symptoms of hyperventilation are light-headedness, carpopedal spasm, and muscle tremors. These symptoms are dramatically halted if the patient rebreathes air in a paper bag, thereby raising the P_{CO_2} of the alveolar air and increasing the denominator of the fraction.

METABOLIC ALKALOSIS

In metabolic alkalosis, the total CO_2 increases because the bicarbonate numerator rises. The initial response to an increased numerator is to decrease respiratory effort and conserve CO_2 so that the denominator can also increase. This compensation is doomed to failure, for respiration can diminish only to a certain point. Beyond that point, the rising P_{CO_2} has a stimulatory effect on the respiratory center. If the respiratory center becomes refractory to CO_2 rise, hypoxia alone can promote respiratory effort.

The Potassium Problem

The causes of metabolic alkalosis are varied. Excess bicarbonate ingestion, by itself, rarely causes significant alkalosis because the properly functioning kidney can excrete enormous amounts of this ion. If something prevents the suitable excretion of bicarbonate and accompanying cations, equilibrium is disturbed and alkalosis may occur. Prolonged bicarbonate excretion forces the urinary loss of abundant potassium as well as sodium. If potassium loss is not compensated by increased intake, potassium deficiency may occur. The kidney, in an effort to conserve potassium, excretes hydrogen ions into the urine, reabsorbing both sodium and potassium. As sodium ions return from the tubular urine into the blood, they carry bicarbonate back with them, thus reversing the direction of bicarbonate flow and defeating the effort to excrete excess bicarbonate. If potassium is lost in the urine, serum levels are repleted from intracellular stores. To replace potassium in the intracellular fluid, hydrogen ions leave the blood stream. This maintains the ionic balance in the cells, but the H^+ loss further raises the serum pH. A primary potassium deficit from unbalanced parenteral feeding, drug-induced diuresis, or gastrointestinal loss, can by itself initiate metabolic alkalosis through this effect.

The Bicarbonate Problem

Loss of gastric contents by prolonged vomiting or gastric suction is the most common cause of metabolic alkalosis. Gastric secretions are acid, containing high levels of hydrogen and chloride ions as well as large amounts of water. Prolonged vomiting leads not only to hydrogen ion deficit, but to hypochloremia and dehydration. Serum bicarbonate rises to compensate chloride loss. Potassium and sodium are also lost with gastric contents, so that cation deficits may additionally complicate the condition. As the kidney attempts to increase bicarbonate excretion, further sodium and potassium loss occurs in the urine. In its attempt to conserve cations and continue excreting bicarbonate, the kidney may excrete hydrogen ions to balance the bicarbonate anions. The seemingly paradoxical result is an acid urine at a time of increasing alkalosis.

Laboratory Findings

The laboratory findings in metabolic alkalosis may be complex. The blood pH and total CO_2 content are increased, but P_{CO_2} cannot rise beyond a certain point. Serum chloride values are low, and sodium and potassium levels may be misleading. The serum potassium and sodium concentrations are affected by dehydration. If water loss exceeds electrolyte loss, hemoconcentration may result in normal or even elevated sodium values.

RESPIRATORY ACIDOSIS

The defect in respiratory acidosis is impaired excretion of carbon dioxide, so that CO_2 retention increases the denominator of the fraction. Normally, there is rapid and complete diffusion of carbon dioxide from capillary blood into alveolar air space. Only the most severe thickening of the alveolar wall can by itself signifcantly impair gaseous exchange. This may occur in hyaline membrane disease in infants; the presence of intraalveolar edema fluid or inflammatory infiltrate can exert a similar effect. Gas exchange is more often impeded by a combination of thickened alveolar wall and loss of capillary blood supply, through scarring, vascular disease, or destructive processes.

Respiratory acidosis is usually a chronic problem occurring in patients with long-standing pulmonary or cardiovascular disease. The respiratory center responds to elevated P_{CO_2} levels (hypercapnea) with increased ventilation. This alone can return the P_{CO_2} to normal if the condition is mild. More often, if the pulmonary problem is a chronic one, increased respiratory effort succeeds only in preventing additional CO_2 buildup, but does not return the CO_2 levels to normal. To compensate for the persistently elevated denominator, the kidney retains bicarbonate and sodium and excretes the excess hydrogen ions as NH_4^+. These cations carry chloride out in the urine, so that serum chloride falls and bicarbonate rises. Both numerator and denominator increase; if the proportion of 20:1 is maintained, pH remains unchanged.

Chronic Hypercapnea

This condition of compensated respiratory acidosis with chronically elevated P_{CO_2} causes the respiratory center to become progressively less sensitive to existing P_{CO_2} elevation. Only an additional rise in P_{CO_2} causes the respiratory center to respond once again to stimulation. This process of accommodation to rising P_{CO_2} levels may reach extreme proportions, so that P_{CO_2} virtually loses its power to affect respiration. At that stage, the effective stimulus to respiratory effort is simply hypoxia, and well-meaning treatment which suddenly restores oxygen values to normal may remove the stimulus left for respiratory effort. Treatment of far-advanced pulmonary disease should be carefully planned, and mechanical respirators are frequently advisable during the period of physiologic readjustment.

Respiratory acidosis is the condition in which P_{CO_2} determination has its greatest value, since the pH and the total CO_2 content may not reflect rapid changes in respiratory state. If compensation is successful, of course, the pH does not change at all. Total CO_2 may be misleading if concomitant metabolic problems also affect the bicarbonate level. In pure respiratory acidosis, the potassium and sodium are approximately normal, the chloride is low, and the total CO_2 and P_{CO_2} are elevated.

WATER AND ELECTROLYTES

Approximately 45 to 70 per cent of the body weight is water, and a variety of substances are dissolved or suspended in this water. The principal electrolytes of the extracellular fluid are sodium, chloride, and bicarbonate; lesser contributions to the anions come from phosphates and organic acids, and to the cations from potassium, calcium, and magnesium. The fluid within cells is quite different, containing potassium as its principal cation, while proteins and bicarbonate markedly affect the anionic content.

FLUID BALANCE

Body water comes from oral intake and from metabolic processes, the so-called water of oxidation. Water is lost through many routes. Insensible loss, amounting to about 400 ml per day, occurs from the skin and the lungs. Increase in body temperature or environmental temperature increases this quantity. A minimum of 500 ml of urine per day is necessary to excrete metabolic end products if the kidneys can exert maximum concentrating power. Fecal losses vary with the state of gastrointestinal physiology, but tend to average about 100 ml per day. Sensible sweating accounts for a variable fluid loss, depending on activity, environmental temperature, and body temperature.

Regulation of fluid and electrolyte balance occurs largely through the kidney, for the losses from skin, lungs, and intestines are under little physiologic control. The kidney regulates sodium, potassium, hydrogen ion, and bicarbonate excretion to maintain electrolyte balance, while regulation of urinary volume and concentration maintains fluid homeostasis. Renal regulation of volume is largely directed by the pituitary hormone vasopressin (antidiuretic hormone), through whose action the kidney can secrete small volumes of concentrated urine when water must be conserved. Sodium is retained and potassium excreted under the influence of the adrenal hormone aldosterone. Bicarbonate, ammonium, and hydrogen ions are regulated by chemical reactions in the tubular epithelium. Phosphate excretion is influenced by the parathyroid hormone. These multiple influences on normal fluid and electrolyte regulation can be challenged by a variety of abnormal states, affecting virtually any organ system.

LABORATORY DETERMINATION

The flame photometer is used to measure serum sodium and potassium concentrations. Chemical reactions are used for measuring chlorides, phosphates and, usually, calcium. Measurement of the bicarbonate-carbon dioxide variables has already been discussed (see pages 148-152). Total plasma osmolality can be directly measured through freezing point determinations.[8] Since sodium chloride principally affects plasma osmolality, the sodium value is often used to estimate osmolality, but high concentrations of glucose, urea, or lipids can alter plasma osmolality without affecting the electrolyte values. High levels of circulating alcohol produce hyperosmolality without changing other values, at least acutely, and the hyperosmolality of lactic acidosis is accompanied by pH change and other abnormalities.

Electrolyte values alone can be misleading unless the overall state of hydration is known. Serum sodium concentration, for example, can be low when edema or congestive heart failure expands the extracellular fluid volume, but the whole-body supply of sodium tends to be greater than normal. In dehydration, the serum sodium concentration may be high, but if both water and electrolytes have been lost, the overall sodium stores may be significantly lower than normal.

In estimating the overall state of fluid and electrolyte equilibrium, a variety of laboratory determinations can supplement serum electrolyte measurements. Examination of urine volume and specific gravity indicates the overall state of hydration, and measurement of urinary electrolyte concentrations may clarify the etiology of the metabolic alterations.

SODIUM

Whole-Body Deficit

If fluid and sodium are lost in proportions equal to that in plasma, isotonic dehydration results with relatively little change in electrolyte concentrations. In diagnosing this state, elevated levels of serum proteins and a high hematocrit indicate hemoconcentration. Consideration of the patient's clinical state is essential in diagnosing and treating dehydration. Severe vomiting, hyperventilation, sweating, or diuresis may cause loss of water in excess of sodium loss, resulting in hypernatremic dehydration, even though total sodium supplies are decreased to some extent. In these cases, serum sodium concentration may be normal or high, along with elevated hematocrit and high serum protein values. The urinary sodium load will be very low, indicating a whole-body need for sodium retention despite normal serum values.

Whole-Body Excess

In states of increased total body water, the whole-body sodium supply may be high, even though the sodium concentration in a serum aliquot is lower than normal. This occurs in cardiac failure, renal insufficiency, cirrhosis, and other conditions in which hypoalbuminemia reduces plasma colloid pressure and decreases renal plasma flow. Low serum sodium concentration may occur in states of water intoxication, which is often iatrogenic, or in conditions of inappropriate secretion of antidiuretic hormone (see p. 384).

POTASSIUM

Whole-Body Deficit

The relation between whole-body potassium and serum potassium concentration is also variable. Since potassium is primarily an intracellular ion, the bulk of the body's stores cannot be measured in routinely available tests. If there is massive loss of extracellular potassium, normally intracellular potassium may leave the cells to support the serum concentration. This process cannot be measured directly and can only be inferred from an understanding of the clinical state and from such signs as dehydration, muscle weakness, tremors, and changes in the electrocardiographic tracing.

Diabetic ketoacidosis is a prime offender in this respect, and primary or secondary hyperaldosteronism may also deplete whole-body potassium stores. In acidosis of any type, potassium ions may enter the blood stream as hydrogen ions enter the cells; administration of insulin produces the opposite effect, causing potassium to leave the plasma and go into the intracellular fluid.

Potassium loss can occur through the urinary or gastrointestinal tracts, due to renal tubular disorders, massive diuresis, hyperaldosteronism, diarrhea, intestinal fistulas, or vomiting. Loss of gastric contents causes massive loss of hydrogen ions, since the gastric juices are highly acidic. Severe vomiting and other conditions associated with alkalosis may be accompanied by hypopotassemia far more severe than the external loss would suggest.

Whole-Body Excess

Hyperkalemia can result from decreased urinary output or from excessive intake. Whenever there is destruction of protein or body tissue, normally intracellular potassium is released into the blood stream. Thus, severe accidental or operative trauma, burns, or wasting diseases impose a potassium load on the body. Usually these very conditions are associated with impaired renal function or impaired renal blood flow, or both, so that with the normal excretory route blocked, severe hyperkalemia may occur. High serum potassium levels may complicate adrenal insufficiency, acute renal failure, and the terminal stages of chronic renal disease.

Artefacts

Artefactual elevation of the serum potassium levels can occur in improperly handled blood samples. Prolonged venous stasis during venepuncture can cause mild changes, and hemolysis of the specimen renders the potassium measurement worthless. Prompt separation of serum from cells is advisable so that intracellular potassium does not diffuse into the serum.

CHLORIDE

Alteration of serum chloride is seldom a primary problem. Chlorides are excreted with cations during massive diuresis from any cause and are lost from the gastrointestinal tract in vomiting, diarrhea, or intestinal fistulas. Measurement of serum chloride is usually done for its inferential value. Serum chlorides are decreased in acidosis when the anionic compartment is invaded by "unmeasured anions" from organic or other acids; in conditions of gastrointestinal loss or obstruction; in conditions of extracellular fluid excess such as edema and congestive heart failure; in conditions of excessive urinary loss such as chronic renal failure or tubular acidosis; and in certain abnormal states of the central nervous system. Hyperchloremia is rare, because sodium and chloride retention is usually accompanied by fluid retention as well. Severe dehydration, complete renal shut-down, and injudicious administration of ammonium chloride may elevate serum chloride concentrations.

BIBLIOGRAPHY

1. ARIEFF, A.I., AND CARROLL, H.J.: Nonketotic hyperosmolar coma with hyperglycemia: Clinical features, pathophysiology, renal functions, acid-base balance, plasma-cerebrospinal fluid equilibria and the effects of therapy in 37 cases. Medicine (Baltimore) 51:73-94, 1972.
2. ASTRUP, P., ENGLE, K., JØRGENSEN, K., AND SIGGAARD-ANDERSEN, O.: Definitions and terminology in blood acid-base chemistry. Ann. N.Y. Acad. Sci. 133:59, 1966.
3. COHEN, J.J.: A new acid-base nomogram featuring hydrogen ion concentration. Ann. Intern. Med. 66:159, 1967.
4. DANOWSKI, T.S.: Non-ketotic coma and diabetes mellitus. Med. Clin. North Am. 55:913, 1971.
5. GAMBINO, S.R.: "pH and Pco_2," In Meites, S. (ed.): Standard Methods of Clinical Chemistry. Academic Press, New York, 1965, vol. 5.
6. GAMBINO, S.R., ASTRUP, P., BATES, R.G. ET AL.: Report of the Ad Hoc Committee on acid-base methodology. Am. J. Clin. Path. 46:376, 1966.
7. HARRINGTON, J.T., AND LEMANN, J.: The metabolic production and disposal of acid and alkali. Med. Clin. North Am. 54:1543, 1970.
8. HENDRY, E.B.: Osmolality of human serum and of chemical solutions of biologic importance. Clin. Chem. 7:156, 1961.
9. HUCKABEE, W.E.: Abnormal resting blood lactate. Am. J. Med. 30:833, 1961.
10. LEVITIN, H.: "Acid-base balance," In Bondy, P.K. (ed.): Duncan's Diseases of Metabolism, ed. 6. W.B. Saunders Company, Philadelphia, 1969.
11. MACCONNACHIE, H.F.: An old-fashioned approach to acid-base balance. Am. J. Med. 49:504, 1970.
12. NUTTALL, F.Q.: Serum electrolytes and their relation to acid-base balance. Arch. Intern. Med. 116:670, 1965.
13. REDETZKI, H.M., HUGHES, J.R., AND REDETZKI, J.E.: Differences between serum and plasma osmolalities and their relationship to lactic acid values. Proc. Soc. Exp. Biol. Med. 139:315, 1972.
14. SIGGAARD-ANDERSEN, O.: An acid-base chart for arterial blood with normal and pathophysiological reference areas. Scand. J. Clin. Lab. Invest. 27:239, 1971.
15. STINEBAUGH, B.J., AND AUSTIN, W.H.: Acid-base balance. Common sense approach. Arch. Intern. Med. 119:182, 1967.
16. TRANQUADA, R.E., GRANT, W.J., AND PETERSON, C.R.: Lactic acidosis. Arch. Intern. Med. 117:192, 1966.
17. WELT, L.G.: "Acidosis and alkalosis," In Wintrobe, M.M., Thorn, G.W., Adams, R.D. et al. (eds.): Harrison's Principles of Internal Medicine, ed. 6. McGraw-Hill Book Company, New York, 1970.
18. WINEGRAD, A.I., AND CLEMENTS, R.S., JR.: Diabetic ketoacidosis. Med. Clin. North Am. 55:899, 1971.

CHAPTER 6

Serum Enzymes of
Diagnostic Importance

Enzymes are catalysts, enhancing the multiple reactions that collectively constitute body metabolism. Enzymes are highly specific in their activity, and all metabolizing cells contain some or many of these essential compounds. Certain tissues contain characteristic enzymes which enter the blood only when the cells to which they are confined are damaged or destroyed. The presence in the blood of significant quantities of these specific enzymes indicates the probable site of tissue damage. Small amounts circulate in the blood at all times. Of the many enzymes known to biochemists, relatively few have widespread diagnostic implications. These will be discussed in alphabetical order.

ALDOLASE

This glycolytic enzyme splits fructose-1,6-diphosphate and is present most significantly in skeletal and heart muscle although all cells contain a small amount and the liver has a moderate concentration. Both colorimetric and spectrophotometric methods are used for measurement. The normal range in adult serum is 1.5 to 7.2 micromoles per minute per liter[43] using the method of Sibley and Lehninger.[38] Because aldolase is present within red blood cells, unhemolyzed serum must be used when enzyme activity is measured. Damage to skeletal muscle produces high serum levels of aldolase, particularly progressive muscular dystrophy in which the level may be ten to fifteen times normal. There is no aldolase elevation in muscle diseases of neural origin such as neurogenic muscular atrophy, poliomyelitis, myasthenia gravis, and multiple sclerosis, but any of the inflammatory conditions involving muscle may cause moderately high values. In progressive muscular dystrophy, the aldolase level subsides as the disease progresses toward pronounced muscular wasting.

Despite the relatively low concentration in the liver, aldolase elevations to 17 to 80 international units (IU) per liter occur in early viral hepatitis. The sharp initial rise dissipates over the ensuing two or three weeks of the disease. Biliary obstruction and cirrhosis do not affect the aldolase level. Myocardial infarction may cause a slight rise, but aldolase determinations offer no advantage over transaminase determinations in diagnosing cardiac or hepatic disease. Serum aldolase may also rise with advanced prostatic carcinoma.

AMYLASE

This enzyme splits starch into its component sugars. Its activity is extracellular, and salivary glands and the pancreas secrete the enzyme into the saliva and pancreatic fluid. Since a quantity of unsecreted enzyme exists within the secretory cells, damage to either the glandular cells or the secretory pathway may cause amylase to enter the blood stream. Amylase activity is measured by its effect upon a starch solution. This can be expressed either as the amount of sugar produced or as the amount of starch altered. In the Somogyi method, the resulting sugars are measured colorimetrically,[19] giving normal values of 40 to 140 units per 100 ml.

The amyloclastic method of Huggins and Russell[21] uses iodine to measure the amount of starch present before and after enzymic digestion. Normal values for this method are 10 to 35 units per 100 ml.

PANCREATIC DISEASE

Serum amylase elevations ordinarily indicate pancreatic disease. In acute pancreatitis, levels may rise to 600 Somogyi units within four hours of onset, reaching levels as high as 2000 units within a relatively short time.[43] The fall, like the rise, is rapid, and values may return to normal within 48 to 72 hours, even though active inflammation persists. Under these circumstances, elevated urinary amylase levels may be diagnostically revealing. In patients with severe abdominal pain, blood should be drawn for amylase levels before diagnostic or therapeutic measures are undertaken. Spasm of the sphincter of Oddi can, even without pancreatic disease, elevate the serum amylase to as much as 600 units. Both morphine and certain radiopaque substances used in cholecystography induce significant spasm of the sphincter.

OTHER DISEASES

Elevated serum amylase may accompany acute abdominal pain in certain cases of perforated peptic ulcer, empyema of the gallbladder, intestinal obstruction, ruptured ectopic pregnancy, or peritonitis from any cause.[30] In these cases, chemical irritation of the pancreas may cause transient pancreatitis, and the engorged permeable capillaries of the inflamed area readily absorb the enzyme from the biliary or intestinal fluid. Chronic pancreatitis produces less marked and rather variable elevations of serum amylase, and carcinoma of the pancreas characteristically does not affect the enzyme. Serum amylase levels as high as 700 to 900 units may follow disease of the parotid gland. Although enzyme determination is rarely needed for diagnosing disease of the salivary glands, it may be helpful in cases of mumps encephalitis or mumps orchitis with little overt salivary gland involvement. Separation of amylase activity into isoenzymes according to the gland of origin is feasible, but presently not of diagnostic use.[30]

Amylase is excreted in the urine, and if the serum level has already declined, the urinary level may be diagnostically useful. Patients with severe renal disease may retain amylase in the serum, and elevation resulting from acute pancreatitis persists for an abnormally long time if the kidneys are diseased.

CHOLINESTERASE

Two different cholinesterases have been identified, both of which hydrolyze acetylcholine and other cholinesters. One acts upon acetylcholine more rapidly than upon other cholinesters, and is called acetylcholinesterase, formerly called "true" cholinesterase. It is present in nearly all tissues, but especially in the gray matter of the central nervous system and in the conducting tissue, and is found in red blood cells but not plasma. The less specific enzyme, formerly called "pseudocholinesterase," acts indiscriminately upon a variety of cholinesters, including succinylcholine. This form, now known as cholinesterase, exists in plasma but not red cells. Manufactured by the liver and present in a variety of organs, its physiologic role is imperfectly understood.

ACETYLCHOLINESTERASE

Both cholinesterases are irreversibly inactivated by organophosphates, but acetylcholinesterase determinations are usually employed to document acute or chronic toxicity from this class of insecticides. The erythrocyte enzyme reflects toxicity more reliably than does the plasma activity,[11] and its regeneration after inhibition is much slower. In a normal population, a rather wide range of activity exists, so that precise normal values are difficult to define, and a single value, measured during an episode of suspected organophosphate toxicity, may be difficult to interpret.

If the individual's pre-exposure level is known, this can be extremely helpful; repeated surveillance of individuals known to be at risk for organophosphate exposure provides highly useful baseline data. Without comparison data for the individual, an activity level below 25 per cent of the mean for the laboratory's normal population is considered diagnostically low.

CHOLINESTERASE

Serum, or plasma, cholinesterase exists in several genetically determined variants. The normal form, assayed by its activity on selected substrates in an appropriate buffer, can be measured as an index of liver function. Levels are decreased in parenchymatous liver disease, especially hepatitis and cirrhosis, and in such other conditions of disordered protein synthesis as malnutrition, carcinomatosis, severe anemia, and so forth. It is reported to be high in patients with nephrotic syndrome.[11] The enzyme is rarely measured for these conditions, since cholinesterase determination provides no information in addition to that supplied by the usual diagnostic tests for these diseases.

Succinylcholine Sensitivity

Although the intended physiologic role of cholinesterase is obscure, its absence can produce serious pharmacologic consequences. When patients lacking normal enzyme levels are exposed to suxamethonium (succinylcholine), protracted apnea and generalized muscle relaxation occur, apparently due to failure to inactivate the ester. This condition constitutes a disease of medical progress, since succinylcholine enters the body only when given as a relaxant prior to anesthesia or electroconvulsive therapy. Individuals with the usual cholinesterase readily inactivate the drug; those with any of the variant enzymes appear unable to overcome the drug, and sustain its exaggerated effects for several hours.

At least three variant genes have been identified, determining forms of cholinesterase described as dibucaine resistant, fluoride resistant, and "silent."[27] Dibucaine resistance has been known for many years, and the *dibucaine number* has long been used to classify heterozygotes and homozygotes for this atypical enzyme. Homozygotes, who number perhaps 0.1 to 0.5 per cent of the white population,[28] are susceptible to succinylcholine apnea, but occasional heterozygotes may also show symptoms. The other forms are still less frequent. Symptomatically, the patients are similar, but the variants are fairly readily distinguished chemically.[16]

Accurate enzymatic determination is the only reliable way to identify patients at risk. A simple kit is available for screening, but its sensitivity appears insufficient to characterize those members of the general population for whom succinylcholine exposure may prove dangerous.[12]

CREATINE PHOSPHOKINASE

This enzyme catalyzes the reversible transfer of high energy phosphate between creatine and phosphocreatine and between the adenosine phosphates ADP and ATP. Its principal sites are skeletal muscle and cardiac muscle, but appreciable amounts are found in the brain. Red cells lack this enzyme, so mild hemolysis does not render a serum useless.[42] Serum levels are measured in several ways. One measures the amount of creatine liberated from a phosphocreatine substrate, and results are expressed as micromoles of creatine per ml of serum per hour. The normal range is 0.2 to 1.42 units.[43] In another method, the phosphocreatine formed from a creatine substrate is hydrolyzed and the liberated inorganic phosphate is measured. Results are expressed as micromoles of creatine phosphorylated per minute per liter. Normal range for this method is 1 to 10 units.[41]

MUSCLE DISEASES

Because creatine phosphokinase (CPK) exists in so few organs, elevated serum levels point rather specifically to certain diseases. In progressive muscular dystrophy, consistent and marked elevation occurs, rising in the early stages of the disease to as much as fifty to one hundred times the normal levels. As the disease progresses, enzyme elevation persists, but at much lower levels. The elevation is higher in young children than in adolescents. Neurogenic muscular disorders do not affect creatine phosphokinase levels, but polymyositis does cause marked elevation.[41] Heterozygous female carriers with the abnormal gene characteristically have moderately elevated CPK levels, but serum studies performed during pregnancy have sometimes proved lower than values found in the same women while not pregnant.[4] Elevated CPK values in asymptomatic male siblings of known cases point strongly to subsequent overt involvement.[39] The CPK level alone does not predict the severity of progressive involvement.[36]

MYOCARDIAL DAMAGE

Myocardial necrosis produces short-lived CPK elevations to ten to twenty-five times the normal level. This rise parallels that of glutamic-oxalacetic transaminase (GOT), occurring early in the course of myocardial infarction and returning to normal within two to four days. Angina and uncomplicated congestive heart failure rarely affect this enzyme, but dissecting aortic aneurysms may produce an elevation.[18] Unlike the transaminases, CPK is absent from the liver, so that hepatic complications of myocardial disease do not alter this enzyme curve. In the differential diagnosis of early myocardial infarction, elevated CPK levels help in ruling out acute disorders of the pancreas and biliary tract.

OTHER CONDITIONS

Less pronounced elevations of CPK have been reported following heavy exercise or surgical procedures which damage skeletal muscle. Cerebral accidents and thyrotoxicosis may be associated with moderately high levels of CPK, and high doses of salicylates have been reported to cause elevation in some patients.[13] In chronic alcoholics, an episode of severe acute intoxication may be accompanied by CPK levels comparable to those found with myocardial infarcts.[41] Mild elevations may occur in hypothyroidism, and return to normal when the endocrine condition is treated.[17]

HYDROXYBUTYRATE DEHYDROGENASE

This enzyme catalyzes the interconversion between alpha-ketobutyric acid and hydroxybutyric acid. Its activity is entirely comparable to that of the fast-moving or cardiac component of lactic dehydrogenase, which has a high relative activity against the butyrate substrates, and discussion is deferred to the section on lactic dehydrogenase (see below).

LACTIC DEHYDROGENASE

This glycolytic enzyme catalyzes the reversible alteration between pyruvate and lactate. The spectrophotometric determination[47] measures consumption of reduced DPN, and normal values are 200 to 450 units. Several colorimetric methods are available with entirely different units and normal values.

As one of the glycolytic enzymes, lactic dehydrogenase (LDH) is present in nearly all metabolizing cells, but highest concentrations occur in liver, heart, skeletal muscle, and erythrocytes, in descending order. Damage to nearly any tissue can cause elevated serum LDH; therefore, the test is a rather nonspecific indicator of tissue destruction but, in conjunction with clinical data and other laboratory determinations, it can provide useful information.

DISEASE STATES

Heart

Serum LDH levels rise relatively slowly after myocardial infarction, attaining levels of five to six times normal after two days. Because the elevation persists as long as six to ten days, LDH determinations may be useful in the late diagnosis of myocardial infarction. Since acute congestive heart failure, pulmonary embolism, and ventricular arrhythmias can also cause LDH elevations, the test is not specific for myocardial necrosis. The cardiac, or heat-stable, form of LDH remains elevated for as long as two weeks after myocardial damage, so even if total levels are within normal limits, differential determinations may point to prior cardiac involvement.[44]

Liver

Variable elevation has been noted in liver disease, and it is more marked if hepatocellular necrosis is present. Thus, acute hepatitis, toxic hepatitis, infectious mononucleosis, and primary or secondary hepatic neoplasms may cause high serum LDH levels, while cirrhosis and obstructive jaundice have less effect. The LDH level in infectious mononucleosis can be extremely high, higher than the apparent degree of liver damage would warrant. Quite possibly this change is due to hematologic or immunologic changes in the white cells, but this has not been proven.

Hematologic Conditions

In acute leukemias, chronic myelocytic leukemia, and many lymphomas, serum LDH may be moderately elevated, and widespread neoplastic disease of any organ may also cause high total LDH. Megaloblastic anemia, whether due to folic acid or vitamin B_{12} deficiency, causes extremely high LDH levels. Moderate elevations occur in sickle cell anemia, but changes are slight in other hemolytic conditions.

Other Diseases

Primary muscle diseases and visceral infarcts may cause LDH elevations, although perforated peptic ulcer, appendicitis, and intestinal obstruction without gangrene appear to cause little change.[40]

ISOENZYME DETERMINATIONS

The lactic dehydrogenase molecule is composed of four subunits, each of which may be one of two basic types. In each tissue, the enzyme has a characteristic composition. In liver all four subunits are of one type, and in cardiac muscle all four are of the other type. Hepatic LDH, therefore, has electrophoretic, chromatographic, and immunologic characteristics very different from cardiac LDH. Three other forms have been identified in which the subunits are variously combined, and these have characteristics between the two extremes. The hepatic type migrates slowly in an electrophoretic field and is heat labile. The cardiac type, which migrates rapidly to the anode and is heat stable, readily removes hydrogen from hydroxybutyrate substrates. Since separation of LDH fractions by physical means may reduce the total quantity of enzyme in the specimen, comparison of hydroxybutyrase levels with total LDH has been suggested as a means of provisional fractionation.

Fractionating the LDH activity sharpens its diagnostic value since, as we have seen, total LDH activity can reflect a multitude of origins. In liver disease the total level of LDH may change relatively little, but the hepatic fraction increases markedly and the proportion of cardiac fraction declines. In pulmonary infarction the proportion of hepatic LDH rises, presumably due more to secondary hepatic damage than to pulmonary necrosis, since the lung contains relatively minor amounts of the enzyme. Myocardial necrosis, of course, causes elevation in the cardiac, or hydroxybutyrase-active, fraction.[15] Erythrocyte LDH presents an electrophoretic pattern intermediate between liver and cardiac muscle, but tending more toward the fast-moving cardiac type. In pernicious anemia, fast-moving LDH is markedly elevated, and hydroxybutyrase activity is greatly increased.[46] The LDH level decreases very rapidly when megaloblastic anemia is treated, the decrease occurring even before the reticulocyte response.[20]

LEUCINE AMINOPEPTIDASE

This proteolytic enzyme is present in pancreas, liver, and small intestine. Early observers[35] suggested its use in distinguishing carcinoma of the pancreas from other forms of obstructive biliary disease. Subsequent studies have shown that many types of hepatic and biliary diseases affect serum and urine levels of this enzyme, and its determination offers no advantages over the more easily obtained transaminase and alkaline phosphatase determinations.[26] When low-grade or confusing enzyme patterns occur, leucine aminopeptidase values may clarify the problem by pinpointing hepatobiliary tract disease, for which it is largely specific.

LIPASE

This hydrolytic enzyme is secreted by the pancreas into the duodenum where, aided by bile salts and calcium ions, it splits fatty acids from triglycerides. Like amylase, lipase exists within the secretory cells and appears in the bloodstream following damage to the pancreas, the only organ known to produce it. Assay methods present certain technical difficulties, since the classic method required 24 hours of incubation.[7] Subsequent modifications permit more rapid analysis, giving the test greater clinical applicability. Normal values depend upon the method used but, in health, serum levels are low.

Acute pancreatitis is the most common cause of lipasemia. The lipase levels usually parallel serum amylase elevations early in the disease, but elevated lipase levels may persist up to a week after the actue episode. This makes lipase determinations helpful in the late diagnosis of acute pancreatitis. The enzyme is less useful in cases of chronic pancreatitis, chronic biliary tract disease, and pancreatic carcinoma. Diseases of the salivary gland do not affect lipase levels.

PHOSPHATASES

These hydrolytic enzymes catalyze the cleavage of phospnate esters with little specificity as to preferred substrate. Two general types are recognized: that with a pH optimum of 4.5 to 5.5, called acid phosphatase; and that with a pH optimum between 9 and 10, called alkaline phosphatase. Although similar in catalytic effect, they are easily separated by altering the pH at which the test is run. Basically similar assays are used for both.

In the Bodansky method, β-glycerophosphate is the substrate, and the liberated inorganic phosphorus is measured. The original King-Armstrong method uses a phenylphosphate substrate and measures milligrams of phenol liberated. Various modifications are employed with each, and by varying the pH of the reaction mixture, each method can be used for either type of phosphatase. One Bodansky unit (BU) is equal to approximately 2.5 King-Armstrong (K-A) units. Normal serum levels for alkaline phosphatase are 1.5 to 4 BU or 3 to 13 K-A units. King and Wooten[24] give 1 to 3

K-A units as the normal range for acid phosphatase. For the Babson-Read method, using α-naphthyl phosphate as the substrate, normal acid phosphatase values are 0.5 to 5 Babson-Read units.[1]

ALKALINE PHOSPHATASE

Alkaline phosphatase activity derives from several different tissues. Isoenzymes have been demonstrated as originating from liver, bone, placenta, and intestine, each with different properties which facilitate identification. That of bone origin is most readily inactivated by heat. Exposure to L-phenylalanine inhibits both the placental and intestinal forms. Electrophoresis, especially on polyacrylamide gel, probably gives the best separation, and immunologic specificity can also be demonstrated.

In normal adults, circulating alkaline phosphatase derives both from bone and liver[6] with children exhibiting significantly higher proportions of the osteoblastic form. The enzyme excreted in bile derives almost entirely from liver,[33] but biliary excretion is probably not the dominant metabolic pathway. Most of the enzyme produced appears to be degraded as part of the general protein pool, and is not excreted.[5] The phosphatase increase seen during pregnancy reflects placental manufacture. High serum levels of alkaline phosphatase have been reported following massive infusions of human albumin.[29] When the specifically placental isoenzyme was identified in these patients, the source was found to be the human placentas from which the albumin was prepared. Albumin preparations of nonplacental origin do not produce this artefact.

Bone Disease

In conditions of pronounced osteoblastic activity, serum alkaline phosphatase activity is high. Prepubertal children have normal levels of 15 to 25 K-A units, and as bone growth ceases, the level declines to adult range. In conditions of retarded bone growth such as childhood hypothyroidism, alkaline phosphatase levels are low. Persistent elevation to childhood levels occurs in older patients whose skeletal growth continues abnormally, due to disorders of skeletal maturation or excessive production of growth hormone.

The highest levels of alkaline phosphatase are found in Paget's disease and in hyperparathyroidism with skeletal involvement. In these conditions, values may reach 200 BU, although more moderate elevations are the rule. Jaffe and Bodansky[22] noted that in Paget's disease a sudden rise from a stable and moderate elevation may signal the development of osteogenic sarcoma. Alkaline phosphatase is not elevated in hypervitaminosis D which, like hyperparathyroidism, is associated with hypercalcemia and hypercalciuria. Vitamin D deficiency (rickets) in children may raise the serum level to 30 to 40 K-A units. Osteoblastic metastatic tumor may produce elevations to 20 to 30 BU[43] while osteolytic metastases and foci of multiple myeloma do not affect the enzyme level.

Hepatobiliary Disease

Both hepatocellular disease and bile duct abnormalities affect the serum alkaline phosphatase level, which may rise to diagnostic levels in early obstructive disease before the serum bilirubin increases. Complete extrahepatic duct obstruction reliably causes elevations to 25 or 35 BU or higher, but much higher levels accompany inflammatory or proliferative changes affecting intrahepatic radicles. Biliary cirrhosis produces exceptionally high levels, but cholangiolitic hepatitis and infiltrative liver disease produce significant elevations. Infectious mononucleosis, even without overt signs of liver damage, may cause mildly elevated levels.[32] Alkaline phosphatase levels may be more sensitive than transaminase levels in indicating infections, particularly granulomatous inflammation, or metastatic tumor infiltration.[5] Cirrhosis produces only mild changes in total alkaline phosphatase activity, but the intestinal isoenzyme may become apparent on electrophoresis, a finding associated almost exclusively with this form of liver disease.[6,8]

ACID PHOSPHATASE

The function of this enzyme is not understood. It occurs primarily in the adult prostate gland and in erythrocytes, and the two organs contain rather different forms of the enzyme. Several methods are in use to separate the two forms. The Babson-Read method[1] uses a substrate specific for the prostatic enzyme, so that the erythrocyte portion does not interfere.[25] Another fairly specific substrate is β-glycerophosphate, but with this method (the Shinowara[37] modification of Bodansky's technique) it is necessary to measure liberated inorganic phosphate which may be affected by pre-existing serum phosphate levels.[2] When phenylphosphate is used as the substrate, the two fractions can be partitioned by addition of L-tartrate.[14] This inhibits the prostatic fraction, so that the difference between the total enzyme activity and the activity after inhibition represents the prostatic portion. The problem here is that the prostatic activity contributes only a small proportion to the total.

Significantly elevated serum acid phosphatase nearly always points to metastatic carcinoma. Both total and prostatic fractions are elevated in approximately 80 per cent of cases of prostatic carcinoma with metastasis to bone[45] and in 10 to 25 per cent of patients with prostatic tumor without metastases. If the tumor is successfully treated, enzyme levels decline within three to four days of surgical castration, or three to four weeks of estrogen therapy.[40] Benign prostatic hyperplasia and prostatitis cause no change in the enzyme level.

Elevation of the nonprostatic fraction occurs in Gaucher's disease.[9] The best substrate for documenting this activity is p-nitrophenylphosphate (the Bessey-Lowry[3] technique) which is much less sensitive to the prostatic fraction than α-naphthyl phosphate or β-glycerophosphate.

TRANSAMINASES

These enzymes catalyze the reversible transfer of amino groups between various acids in the glycolytic cycle. In human tissues, two have been recognized, and both have glutamic acid as one of the substrates. Glutamic-oxalacetic transaminase (GOT) mediates between glutamic and oxalacetic acid, and glutamic-pyruvic transaminase (GPT) has pyruvic acid as the other substrate. Very high concentrations of GOT occur in the heart and liver, and moderately large amounts are in skeletal muscle, kidney, and pancreas. Kidney, heart, and skeletal muscle, in decreasing order, have significant concentrations of GPT. Liver contains the highest concentrations of GPT, but even liver has three and one-half times as much GOT as GPT. Both colorimetric and spectrophotometric methods of assay are used, and normal serum values vary from laboratory to laboratory, depending upon the technique.

MYOCARDIAL INFARCTION

Because intact myocardium contains abundant GOT, myocardial necrosis releases large quantities of the enzyme into the circulation. Within 6 to 10 hours after an acute infarction, significant elevation of the serum GOT occurs, reaching a maximum at 24 to 48 hours.[31] In the absence of liver damage, recurrent elevation after the first peak has subsided indicates additional fresh necrosis. Numerous studies indicate correlation as high as 96 to 98 per cent between myocardial infarction and elevated serum GOT.

Elevated serum GOT does not always indicate myocardial infarction, since severe arrhythmias and severe angina have also been reported to cause elevations. Uncomplicated congestive failure and uncomplicated pulmonary infarction probably cause little change, but secondary liver damage tends to complicate both clinical and enzyme diagnosis. Serum

GPT levels rise less markedly and less consistently than GOT following myocardial infarction, perhaps due to initially lower concentration in the intact muscle.

LIVER DISEASE

When hepatic cells are damaged, serum GOT and GPT levels rise. These enzyme changes occur early in the disease, whether damage is due to infectious or toxic hepatitis, central congestion, biliary obstruction, or active cirrhosis. The enzyme levels are especially useful in assessing subtle or early changes. In hepatitis, for example, transaminase levels rise several days before jaundice begins. The enzyme levels also fall rather rapidly and may return to normal while parenchymal changes are still active. A second rise tends to indicate a relapse. The serum GPT level returns to normal more slowly than does the GOT. In obstructive jaundice, there may be mild to moderate elevation, less striking than the change following hepatocellular disease. Mild elevation occurs in cases of active cirrhosis and metastatic tumor. While nonicteric cholecystitis does not alter the GOT and GPT levels, acute pancreatitis may cause some rise. Infectious mononucleosis often causes transaminase elevations, but the changes are less pronounced than the rise in LDH. Such muscle diseases as progressive muscular dystrophy and dermatomyositis may cause elevations in GOT with only minimal change in GPT, whereas myasthenia gravis and rheumatoid arthritis have no effect on either.

BIBLIOGRAPHY

1. BABSON, A.L., AND READ, P.A.: A new assay for prostatic acid phosphatase in serum. Am. J. Clin. Pathol. 32:88, 1959.
2. BABSON, A.L., READ, P.A., AND PHILLIPS, G.E.: The importance of the substrate in assays of acid phosphatase in serum. Am. J. Clin. Pathol. 32:83, 1959.
3. BESSEY, O.A., LOWRY, O.H., AND BROCK, M.J.: A method for the rapid determination of alkaline phosphatase with five cubic millimeters of serum. J. Biol. Chem. 164:321, 1946.
4. BLYTHE, H., AND HUGHES, B.P.: Pregnancy and serum-C.P.K. levels in potential carriers of "severe" X-linked muscular dystrophy. Lancet 1:855, 1971.
5. BREEN, K.J.: Liver function tests. Crit. Rev. Clin. Lab. Sci. 2:573, 1971.
6. CANAPA-ANSON, R. AND ROWE, J.F.: Electrophoretic separation of tissue-specific serum alkaline phosphatases. J. Clin. Pathol. 23:499, 1970.
7. CHERRY, I.S., AND CRANDALL, L.A.: The specificity of pancreatic lipase: its appearance in the blood after pancreatic injury. Am. J. Physiol. 100:266, 1932.
8. CONNELL, M.D. AND DINWOODIE, A.J.: Diagnostic use of serum alkaline phosphatase isoenzymes and 5-nucleotidase. Clin. Chim. Acta 30:235, 1970.
9. CROCKER, A.C., AND LANDING, B.H.: Phosphatase studies in Gaucher's disease. Metabolism 9:341, 1960.
10. DAWSON, D.M., AND FINE, I.H.: Creatine kinase in human tissue. Arch. Neurol. 16:175, 1967.
11. DE LA HUERGA, J., PETRUS, E.A., AND SHERRICK. J.C.: "Detection of cholinesterase

inhibition," *In* Sunderman, F.W., and Sunderman, F.W., Jr. (eds.): Laboratory Diagnosis of Diseases Caused by Toxic Agents. Warren H. Green, Inc., St. Louis, 1970.

12. DIETZ, A.A., RUBINSTEIN, H., AND LUBRANO, T.: Detection of patients with low serum cholinesterase activity: inadequacy of "Acholest" method. Clin. Chem. 18:565, 1972.

13. DRIVSHOLM, A., AND MADSEN, S.: The influence of treatment with sodium salicylate on the serum glutamic oxalacetic transaminase activity. Scand. J. Clin. Lab. Invest. 13:442, 1961.

14. FISHMAN, W.H., AND LERNER, F.: A method for estimating serum acid phosphatase of prostatic origin. J. Biol. Chem. 200:89, 1953.

15. FREEMAN, I., AND OPHER, A.W.: Lactic dehydrogenase isoenzymes in myocardial infarction. Am. J. Med. Sci. 250:131, 1965.

16. GARRY, P.J., OWEN, G.M., AND LUBIN, A.H.: Identification of serum cholinesterase fluoride variants by differential inhibition in tris and phosphate buffers. Clin. Chem. 18:105, 1972.

17. GRAIG, F.A., AND ROSS, G.: Serum creatine-phosphokinase in thyroid disease. Metabolism 12:57, 1963.

18. GRIFFITHS, P.D.: ATP: Creatine phosphotransferase in the diagnosis of acute chest pain. Br. Heart J. 28:199, 1966.

19. HENRY, R.J., AND CHIAMORI, N.: Study of the saccharogenic method for the determination of serum and urine amylase. Clin. Chem. 6:434, 1960.

20. HESS, B.: Enzymes in Blood Plasma, trans. K.S. Henley. Academic Press, New York, 1963.

21. HUGGINS, C., AND RUSSELL, P.S.: Colorimetric determination of amylase. Ann. Surg. 128:668, 1948.

22. JAFFE, H.L., AND BODANSKY, A.: Diagnostic significance of serum alkaline and acid phosphatase values in relation to bone disease. Bull. N.Y. Acad. Med. 19:831, 1943.

23. JENNINGS, R.C., BROCKLEHURST, D., AND HIRST, M.: A rapid, automated screening technique for the detection of placental-like alkaline phosphatase in malignant disease. J. Clin. Pathol. 25:349, 1972.

24. KING, E.J., AND WOOTEN, I.D.P.: Micro-Analysis in Medical Biochemistry, ed. 3. Grune & Stratton, New York, 1956.

25. KLEIN, B., AND AUERBACH, J.: Automated determination of acid phosphatase. III. An evaluation of the alpha-naphthyl-phosphate substrate for serum prostatic acid phosphatase. Clin. Chem. 12:289, 1966.

26. KOWLESSAR, O.D., HAEFFNER, L.J., RILEY, E.M., AND SLEISENGER, M.H.: Comparative study of serum leucine aminopeptidase, 5-nucleotidase, and non-specific alkaline phosphatase in diseases affecting the pancreas, hepatobiliary tree, and bone. Am. J. Med. 31:231, 1961.

27. LEHMANN, H. AND LIDDELL, J.: "The cholinesterase variants," *In* Stanbury, J.B., Wyngaarden, J.B., and Frederickson, D.S. (eds.): The Metabolic Basis of Inherited Disease, ed. 3. McGraw-Hill Book Company, New York, 1972.

28. LUBIN, A.H., GARRY, P.J., AND OWEN, G.M.: Sex and population differences in the incidence of a plasma cholinesterase variant. Science 173:161, 1971.

29. MACKIE, J.A., ARVAN, D.A., MULLEN, J.L., AND RAWNSLEY, H.M.: Elevated serum alkaline phosphatase levels after the administration of certain preparations of human albumin. Am. J. Surg. 121:57, 1971.

30. MEITES, S.: Amylase isoenzymes. Crit. Rev. Clin. Lab. Sci. 2:103, 1971.

31. NISSEN, N.I., RANLOV, P., AND WEIS-FOGH, J.: Evaluation of four serum enzymes in the diagnosis of acute myocardial infarction. Br. Heart J. 27:520, 1965.

32. POPPER, H.P., AND SCHAFFNER, F.: Liver: Structure and Function. McGraw-Hill Book Company, New York, 1957.

33. PRICE, C.P., HILL, P.G., AND SAMMONS, H.G.: The nature of the alkaline phosphatases of bile. J. Clin. Pathol. 25:149, 1972.

34. RAMDEO, I.N., AND JOSHI, K.C.: Serum lactic dehydrogenase and its isoenzymes in hepatic disorders. Am. J. Gastroenterol. 55:459, 1971.

35. RUTENBERG, A.M., GOLDBARG, J.A., AND PINEDA, E.P.: Leucine aminopeptidase activity, observations in patients with cancer of the pancreas and other diseases. N. Engl. J. Med. 259:469, 1958.
36. SHAW, R.F.: Serum enzymes and prognosis in muscular dystrophy. Lancet 1:856, 1971.
37. SHINOWARA, G.Y., JONES, L.M., AND REINHART, H.L.: The estimation of serum inorganic phosphate and "acid" and "alkaline" phosphatase activity. J. Biol. Chem. 142:921, 1942.
38. SIBLEY, J.A., AND LEHNINGER, A.L.: Determination of aldolase in animal tissues. J. Biol. Chem. 177:859, 1949.
39. SMITH, H.L., AMICK, L.D., AND JOHNSON, W.W.: Detection of sub-clinical and carrier states in Duchenne muscular dystrophy. J. Pediatr. 69:67, 1966.
40. TICKTIN, H.E., AND TRUJILLO, N.P.: Serum enzymes in diagnosis. Disease-a-Month, June, 1966.
41. VELEZ-GARCIA, E., HARDY, P., DIOSO, M., AND PERKOFF, G.T.: Cysteine-stimulated serum creatine phosphokinase: Unexpected results. J. Lab. Clin. Med. 68:636, 1966.
42. WARBURTON, F.G., BERNSTEIN, A., AND WRIGHT, A.C.: Serum creatine phosphokinase estimations in myocardial infarction. Br. Heart J. 27:740, 1965.
43. WILKINSON, J.H.: An Introduction to Diagnostic Enzymology. Williams & Wilkins, Baltimore, 1962.
44. WILKINSON, J.H.: Clinical significance of enzyme activity measurements. Clin. Chem. 16:882, 1970.
45. WOODARD, H.Q.: The clinical significance of serum acid phosphatase. Am. J. Med. 27:902, 1959.
46. WRIGHT, E.J., CAWLEY, L.P., AND EBERHARDT, L.: Clinical application and interpretation of the serum LDH zymogram. Am. J. Clin. Path. 45:737, 1966.
47. WROBLEWSKI, F., AND LADUE, J.S.: Lactic dehydrogenase activity in blood. Proc. Soc. Exp. Biol. Med. 90:210, 1955.
48. ZAVON, M.R.: Treatment of organophosphorus and chlorinated hydrocarbon insecticide intoxications. Mod. Treat. 8:503, 1971.

CHAPTER 7

Microbiologic Examinations

The exogenous invaders producing human disease are legion, ranging from viruses, the smallest known living entities, to worms and flukes of really substantial size. By convention, microbiology concerns itself with the plant kingdom, while animal parasitology occupies a separate niche. Most clinical microbiology laboratories isolate, identify, and cultivate bacteria and fungi, leaving to specialized laboratories the demanding techniques of virus and rickettsial cultivation.

BACTERIAL PROPERTIES

To some extent, certain pathologic processes can be correlated with the characteristics of the inciting organism. This kind of information is interesting, and useful to a point, but cannot fully explain the course of any one patient's disease. Nevertheless, we may profitably consider some elements determining the scope and nature of bacterial disease. The disease-producing organism must achieve an ecologic relationship with its hosts such that its continuation, as a species, is assured. This means that the agent must enter a host, multiply itself, leave the primary host, and then enter another host immediately or be able to survive independently. Although the cycle can be interrupted in an individual, by death or cure of the disease, no means have been found for deliberate eradication of disease-producing species. Techniques of sanitation, asepsis, and sterilization attempt to prevent entry into hosts and transmission to other hosts, while therapeutic agents attempt to prevent multiplication of the organisms and prevent or correct deleterious effects of this multiplication.

HOST-INVADER INTERACTIONS

The body copes with bacterial invaders by cellular and humoral defenses. Both mononuclear and polymorphonuclear cells can attack invading organisms by engulfment or phagocytosis. Granulocytic leukocytes produce lytic substances which attack extracellular organisms as well as mediating intracellular destruction of the bacteria. Antibodies, both circulating and those on cell surfaces, may destroy the organism directly, or alter its properties so that other cell-mediated defenses are more effective. The structure of certain tissues, like the alveolar walls in the lungs, the fascial planes in muscle, and collagenous barriers in skin, contribute to mechanical confinement of the invader, thus concentrating and enhancing the body's other defenses. Bacteria, on the other hand, have various properties which protect them against the host's attacks and the course of disease is the balance between these opposing forces.

Surface Characteristics

The bacterial cell surface significantly affects the host-invader balance. Capsules or other surface characteristics may resist phagocytosis, thereby promoting bacterial multiplication. Pneumococcus, H. influenzae, and Klebsiella have capsules; the surface proteins of group A streptococcus, although not a capsule, have antiphagocytic properties. This advantage to the bacteria is offset by the antigenic nature of capsular material and surface proteins, that is, they stimulate the host to produce antibodies which inactivate or neutralize the antiphagocytic effect. The antigenic strength of these surface elements varies with different organisms, and different strains of the same organism. The host's capacity to approach, engulf, and destroy the bacterial invader depends on individual factors as well. Immunologic competence, the numbers and functions of the leukocytes, the general state of protein metabolism, and the existence of adequate circulation and blood supply to the infected area all contribute to the outcome of the battle.

Immunologic stimulation and response are not the only determinants. Other bacterial products exert other effects. Many pathogenic staphylococci possess a coagulase which converts fibrinogen to fibrin. This deposits on the bacterial cell as an envelope which makes phagocytosis difficult. Although it is tempting to assign teleologic significance to this property, the role of coagulase in promoting staphylococcal infection is unproved. Hyaluronic acid, in the capsules of group A and C streptococci, is too similar to human polysaccharides to evoke antibodies, but it nonetheless interferes with phagocytosis.

Bacterial Toxins

Bacteria produce a wide variety of extracellular substances with physiologic activity. Some of these produce disease directly, while others may enhance pathogenicity or be indifferent. For example, clostridial proteolytic enzymes and streptococcal hemolysins and proteases are not inherently pathogenic, but assist bacterial multiplication or spread. Bacterial products which directly damage the host are called toxins. These are of two kinds. Exotoxins, produced by the cells, are secreted into the host's tissues or fluids and exert their effect independent of the presence or multiplication of the organism. Endotoxins are intrinsic to the organism, usually a lipopolysaccharide structural component, and these damage the host only when bacterial death or lysis liberates them into direct contact with host tissue.

Exotoxins. Exotoxins, not bacterial multiplication, mediate the harmful effects of such diseases as diphtheria, tetanus, botulism, and a variety of diarrheal syndromes ranging from "traveller's tummy" through staphylococcal food poisoning to cholera. Although the proteins are highly antigenic, they act so promptly that the patient usually dies or recovers before he can mount an antibody response. Exogenous antitoxins are used against the catastrophic effects of Cl. tetani and Cl. botulinum toxins. In cholera, diphtheria, and the gram-negative bacillary diseases, therapy aims more toward eradicating the organism than toward neutralizing the specific toxin.

Endotoxins. The role of endotoxin depends partly on its quantity and mode of entry, and partly on the biologic and immunologic condition of the patient. Endotoxins produce a generalized "toxic" state which may include fever, leukopenia, intravascular coagulation, and vascular and hemodynamic changes leading, in severe cases, to shock and death. On a weight-for-weight basis, exotoxins are far more potent than endotoxins, but a larger volume of morbidity and mortality derives from endotoxin effects, notably those of gram-negative bacilli. These multifarious systemic effects cannot be neutralized by specific antitoxins. The cell wall lipopolysaccharides mediate the antigenic identity of the organisms as the O (or somatic) antigens of the gram-negative rods, but diseases result from highly complex interactions of bacteria, host tissues, and immune response, rather than from chemical toxins alone.

ANTIBIOTICS

Antimicrobial agents have, in the last 30 years, radically altered the age-long battle between host and microbial invader. Bacterial growth can be altered by changes in pH, temperature, nutrient environment, and so forth, but antibacterial chemotherapy implies a different attack. Antibiotics are chemical substances, produced by microorganisms, with the capacity to inhibit or destroy other microorganisms in dilute solution. To be medically useful, the substance must selectively attack invading organisms without seriously impairing the host. Many bacteria, fungi, and actinomycetes produce antibacterial metabolites, but most are too toxic to human or other hosts, or else too weakly active against other organisms to be therapeutically effective. Perhaps 50 or fewer[20] have found medical employment, reflecting their ability selectively to damage or destroy the invader (usually a bacterial one) at reasonable pharmacologic dosage levels.

The ideal therapeutic agent should selectively interrupt some process vital to the invader, but absent or nonessential in the host's metabolism. The secondary results of such attack should not damage the host. There should, additionally, be no harmful secondary effects from the metabolic alteration, such as accumulation of toxic waste products or overgrowth by other invaders. No known drug or therapeutic agent achieves this ideal completely.

Bacterial Cell Walls

Certain morphologic and metabolic characteristics of bacteria do permit fruitful avenues of attack. All living cells are surrounded by a cytoplasmic membrane, but bacterial cells are unique in the plant and animal kingdoms in possessing a rigid layer external to this. The cell wall gives the organism its shape and permits its survival in the usual vegetative form. Under suitable culture conditions, some bacteria survive without cell walls, in a spherical form called protoplast or L-form. Under ordinary growing conditions, however, the wall is essential for survival.

The necessity for bacteria to synthesize and retain the cell wall renders them liable to toxic agents and reactants which do not affect other living creatures. Bacteria differ from one another in details of cell wall composition and in the metabolic steps involved in synthesizing the cell wall. Penicillin, the first practical antibiotic isolated and accepted into clinical use, interferes with a late phase in cell wall synthesis. Other comparable interfering agents are bacitracin, vancomycin, ristocetin, and cycloserine, but the site of interference and mode of action almost certainly varies among these antibacterial substances. Of these, perhaps the best understood is D-cycloserine, which is structurally analogous to D-alanine; if sufficient quantities of D-alanine are present in the medium, its antibacterial activity can be reversed.

Other Sites of Activity

Not all antibacterial agents attack the cell wall. Like other dividing cells, bacteria must transcribe the genetic message, replicate DNA, activate messenger and transfer RNA, and synthesize proteins. All these steps are susceptible to interruption, as are some phases of mature metabolic functioning, especially cytoplasmic membrane activities. The bewildering array of antibiotics reflects these multiple potential attack sites. In broad terms, antibiotic activity can be grouped as follows:[20] (1) Membrane function, a term which covers a multitude of discrete reactions, is inhibited by bacitracin, colistin, polymyxin, and probably, streptomycin. Streptomycin has additional sites of action, among them the functions leading to RNA synthesis and activity. (2) The processes of replication, transfer of specific information, and ribosomal protein synthesis are inter-related and subject to attack by a broad group of compounds, notably chloramphenicol, the tetracyclines, and a variety of "-mycins" (kanamycin, neomycin, gentamicin, erythromycin, and the streptomycins). (3) Griseofulvin acts on nucleic acid metabolism. (4) The sulfonamides, which are bacteriostatic rather than bactericidal, interfere with intermediary metabolism by competitively inhibiting reactions requiring para-amino benzoic acid.

Host-Invader-Drug Interactions

Antibacterial agents, effective as they are in altering the course of infections, do not work miracles unaided. The host must still mobilize appropriate defenses. By slowing or halting bacterial spread, antibiotics enhance the effectiveness of the host's efforts. Their efficacy is affected by such considerations as circulatory adequacy, location of the infectious process, host hypersensitivity to the drug, dilution or inactivation by tissue fluids or metabolic processes, and so forth. For these reasons, a drug's in vitro effectiveness may not be translated, in vivo, into the desired therapeutic effect. Clinical efficacy almost never exceeds the in vitro findings, but it often falls short.

When an infectious agent has been identified, therapy should be selected to be optimally effective against the specific organism. Bacteria constantly grow and change; as antibiotic drugs alter epidemiologic patterns, bacterial patterns may alter responsively. This does not imply a teleologic or purposeful approach by the bacteria. Mutation and adaptation occur continually; the enormous numbers of bacteria and the rapidity of growth cycles permit expression of various spontaneous alterations. Some changes are maladaptive, and extinguish themselves. Most confer no particular benefit or handicap, and are perpetuated on a random basis.

ANTIBIOTIC RESISTANCE

If some alteration in bacterial metabolism or structure enhances survival, the change will persist and the better endowed organisms may come to outnumber other forms. Antibiotic resistance naturally confers rather marked advantages to those strains possessing it, but concomitant alterations in pathogenicity, metabolic requirements, reproductive rate, and so on may offset the overall competitive advantage. Emergence of antibiotic-resistant organisms, however, severely threatens clinical practice, both in treating specific patients and in preventing or controlling spread within susceptible populations.

Antibiotic resistance may occur by chemically inactivating the drug, as with the penicillinase-producing staphylococci. Bacteria may evolve alternate metabolic pathways which by-pass the effect of the drug, or increase the efficiency of the drug-inhibited activity. Changes in surface metabolism may prevent the entry of drugs whose action must be intracellular to be effective. None of these result from purposeful adaptation following exposure to the drug. The drug merely exerts a selective effect upon organisms undergoing spontaneous changes.

Mutation

The mechanisms of bacterial change are complex. Mutation occurs continuously, at rates which vary enormously among different organisms. Mutational pathways may include the development of new enzymes which alter the drug or the elimination of some chemical or structural component necessary for drug activity. The incidence of change depends, as far as can be determined, neither on the drug nor the organism. Group A streptococci, for example, have remained highly sensitive to penicillin for a quarter of a century, but many strains became sulfonamide resistant shortly after the drug achieved wide usage. Penicillin resistance, on the other hand, is widespread among other gram-positive organisms.

Transmission

Presumably, all forms of drug resistance arise through mutation. Perpetuation, however, can occur by other mechanisms once the heritable information has been coded. Offspring of a mutant will be the same organism and will perpetuate the mutation. The DNA carrying this information can, however, be transferred to another organism, thus transmitting the trait. This introduction of DNA may occur in several ways, most often by virus-mediated transduction or by conjugation between organisms. In transduction, the invading phage may integrate its genetic material with the chromosome of the host. Subsequent phage multiplication leads to replication of some specific portion of host DNA, which enters another cell when the multiplying phage invades a new host. Thus genetic material from the first organism is introduced into a second host, which incorporates this into its own genetic material and perpetuates the change in its offspring. Transduction of this sort occurs in both gram-positive and gram-negative organisms. The capacity to produce penicillinase can be transferred between various staphylococcal strains by this method.[5]

Conjugation, on the other hand, involves the direct transfer of intracellular material from one organism to another, always gram-negative, as far as we know.[20] Conjugation requires threadlike surface protrusions through which material is passed. Development of these pili occurs under the influence of so-called sex factors, which are, themselves, transmissible units of genetic information. Possession of sex factors permits the organism to pass this, and other, material to recipient cells. The transmitted material is independent of the host chromosomes, and does not alter the identity of host or recipient, so the exchange is not due to sexual recombination.

Resistance Factors

Among the other information that can be passed from cell to cell are Resistance, or R, factors. Bacteria possessing an R-factor become insensitive to specific drugs, either a single drug or a group of drugs, which may be related or unrelated. That a bacterium has R-factor activity against a specific drug need not mean it has been exposed to that drug; a strain of E. coli lyophilized since 1946 has been found to have R-factor-mediated resistance to streptomycin and tetracycline.[27] R-factors can be transmitted from one strain to another of the same organism, sometimes from nonpathogenic strains to those producing disease in man or animals. R-factor transference also occurs between different organisms, as from P. vulgaris to E. coli,[28] or from S. choleraesuis to E. coli.[18] Among the drugs implicated have been streptomycin, tetracyclines, chloramphenicol, sulfonamides, penicillins, and cephalosporins. The capacity to transmit R-factors is distinct from the R-factors themselves; resistance transfer factor (RTF) appears to determine replication and transmission of the separate unit (r-determinant) which harbors the actual drug-resistant genes.[7] Both are extrachromosomal genetic elements which replicate themselves independently of the host cell's chromosomes, and which can be affected by certain dyes which affect the intracellular environment.[5]

The gram-negative Enterobacteriaceae are the only organisms known to be implicated in this process. This group contains enough worrisome pathogens, including E. coli, pseudomonas, salmonella, and shigella, that the prospect of rampant *infectious drug resistance* is alarming. The clinical significance of the phenomenon, however, is far from clear. Particularly in Japan, R-factor transmission in shigella species has posed both clinical and epidemiologic problems.[32] Other evidence indicates[20] that the clinical occurrence is far lower than the laboratory results might suggest. Still under investigation are the incidence of transmission, the necessary conditions for transfer, the possibility that R-factors induce intracellular repressors, and the suggestion that R-factors may sometimes be associated with reduced pathogenicity. The entire field should be considered unsettled.

MICROBIOLOGIC TECHNIQUES

One vitally important function of diagnostic microbiology is the documentation of patterns of drug sensitivity and resistance in clinical pathogens. Before discussing these techniques, we must consider how pathogens are identified and implicated in clinical situations.

Bacteria are ubiquitous. They can be present in or on diseased tissue without causing the disease. Some bacteria cause disease in one site but grow harmlessly at some other. Some bacteria cause disease, but are difficult to culture. Identifying a significant pathogen requires that suitable clinical material be examined, that suitable microbiologic techniques be followed, and that resulting findings be interpreted in the light of general principles and individual circumstance.

SPECIMEN COLLECTION

Selection and handling of clinical material for examination seems to be simpler in theory than in practice. The principles are obvious. The specimen should be taken when viable organisms are numerous, from a site where organisms are likely to be found. It should be collected before instituting antibacterial therapy, and be handled without contaminating the specimen with outside organisms or spreading the patient's organisms to others. The specimen should be transported promptly to the laboratory and processed before relevant organisms have died or multiplied to levels which distort the true clinical picture. Any and all of these goals may fall short of achievement, either by inadequate patient care, laboratory failure, poor cooperation from the patient himself, or plain bad luck.

Time of Collection

The phase of the disease may be particularly critical, and particularly difficult to control. Salmonella and shigella are more easily cultured from stool specimens early in the illness, but the patient may not come for help until the process is well established. Brucella infections produce chronic, relapsing symptoms for months after cultures become negative. Recurrent bacteremias can produce persistent illness, but blood cultures taken between so-called showers may be negative. Tularemia and plague produce short-lived, early bacteremias, but once the organisms enter fixed tissue, they become extremely difficult to culture.

Site of Collection

The site for culture is obvious when symptoms are localized, as with meningitis, abscesses, wound infections, or purulent pneumonias. More diffuse processes require greater selectivity, as, for example, in choosing among nasopharyngeal, throat, or sputum cultures for respiratory tract symptoms or in discriminating between the urinary tract and the genital tract as the origin of dysuria. When infection is deep-seated, culture material should come from deep in the tissue, to avoid contamination with superficial organisms.

Effect of Medication

It may prove impossible to obtain a specimen before antibacterial therapy has begun. Ideally, therapy should await accurate diagnosis, or, when the need is acute, cultures should be taken just before medication is given. In practice, the patient may have been medicating himself, and come to medical attention only when his own efforts have failed. Or the need for bacteriologic study may become urgent only after initial therapy has proved unsuccessful. Or complications may occur which alter the initial diagnosis and require additional diagnostic study.

Antibiotic therapy does not always invalidate subsequent cultures. Sometimes penicillinase or some other anti-antibiotic is added to the culture medium; sometimes diluting the specimen will diminish the drug effect without suppressing the growth of significant organisms. If cultures must be taken after drugs have been given, laboratory personnel should be informed so they can make suitable changes in culture techniques.

Avoiding Contamination

Bacterial contamination may go in several directions. Organisms may spread from specimen to personnel, from personnel to specimen, or from one specimen to another. Contamination of personnel usually results from carelessness or from inadequate containers. Sputum and feces containers tend to be the worst offenders, although urine collections, drainage tubes, and wound dressings are fertile sources of infection for the unwary. Spinal fluids and blood cultures are seldom handled sloppily, probably because the precautions necessary for obtaining the specimen are applied to the material throughout its processing.

Specimens should be collected with due concern for the desired results. This means meticulous cleansing of the skin before taking blood cultures or of the urethral meatus before taking urine samples. It also means excluding saliva from sputum specimens, and avoiding admixture of urine with feces for stool culture. In these two latter instances, the cooperation of the patient is highly desirable; the extra time invested in instructing the patient may be rewarded by vastly improved specimen quality.

Delay Before Culturing

A specimen may be examined immediately, or be transported down a corridor, or may have to spend several days in the mail. Depending on the organism involved and the transport medium used, any of these can give excellent results. If delay must occur between collection and processing, the organisms must be protected from drying, from pH change, and from inimical temperatures. The bacterial population should also be held near its original proportions, without unduly encouraging or discouraging certain strains.

Material on cotton swabs is particularly likely to dry, so nonnutrient broth or holding medium is frequently used, even for short-term delays. Pathogens in urine, feces, and sputum specimens can survive refrigeration for a number of hours. Specimens with suspected shigella, however, should be rapidly processed to avoid overgrowth by hardier, nonpathogenic organisms. Shigella and salmonella will survive for long periods if the fecal sample is smeared thinly on filter paper and air-dried. Such samples can be mailed, and the dried material later reconstituted in suitable medium.

Urine for cultures can be held at refrigerator temperatures for several days without affecting the validity of the results.[24] Spinal fluid, on the other hand, should be examined as soon as possible after lumbar puncture, partly because the clinical situation may be urgent, but also because such organisms as H. influenzae and meningococci are sensitive to environmental changes.

DIRECT EXAMINATION

Specimens are sent to the microbiology laboratory to answer several questions: Are any organisms present? If present, what are they? Are they causally related to the patient's disease? If they are pathogenic, what therapeutic agents can best be employed? Cultivating the organisms on culture medium gives the most accurate answers to these questions. Successful cultures require time for bacterial growth and depend upon the presence of viable organisms in the specimen as received. If time is short, or if the organisms may not be viable, direct microscopic examination of the material may be helpful.

Wet Mounts

Most clinical specimens are stained and fixed for examination, but wet mounts are used to identify fungi and to demonstrate motile protozoa in, for example, trichomonal vaginitis or parasitic diarrheas. A classic technique is the demonstration of cryptococcus (torula) in spinal fluids by adding India ink to the fluid. To find parasites or their ova, stool specimens can be emulsified, sometimes with added iodine, and examined in as fresh a condition as possible. Dark-field illumination enhances the visibility of motile organisms, notably spirochetes. All these techniques are excellent for immediate diagnosis, but their usefulness depends on the skill of the examiner, the presence of sufficient organisms to make detection feasible, and upon the morphologic features of these organisms which render them visible with relatively little processing.

Stains

Gram Stain. Most bacteria are small and difficult to examine unstained. Their surface chemistry, however, permits combination with various stains to enhance visibility; differing chemical compositions permit differential staining reactions. The Gram stain and the acid-fast stain are the two most widely used. In the Gram stain, a purple-blue dye complex enters the organism when the smeared material is flooded with crystal violet and iodine. Once the dye complex has entered the cell, alcohol or acetone is added as a decolorizer. The alcohol dehydrates some bacterial walls, rendering them impermeable and preventing the escape of intracellular dye complex. In other organisms, presumably those with high lipid content, the organic solvent removes much of the cell-wall lipid, increasing permeability and permitting the dye complex to wash out of the interior.[22] Bacteria which retain the blue-purple stain are called gram-positive, while those which alcohol decolorizes are called gram-negative. A contrasting counter stain (usually carbolfuchsin or safranin) is used to color the gram-negative organisms so they can be seen and their morphology noted. Since retention of the dye complex depends on intact cell walls, organisms with absent or damaged walls will appear gram-negative, even if intact members of the species are gram-positive.

Besides differentiating organisms according to their cell wall composition, the Gram stain permits excellent visualization of bacteria, so their morphology can be studied with some precision. Shape, relative size, and growth configuration all contribute to identification. Sputum, spinal fluid, urine, exudates, and other clinical specimens can be smeared, Gram-stained, and examined directly, in many cases permitting rapid presumptive diagnosis of bacterial infection. Centrifugation, with subsequent examination of the sediment, can be used to concentrate the organisms to readily detectible levels. The presence and nature of cells and the relation of organisms to the cell are additional diagnostic data available from properly made Gram-stained material. Gram stains are also used after organisms have been cultivated, to demonstrate the morphology of organisms comprising colonies seen on culture. Modifications of the Gram stain are used to demonstrate bacteria in sections of fixed tissue, but morphologic detail may be altered by processing and sectioning.

Acid-Fast Stain. The acid-fast stain also relies on cell wall properties, probably the lipid content, but the principle is less well understood than that of the Gram stain. Again, the result is that intracellular dye resists decolorization, and acid-fast organisms are also gram-positive. In the acid-fast procedure, carbolfuchsin is introduced into the cell with heat and acid. The cells accept the stain only with difficulty, but once in, the stain remains despite further acid treatment. Organisms which lack appropriate cell wall characteristics have no color after acid washing, and can be seen only if counterstain is applied. The acid-fast technique, like Gram staining, can be used for direct examination of clinical material, for studying cultivated colonies, and for documenting organisms in fixed tissue. Mycobacteria are most often sought with acid-fast staining procedures, but certain nocardia are variably acid-fast, and brucella can sometimes be identified in tissue sections by an appropriately modified acid-fast technique.

Fluorescence Techniques

Fluorescent Antibodies. A fairly new but increasingly useful technique for direct examination is fluorescence microscopy. The organisms are localized and identified by their reaction with a specific, fluorescein-labelled antibody. The theory is simple. If the appropriate organisms are present in the preparation, labelled antibody attaches to them, resulting in localized fluorescence. The antibody just rinses off if no bacteria are present, or if the material contains bacteria of other specificities. The success of this technique depends on having a labelled, specific antiserum, and on the presence of the specific organism. This cannot be used as an initial search tool for unknown bacteria. If the presence of a specific organism is suspected, for example in suspected diphtherial pharyngitis, gonorrheal urethritis, or H. influenzae meningitis, direct immunofluorescent examination can give a very rapid answer. The technique can also be used to identify strains and subspecies of organisms, if appropriate antibodies are available. Both the fluorescent dye and the antibody must be pure and of high quality, and the conjugation must be specific and firm.

Indirect Immunofluorescence. Using indirect immunofluorescence is somewhat more flexible than using labelled specific antiserums. In the indirect technique, a battery of unlabelled specific antibodies can be used, and only a single serum, an anti-immunoglobulin or anti-antibody, need be labelled. Smears of clinical material are incubated with antibodies directed against the organisms suspected to be present. If the organism is present, the unlabelled antibody attaches to it, and subsequent addition of fluorescent antiglobulin serum produces fluorescence. If the antibody does not find its antigen, the subsequent fluorescent antiglobulin serum has nothing to attach to, and no fluorescence remains when the specimen is rinsed. In this way, a single conjugated serum can be used to demonstrate a variety of antigenic specificities, as long as all the specific, unlabelled antibodies react similarly with the conjugated antiglobulin serum. The antiglobulin serum must not, itself, react with the organisms or with any other material present on the slide.

CULTURES

Ultimate diagnosis of infectious diseases depends on isolating, cultivating, and characterizing the organism. Most of clinical microbiology involves general and differential cultural techniques, exploiting the wide range of biochemical and morphologic characteristics of pathogenic flora. A chapter like this cannot detail the many media and techniques available but we can profitably consider some general principles of culturing and show their clinical applications.

Different culture media may promote or discourage individual bacteria, and their use is dictated by the organisms likely to be found in a specimen. To some extent, the source of the specimen suggests the probable organisms and the manner in which the material should be handled. In anything but highly routine situations, however, the more information the microbiologist has about the clinical problem, the more directly he can achieve diagnostically significant results. Among the major considerations for the laboratory are whether or not to do anaerobic cultures, whether fast-growing contaminants or commensals are likely to be present and obscure the pathogen, and whether the suspected organism requires special culture media. The time devoted to a brief clinical note on microbiology requests can result in much faster and better culture interpretations.

BLOOD CULTURES

Blood is one of the few specimens routinely cultured in broth rather than on a solid medium. One major advantage of solid over liquid media is that they permit colonies to grow distinct from one another, so that mixed flora can be discriminated. Bacteremias are rarely mixed, so blood culture does not require colony separation. An advantage of broth culture is that dilution disperses the bactericidal effects of blood itself and of whatever drugs the patient may have received.

Routine cultures are placed in thioglycollate broth to permit growth of anaerobic or microaerophilic organisms, as well as in standard nutrient broths. Since growth may be slow, negative-appearing cultures are kept for 15 days before the final verdict. Most growth occurs much earlier, and bacteria are encouraged to show themselves as early as possible. Initial broth cultures are subcultured quite early onto several aerobic and anaerobic media. Gram stain of the broth after overnight incubation may demonstrate early significant growth, but both Gram staining and subculturing must be done carefully to avoid contaminating the remaining material.

Contaminants

Contamination of blood cultures is by no means uncommon, but usually occurs as the specimen is collected. The blood sample must be drawn through the skin, a fertile source of contaminants. Meticulous skin asepsis is essential; the detergents, alcohol sponges, or other cleansers used before most injections are not adequate. After superficial cleansing the area should be treated with 3.5 per cent tincture of iodine, unless severe iodine sensitivity is present. Although everyone knows that the cleansed area should not be touched, it is amazing how often the venipuncturist palpates the vein "just one last time, to be sure." When Staphylococcus epidermidis or diphtheroids are found in blood cultures, as they are frequently, the inclination is to consider them contaminants. S. epidermidis may, however, be a blood stream invader in patients with endocarditis or prosthetic heart valves; in debilitated or immunosuppressed patients, it may be rash to consider any organism nonpathogenic.

Since blood stream invasion tends to be episodic, repeated blood cultures are desirable if bacteremia is suspected. Three to five cultures taken over a 24 to 48 hour period usually provide an adequate sampling, although if antibiotics are present, the number should be doubled. Drawing several samples also aids in evaluating contaminants. If the same organism is grown from several different cultures taken at several different times, then it probably has clinical significance.

SPINAL FLUID

Cerebrospinal fluid normally contains no organisms and very few cells. Meningeal inflammation of any sort may increase the cell content and alter the chemical findings, but the demonstration of organisms signals particular clinical urgency. Because meningitis should be treated as promptly as possible, even the delay of primary culturing may be dangerous. Examining a Gram-stained spinal fluid smear may give a presumptive diagnosis, to be later confirmed after cultures have grown. Naked-eye examination can differentiate grossly purulent from clear fluid, but even a seemingly clear fluid can harbor organisms and increased numbers of mononuclear or neutrophilic leukocytes.

Immediate Examination

Spinal fluid specimens are ordinarily submitted to the laboratory in several aliquots. The cell count must be done on uncentrifuged material. Bacterial cultures must come from material handled under sterile conditions, and the centrifuged sediment may be preferable, since organisms and cells are concentrated into a small volume. The sediment is Gram stained and examined after cultures have been taken. The shape and staining properties of several common organisms are fairly characteristic, so presumptive diagnosis can be very rapid. H. influenzae, an increasingly frequent cause of meningitis in small children, may be difficult to find; its pleomorphic nature may be hard to distinguish from debris or nonviable organisms on the slide, since these, too, would be gram-negative. Another possible artefact is the presence of gram-positive or gram-negative rounded bodies resembling yeasts, which may be seen in spinal fluids shortly after performance of a myelogram.[1]

Bacterial Infection. The other common invaders, if present in large enough numbers, can readily be identified. Neisseria meningitidis (meningococcus) is a gram-negative diplococcus, while the pneumococcus is a gram-positive diplococcus. The clustered or chain-like patterns of staphylo-coccal and streptococcal growth are seldom appreciated in this kind of preparation. The distinction does not, however, affect the immediate ther-apy initiated. Coliform bacilli are gram-negative rods, while Mycobacter-ium tuberculosis is a gram-positive rod. Acid-fast stain of the smeared sediment should be done whenever clinically indicated, especially if the meningeal symptoms have been long-standing or vaguely defined or have not responded to therapy.

Cryptococcus. Cryptococcus neoformans needs special treatment, since it may cause rather prolonged illness with very little cellular reaction. Being round, uniform cells the size of lymphocytes, they may be considered lymphocytes by the unwary examiner performing a cell count. Their diag-nostic feature, however, is a large, clear capsule which stands in brilliant contrast to the carbon particles of added India ink. India ink examination is routine in many laboratories which examine spinal fluids, but the or-ganisms may be sparse and difficult to demonstrate. A recently developed immunologic procedure can demonstrate cryptococcal antigen in spinal fluids even if direct examination and culture have been negative.[15]

Culture Media

Spinal fluid sediments are routinely cultured in several media. Since meningococci are sensitive to cold temperature, spinal fluid specimens should not be refrigerated if any delay occurs before culturing. Blood agar plates are useful for gram-positive cocci and gram-negative bacilli. Choco-late agar, in which prior heating renders the hemoglobin more accessible, is used for growing H. influenzae and meningococcus. All these organisms are aerobes, but 2 to 10 per cent carbon dioxide enhances initial growth, so these, like primary cultures from many other sources, are incubated in a CO_2-enriched atmosphere. Thioglycollate fluid medium permits isolation of bacteroides and other anaerobes. Individual laboratories have other media as part of their preferred protocol for spinal fluids. Special media for mycobacteria are inoculated if tuberculous meningitis is suspected, and the same applies to suspected fungal disease.

RESPIRATORY TRACT

The respiratory tract harbors a variety of organisms in the upper portion, but secretions from below the larynx normally contain few, if any, organisms. Lower respiratory secretions must, however, traverse the throat, tonsillar area, and mouth, and material from the posterior nasopharynx may drip down into the oropharynx or deeper.

THROAT CULTURES

The normal individual routinely carries in his throat substantial numbers of alpha hemolytic streptococci and nonpathogenic neisseria as well as varying populations of coagulase-negative staphylococci or even Staphylococcus aureus. Other organisms which may inhabit the normal throat include Hemophilus hemolyticus, small numbers of pneumococci, gramnegative bacilli, yeasts, diphtheroids, occasional anaerobes, and gamma streptococci. Under suitable conditions many of these organisms can be pathogens, or be difficult to distinguish from pathogenic species of the same genus. While nonpathogenic neisseria may abound and must be distinguished from N. meningitidis, it must be remembered that healthy carriers may have N. meningitidis in the nasopharynx, or carry pathogenic staphylococci without ill effect. Obtaining and interpreting culture material from the respiratory tract requires both skill and judgment.

Nasopharyngeal Examination

Personnel obtaining nasopharyngeal cultures should be careful to avoid contact between the tip of the swab and the proximal nasal mucosa. In adults, nasopharyngeal cultures are useful in detecting asymptomatic carriers of pathogenic flora. In small children, who frequently cannot produce sputum, nasopharyngeal culture is often used as an index of the bacteriologic condition of the bronchial tree. Pneumococcus, H. influenzae, and N. meningitidis can frequently be grown from nasopharyngeal specimens in children with meningitis from these organisms. Although cough plates are often recommended to isolate Bordetella pertussis from patients with whooping cough, nasopharyngeal cultures probably produce more positives. If bordetella is suspected, Bordet-Gengou medium with added penicillin is used to inhibit the usual flora.

CLASSIFICATION OF STREPTOCOCCI

Throat cultures most often reveal acute streptococcal infections, but other forms of pharyngitis and tonsillitis must be considered. A word about classification of streptococci is in order here. Streptococci are gram-positive cocci which characteristically grow in chains. They thrive in animal and plant environments and are found in dust and water as well. Although several classifications are based on biologic or biochemical behavior, current practice leans toward serologic description. The antigenic characteristics of the polysaccharide C-substance are the basis for classification as being group A,B,C,D, and so on through O in the Lancefield system. Other antigenic classifications are available for distinctions within Group A, of which M-precipitation and T-agglutination are examples. Most acute streptococcal diseases in humans result from group A organisms, although enterococci, which are group D, produce a spectrum of human disorders, and puerperal and neonatal infections have been caused by group B.

Hemolytic Properties

Another diagnostic feature of streptococci is their capacity to hemolyze red blood cells in the culture medium. The type and amount of hemolysis varies not only with the organism but also with the species of red cell. The following brief description relates to sheep blood agar. In alpha hemolysis a few cells immediately beneath the colony remain unhemolysed, with the surrounding medium becoming "green" from partial hemolysis. Beta-hemolysis produces a clear, cell-free zone beneath and around the colony. The term *gamma* is applied to those streptococci which do not hemolyze at all.

Distinguishing Beta-Hemolytic Organisms. Although nearly all group A organisms are beta-hemolytic, organisms of other groups may also exhibit beta-hemolysis. Group A organisms can be distinguished from other beta-hemolytic colonies by their sensitivity to bacitracin, which does not inhibit growth of other groups. Group D organisms, only some of which produce beta-hemolysis, are distinctive in their ability to grow at 45° C and to grow in the presence of sodium azide.

Distinguishing Streptococci from Pneumococci. All streptococci resist dissolution by bile salts, and grow on blood agar despite the presence of added ethylhydrocupreine (Optochin). These features do not help to discriminate among streptococcal groups, but are useful in distinguishing streptococci from pneumococci in throat cultures and other sources where nonpathogenic streptococci and pneumococci may coexist.

Nonstreptococcal Pharyngitis

Acute streptococcal pharyngitis lends itself to prompt bacteriologic diagnosis, since the organisms grow rapidly on agar plates and produce characteristic beta-hemolysis. Other causes of acute pharyngitis may be S. aureus, H. influenzae, various coliform bacilli, or pneumococci. To distinguish these as rapidly as possible on primary cultures a variety of media are used to reveal differences in growth patterns, oxygen requirements, and colony morphology. If exudate is abundant or pseudomembranes are present, necrotizing streptococcal inflammation must be distinguished from diphtheria, candidiasis (thrush), or Vincent's angina, and examining stained smears may be most helpful. C. diphtheriae can occasionally be seen as gram-positive rods which are often somewhat pleomorphic, while candida presents with budding yeast forms and occasional hyphal fragments. The organisms causing Vincent's angina are thought to be the gram-negative spirochete Borrelia vincentii and the pointed gram-negative rod Fusobacterium fusiforme. Cultivation of C. diphtheriae requires special media, usually Loeffler's (which includes coagulated serum) or Pai's (coagulated egg). Candida should be cultured on Sabouraud's medium. Morphologic examination of the smear or pseudomembrane gives better diagnostic results than cultures for Vincent's angina, whereas direct smears tend to be less revealing than cultures for diphtheria.

SPUTUM CULTURE

Lower respiratory tract disease is more complex than upper airway infection because the lungs can undergo such a variety of anatomic and physiologic changes, due to so many different invaders. The usual specimen subjected to microbiologic examination is sputum, but tracheal aspirates, bronchial washings, pleural fluid, and excised tissue all have a place in diagnosing intrathoracic disease. We will briefly consider tuberculosis and the fungus diseases in a later section, and cannot give viral disease more than a passing nod.

Sputum remains the most frequent and most useful source for bacteriologic diagnosis. Sputum is, by definition, the secretions of the tracheobronchial tree. Admixture with saliva or nasopharyngeal material is unfortunately common, especially if the patient has been poorly instructed in coughing, and this severely impairs the diagnostic usefulness. In general, acute bacterial pneumonias are associated with abundant sputum, as is bronchiectasis and certain phases of lung abscess, but scant production in no way rules out these diagnoses. Flecks of mucus, blood, or pus are especially likely to contain organisms, and should be included in the material cultured.

Common Organisms

The pneumococcus continues to be a common cause of acute pneumonia, but H. influenzae is isolated from large numbers of adults,[29] as well as from the pediatric population. The gram-negative rods are increasingly associated with severe pneumonias, particularly in the elderly and debilitated, and in hospital-acquired infections. E. coli, klebsiella, proteus, and pseudomonas are the prime offenders. Staphylococcus aureus often complicates the course of disease in children with mucoviscidosis or patients with bronchiectasis from any cause, and may cause multiple abscesses as an opportunistic invader. Anaerobic organisms may be found in abscesses or empyema and should always be considered when sputum cultures are processed.

Special Considerations

Hospitalized patients, those receiving antibiotics, and patients with altered physiologic responses are susceptible to innumerable insults. The isolation, from sputum, of unusual organisms or of possible pathogens in small numbers only must be interpreted in the light of the patient's total condition. The existence and spread of nosocomial (hospital-induced) infection should always be an important consideration in evaluating sputum cultures.

URINARY TRACT

The urinary tract does not have a normal flora. The kidneys, ureters, and bladder are sterile, and the bacteria present at the urethral meatus ordinarily do not invade the deeper tissues. Urinary tract infection, however, is extremely common, and the range of recovered organisms is broad. The majority of urinary tract pathogens derive from the intestinal flora. Adequate understanding of urine cultures requires some understanding of the gram-negative bacilli, which includes the enormously complex family Enterobacteriaceae, the family Bacteroidaceae, and the pseudomonads. Brucellaceae, a family which includes brucella, haemophilus, pasteurella, and bordetella, are also gram-negative rods, but rarely invade the urinary tract.

CLASSIFICATION OF ENTEROBACTERIACEAE

The term *gram-negative enteric bacteria* by custom refers to the Enterobacteriaceae. One of the major large bowel inhabitants is bacteroides, an anaerobic gram-negative rod, but this group is not commonly considered in this context. The Enterobacteriaceae are gram-negative, nonspore-forming rods which grow well on a variety of artificial media. All ferment glucose and reduce nitrates to nitrites. Beyond these common attributes, they vary in motility, in carbohydrate and amino acid metabolism, in enzyme production, and in the antigenic characteristics of somatic (O) and flagellar (H) composition. Subdivision of the family into five tribes is based on both biochemical and antigenic features, and recent naming and classification of genera differs from older usage. Current taxonomy is based largely on the work of W. H. Ewing.[12, 13] The tribes and genera[23] are shown below.

Tribe	Genera
Escherichieae	Escherichia
	Shigella
Edwardsielleae	Edwardsiella
Salmonelleae	Salmonella
	Arizona
	Citrobacter (formerly E. freundii)
Klebsielleae	Klebsiella
	Enterobacter (formerly Aerobacter)
	Pectobacterium
Proteae	Serratia
	Proteus
	Providence

We cannot detail the distinctions among all the various species, serotypes, and bioserotypes subsumed in these genera. We must, however, consider some of the special purpose media used as initial diagnostic tests when enteric bacilli are isolated or suspected. Enteric bacilli grow well on most media, including blood agar, but gram-positive contaminants or nonpathogens often grow better, making isolation of the desired gram-negative organism more difficult.

Primary Cultures

Urine specimens are often inoculated onto an inhibitory medium, such as MacConkey's or eosin methylene blue (EMB) to encourage gram-negative isolates, and onto one or several general purpose or partially anaerobic media to demonstrate additional organisms. Both MacConkey's medium and EMB contain lactose in addition to other nutrients and a colored indicator. The coliform bacilli ferment lactose, thereby altering the indicator color, while salmonella, shigella, and proteus do not. Thus the primary growth can supply prompt diagnostic clues.

Once primary cultures are available, each separate organism isolated should be subcultured on differential media. The critical step here is achieving pure cultures from the initial growth. Among the enormous range of possible biochemical distinctions, a few are regularly used for preliminary screening. If more detailed differentiation is necessary, further cultures can be made later.

Carbohydrate Utilization

The most rapidly useful observations relate to carbohydrate utilization, motility, urea-splitting capacity, and some preliminary metabolic characteristics. Inoculation of double or triple sugar medium in a slanted tube permits rapid evaluation of carbohydrate utilization. The slanted tube contains a low concentration of glucose and high concentration of lactose or sucrose or both. Fermentation of small or large amounts of sugar produces pH changes which impart characteristic color patterns. The pattern of growth and location of color changes reveal not only which sugars the organism ferments, but also the speed of fermentation and presence or absence of gas production as a by-product. In general terms, the escherichia, klebsiella, enterobacter, and some proteus-providence groups rapidly ferment both lactose and glucose, with gas production. Glucose fermentation without lactose suggests salmonella, shigella, some proteus, some citrobacter, and serratia. No color change occurs with pseudomonas or herellea, because these gram-negative rods are not Enterobacteriaceae and do not ferment glucose.

Urease Production and Motility

Comparable pH-mediated color change is used to document urease production. If the organisms split urea, incorporated into the medium, the resulting alkaline pH converts the phenol red indicator from yellow to red. Again, the speed with which the change occurs has diagnostic implications. Proteus produces urease within a few hours; klebsiella, enterobacter and serratia split urea more slowly; with the others, no color change occurs. The presence of motility can be estimated in some cases by the degree of spreading growth from a straight-line inoculation, while especially "stiff" media can be used to measure the degree of motility. While proteus is considered the classic "spreader," nearly all the genera except shigella and klebsiella exhibit some motility.

The series of four biochemical reactions referred to as IMViC (indole, methyl red, Voges-Proskauer, and citrate) often helps distinguish E. coli from klebsiella and enterobacter, which also ferment lactose rapidly. The use of other diagnostic biochemical tests depends on the magnitude of the clinical problem, and diagnostic charts and flow sheets are available for discriminating different species and variant behaviors.

OTHER ORGANISMS

Not all urinary tract infections are due to gram-negative rods. Staphylococcus and enterococcus not uncommonly produce urinary tract disease. These can often be identified from their appearance in mixed cultures, or they may be isolated from cultures on media which partially inhibit gram-negative organisms. Contaminants, deriving from the periurethral tissues, tend to resemble skin flora—largely coagulase-negative staphylococci and diphtheroids, but organisms of fecal origin may appear in urine of noninfected individuals. Good technique in collecting the specimen reduces this problem, but the kind of perfunctory instructions given many patients makes a really "clean" voided specimen highly unlikely. If well-trained personnel perform the cleansing and the specimen is collected into a sterile container, results may be excellent.

QUANTITATION

The simple presence of bacteria need not imply clinical infection. It is generally agreed that 10^5 organisms per ml constitutes a clinically significant degree of bacteriuria. To some extent, this depends on the patient's physiologic condition. Urine that has remained in the bladder several hours will have a larger population, and very dilute urine will have a lower population, given the same degree of infection. It is preferable to collect and culture urine that has been in the bladder at least two hours; some laboratories recommend culturing the first morning specimen after overnight accumulation. Bacteria multiply in the voided urine as well as in the bladder, so prompt refrigeration is necessary if the specimen will not be processed immediately. At 4°C, multiplication is adequately inhibited for several days.

Quantitation is achieved by culturing a suitably measured or diluted volume of urine. Calibrated loops, delivering approximately 0.1 ml of urine on a streak plate, permit rough estimation by counting the colonies that grow on the single plate. Greater accuracy results from making pour plates with serial dilutions. The colonies are evenly distributed, and the count can be made from that dilution giving the most legible plate. Although more accurate, this is far more time and space consuming than streaking a calibrated-loop specimen, so each technique may be appropriate for different clinical situations.

Quick Quantitation

A very quick, almost bedside screening procedure for significant bacteriuria is examination by Gram stain of uncentrifuged urine. If several bacteria can be seen on most of the oil-immersion fields, then the colony count will probably be 10^5 per ml or more.[24]

Chemical Indicators. Several screening techniques detect significant bacteriuria by the metabolic effect of large numbers of bacteria on an indicator. These vary in efficacy with the conditions of urine collection, the preservation of the reagents, the types of organisms present, and the need for rapid identification of the organism. When treating individual patients, quantitative or semiquantitative culture methods probably provide more information in a shorter period of time than application of biochemical screening tests. For large-scale population studies, the biochemical tests may yield a high rate of information relative to the investment of skill, time, and equipment. The triphenyltetrazolium chloride (TTC) technique is both sensitive and reproducible if adequately controlled.[25] Bacteriuria is better demonstrated by specific tests for bacteria than by inference from urinalysis results since the presence of white cells or proteinuria correlate rather poorly with significant levels of bacterial invasion.

GASTROINTESTINAL TRACT

Microbiologic examination of the gastrointestinal tract is complicated by the normal presence of innumerable organisms. The normal flora consists largely of bacteroides species (gram-negative anaerobic rods); the enteric bacilli, mostly E. coli and proteus species; intestinal streptococci (commonly called enterococci, Lancefield group D); and occasional yeasts, clostridia, and so forth. All of these organisms can produce disease at sites other than their normal habitat, and pathogenic strains of usual commensals can produce significant gastrointestinal disease. Stool culture in diarrhea or proctoscopic swab in dysentery are the usual examinations requested, although gastric aspirate or duodenal or small intestinal specimens may be cultured under particular circumstances.

SALMONELLA AND SHIGELLA

Salmonella and shigella are the usual offenders in acute or chronic diarrheal disease in otherwise healthy adults.[16] While fairly numerous in acute infections, the organisms become difficult to find after several days of illness. The differential media described above may be useful for stool specimens, since gram-positive inhibition is desirable. More selective media, which suppress E. coli and proteus on appropriately prepared plates, are used when salmonella or shigella are suspected. Another useful technique is to incubate a fecal sample in an enrichment broth, which permits salmonella and shigella to grow but temporarily suppresses E. coli and proteus as well as gram-positive organisms. After 12-hours incubation, the presumed pathogens would have a head start, so subcultures onto selective or differential media tend to yield maximal results. Shigella are rather fragile, and may die if specimens are not processed promptly. They may sometimes be overwhelmed by the agents that suppress coliforms.

Characterization of salmonella and shigella, whether from stool, urine, blood, or other sources, is exceedingly complex. Following biochemical identification, serologic typing and subtyping can be done if suitable antisera are available. The techniques of serotyping are fairly simple, but the taxonomy and terminology are in a transitional state.

PATHOGENIC E. COLI

Although E. coli inhabits the normal colon, certain strains may cause disease, especially in infants. As serotyping of E. coli has been standardized, certain serotypes have been observed to cause disease, while others do not. Morphology and biochemical reactions do not distinguish these, so diagnosis of enteropathogenic E. coli rests on accurate serotyping. The diagnosis may be suspected by the epidemic nature of the disease and failure to isolate any other pathogen. In these cases, the E. coli isolated from primary cultures can be serotyped directly. Some of the enteropathogenic E. coli produce exotoxins, with activity similar to that of the cholera vibrio.[11] These toxigenic strains predominantly affect adults and are distinct from the strains which produce invasive, inflammatory changes and largely affect infants.[12]

VIBRIO CHOLERAE

In cholera cases, the Vibrio cholerae, a small, motile gram-negative rod can readily be isolated from stool specimens. Since the vibrios are inhibited by most differential media and selective salmonella-shigella media, their cultivation depends upon prior suspicion and suitable plating. These organisms are bile resistant and enjoy an alkaline medium, although they will also grow at neutral pH.

STAPHYLOCOCCAL DISEASE

Staphylococci produce gastrointestinal disease in two ways. Hemolytic Staphylococcus aureus and other staph organisms produce a highly potent exotoxin, which is heat stable, tasteless, and odorless. When bacteria multiply in prepared food the resulting toxins may attain sufficient levels to produce the rapid onset of gastric and intestinal symptoms. Organisms cannot be grown from stool or vomitus in these cases, but culturing the contaminated foodstuffs permits rapid bacterial diagnosis.

Less dramatically acute, but clinically more worrisome, is the colitis produced by staphylococcal multiplication within the gut, often in patients whose normal flora has been altered by antibiotic therapy. Coagulase-positive staphylococci may be grown from normal stools on media that suppress enterococcal growth, but large numbers of these organisms on a nonselective medium have pathogenic significance.[1] The staphylococci in these conditions are often resistant to the antibiotics previously given the patient.[16]

GENITAL TRACT

Suspected venereal disease usually provokes microbiologic examination of the male or female genital tract. The causative agent of gonorrhea, Neisseria gonorrhoeae, can often be isolated from the male urethra and from the female cervix uteri. In acute gonorrheal urethritis or cervicitis, Gram-stained smears of the exudate reveal intracellular gram-negative diplococci, a finding sufficiently pathognomonic that definitive treatment should be initiated without awaiting culture results. In chronic infections, the organisms may be sparse, but when there are systemic complications, prostatic secretions, joint fluid, or conjunctival exudate often contain readily visible organisms. Failure to culture gonococcus, when clinical gonorrhea is suspected, may mean that the patient has been partially treated or has received antibiotics for some other condition.[26]

GONOCOCCUS

N. gonorrhoeae, the gonococcus, is moderately fastidious and rather fragile. Specimens should be inoculated as soon as possible, since the organisms will not long survive at room temperature or warmer conditions without suitable nutrients. A transport medium may be used if delay is inevitable, and a few hours of refrigeration will not prevent subsequent growth. Both urethral and cervical specimens may contain nonpathogenic contaminants, so the material should be collected with care. Lubricating jellies used to insert the vaginal speculum may damage gonococci, so sterile saline or water should be used to moisten the instrument.[1] Thayer-Martin medium, a chemically enriched blood or chocolate agar with added antibiotics, is the culture medium of choice. This is incubated in a high carbon dioxide atmosphere.

Chemical Tests

Growth from primary cultures can be identified as gonococcus by carbohydrate fermentation reactions on secondary media. The oxidase test, in which a colored indicator reveals the presence of the bacterial oxidizing enzyme, is characteristic of all neisseria. Although it does not identify gonococcus specifically, in appropriate clinical conditions the results may be strongly suggestive. Fluorescent antibody tests offer the most rapid and accurate means of identification and can be used on colonies or directly on smears from the infected tissue.

SYPHILIS

Treponema pallidum, the causative agent of syphilis, cannot be cultivated on artificial media. Scrapings from primary, and especially secondary, lesions may profitably be examined under dark-field microscopy. When present, the treponemes are actively motile, spiral organisms. Dark-field examination often fails to reveal spirochetes, even when performed by experienced examiners; serologic diagnosis of syphilis is easier and more reliable.

NONBACTERIAL VAGINITIS

Two extremely common microbiologic agents involved in genital tract disease are Trichomonas hominis and Candida albicans. Trichomonas are protozoa. In saline-suspended material from vagina or urethra, they are swiftly moving, flagellated cells. Venereal transmission is common. The sexual partners of a woman with trichomonal vaginitis should also be examined and, if necessary, treated to prevent recurrent infestation. Monilial (candida) vaginitis is also extremely common. It is diagnosed by observing characteristic budding or oval cells in KOH-suspended material from the vagina. When this organism invades the tissue, true hyphae can be identified, but vaginitis is usually a superficial infection.

ANAEROBIC ORGANISMS

Clinical circumstances often dictate microbiologic procedures in specimens from wounds and body cavities. While anaerobic pathogens may occasionally infect spinal fluid, gastrointestinal tract, or deep tissues, they occur far more often in wounds, infected operative sites, and deeply-sited abscesses. Specimens from these areas should be cultured immediately, since atmospheric oxygen may be fatal to the strictest anaerobes. If this is not practical, the swab or specimen must be placed in a non-nutrient, nonoxidative holding medium, and plated as soon as possible. More than one pathogen is often involved, so both aerobic and anaerobic primary cultures should be made. Bacteroides, clostridia, and anaerobic cocci are the usual anaerobes isolated from wounds and abscesses, along with assorted gram-positive and gram-negative aerobes.

ANAEROBIC TECHNIQUE

Achievement and maintenance of anaerobiosis require careful attention. Liquid thioglycollate medium offers a range of oxygenation, with moderately complete anaerobiosis in its depth and sufficient oxygen for aerobic growth just below the air-fluid interface. To grow fastidious strict anaerobes, however, incubation in a closed, specially prepared environment is essential. The medium, moreover, should either be freshly prepared or be stored anaerobically, since solid media absorb atmospheric oxygen. Liquid or semisolid media should be boiled (and then cooled!) before use, to drive out absorbed oxygen. Many laboratories use anaerobic jars, of which the simplest employ hydrogen, generated by a self-contained pack, to combine catalytically with the oxygen in the closed space to produce water. This and all other anaerobic containers must be monitored for oxygen exclusion. A favorite indicator is methylene blue, which turns from colorless to blue when oxygen is present.

MYCOBACTERIA

Mycobacteria deserve separate discussion, even though these organisms can cause disease in all of the sites and tissues already mentioned. Mycobacteria are nonmotile, nonspore-forming, aerobic or microaerophilic bacilli with a high lipid content. Although gram-positive, they take the stain only with difficulty but are then exceedingly resistant to decolorizing. Their most salient staining characteristic is acid-fastness. Once a dye or staining agent enters the cell, it remains there despite vigorous treatment with acid-alcohol. The classic stains use carbolfuchsin with or without heating to encourage dye penetration.

FLUORESCENT STAINING

The auramine-rhodamine technique[30] of fluorescent staining employs the same principle as classic acid-fast staining. The fluorescent auramine-rhodamine solution, once attached to the mycobacteria, resists acid-alcohol decolorization. The end-point, fluorescence as opposed to simple staining, is far easier to observe, so that lower-power objectives can be used for scanning. In this way, more material can be examined more thoroughly. The number of organisms found tends to be higher, so that the quantitation code of the National Tuberculosis Association (3 to 9 organisms per slide = rare; 10 or more per slide = few; more than 1 in each oil-immersion field = numerous) may need reinterpretation. In any laboratory which uses a consistent method and code, the clinical importance of the results is unchanged.

In both carbolfuchsin and fluorescent-stained smears, the finding of one or two stained bodies requires cautious interpretation, since artefacts and false positives are not infrequent. When one or two are found after 15 minutes examination additional material should be collected and examined.

CULTURE TECHNIQUES

Finding stained organisms offers rapid, presumptive evidence of myco-bacterial infection. It says nothing about the viability, the clinical significance, or even the identity of the organism. Accurate diagnosis requires meticulous technique, since the identity and drug susceptibility of infecting organisms have serious clinical implications. The mycobacteria are slow-growing, requiring complex media and freedom from more rapidly growing, competing organisms.

Danger to Personnel. Prior to culture inoculation, most specimens are *decontaminated.* This does not mean rendering the specimen harmless to those who handle it. Mycobacteria constitute an ever-present threat to those who work with them. To avoid contagion, the conditions under which mycobacteria are processed, grown, and identified should be carefully regulated. Often, less care is used in handling specimens from patients in whom tuberculous infection is not suspected and these materials probably pose a greater danger than material in the specialized laboratory.

Processing the Specimen

Decontamination attempts to kill off other organisms which might interfere with or overshadow mycobacterial growth. Sputum, bronchial secretions, and gastric washings are treated with strong alkali, which destroys other organisms but not the alkali-resistant mycobacteria. This resistance is only relative, and mycobacteria almost certainly sustain some damage during the process.

Decontamination is usually combined with liquefaction, to permit adequate mixing and sampling of tissue material. If shreds of tissue or purulent particles are visible, these should be separated and cultured directly, since they often harbor a high concentration of organisms. Specimens in which fewer organisms occur, urine, spinal fluid, or joint fluid, for example, should not be subjected to harsh treatment. These materials are often concentrated, either by centrifugation or bacteria-trapping filtration.

Because other organisms are so frequently present, urine may present a particular problem. An early-morning specimen should be collected under clean conditions. If urine volume and concentration are good, centrifuging the whole specimen may concentrate the mycobacteria sufficiently that the sediment can be decontaminated without completely losing the mycobacteria.

Growth Characteristics

Mycobacteria can grow on simple media if the inoculum is really large, but cultivation from clinical material requires complex media and carefully regulated conditions. In differentiating mycobacteria, the rate of growth, colony characteristics, preferred temperature, and presence or absence of pigmentation provide important diagnostic clues. M. tuberculosis takes two or more weeks to grow at 37°C, and fails to grow at higher or lower temperatures. Although mature colonies are cream-colored or buff, there is no distinct pigmentation; the warty, cauliflower-like appearance is quite characteristic. Because growth is so slow, cultures are kept for six weeks before "no growth" is reported.

Beyond the scope of this chapter is discussion of biochemical tests and differential growth-promoting materials available for discriminating among mycobacteria. Culturing a mycobacterium does not always mean tuberculous disease. If M. tuberculosis is isolated or suspected, however, drug sensitivity studies should be initiated promptly. Drug resistance is increasingly prevalent, and patients may simultaneously harbor more than one strain, with various susceptibility patterns.

ANTIBIOTIC RESISTANCE

Some strains of M. tuberculosis resistant to isoniazid have aberrant biochemical reactions; the catalase or peroxidase tests may serve as quick screening procedures for isoniazid resistance. Complete sensitivity testing is very time consuming because the organisms are slow growing to begin with. The primary culture must have sufficient growth to permit subculturing, and the subcultures must have enough growing time to reveal the drug effects. Cultures on drug-containing media must be compared with cultures plated onto drug-free medium of the same composition, and strains of known susceptibility should be included for comparison. Ordinarily two different concentrations of the three commonly used drugs (isoniazid, *p*-aminosalicylic acid, and streptomycin) gives sufficient information.

More extensive testing is necessary only with chronic, complicated, or highly resistant cases. The growth of partially resistant strains may be slow but highly significant, so neither the microbiologist nor the clinician should lose patience after two or three weeks. When many organisms are found on direct smears, sensitivity testing can be initiated simultaneously with primary cultures. If the presence of organisms is doubtful, the longer, indirect method is necessary. As a patient undergoes treatment, repeated cultures and repeated sensitivity trials are desirable, since changes in growth pattern and resistance are prognostically as well as therapeutically significant.

ANTIBIOTIC SENSITIVITY TESTING

Most bacteria grow much faster than mycobacteria, and sensitivity testing can be done rapidly and accurately. When optimum growth occurs in 12 to 18 hours, the effect of the drug on the organism becomes apparent as growth inhibition occurs around a central deposit of the drug. Because the process is brief, the zone of drug diffusion into the medium is finite, and easily measured and reproduced. When growth takes up to six weeks, diffusion would involve the entire culture medium, but to an unstandardized, unreproducible degree. Incorporating a known concentration of drug into the medium avoids this problem, but requires inoculating as many different plates (or segments of plates) as there are drug concentrations to be tested.

SINGLE-PLATE TESTS

Many clinical microbiology laboratories use the Kirby-Bauer technique,[3] a reliable, single-plate method for measuring drug sensitivities of bacteria other than mycobacteria. In this method, paper disks impregnated with the desired drugs are placed on a standardized growth medium inoculated with a uniformly distributed bacterial suspension. The drugs diffuse out of the disks into the agar, at concentrations varying with the initial concentration in the disk and the drug's diffusability. When the disks and the growth conditions are properly standardized, the diameter of the zone of growth inhibition reproducibly reflects the organism's sensitivity to usual therapeutic serum levels of the drug.

This technique requires that the organism grow evenly and almost confluently on drug-free portions of the agar. In the original method a broth suspension of culture was spread over the plate with a cotton swab, the density of suspension being adjusted to match the turbidity of a BaSO₄ standard. Variants of the technique employ different means for standardizing the suspension and spreading it uniformly on the plate.[2] The broth culture must, of course, be pure, for mixed cultures may give overlapping patterns of sensitivity and resistance, rendering the plate uninterpretable.

Interpretation

Changes in incubation temperature, in pH, in atmospheric composition all influence the results, and zone size must be measured accurately, especially with such drugs as polymyxin B and colistin, which diffuse rather slowly. Controls must be run frequently, using strains of known resistance, to insure that the disks remain potent and the medium is satisfactory.

Another problem relates to interpretation. Complete inhibition is easy to measure; so is complete drug resistance when the organism attains confluent growth up to and under the disk. In some cases, however, the results are equivocal and must be reported as such. The clinician must also remember that in vitro inhibition does not always mean clinical effectiveness. Among other determinants are the site and type of infection, the patient's cardiovascular, hepatic, and renal status, and the presence of steroids or other drugs.[33]

DRUG DILUTION METHODS

Sometimes drug concentration is critical, or the growth pattern is not adaptable to the plate and disk method. Sensitivity can then be tested by drug dilution. One method is comparable to that described for mycobacteria in which various concentrations of drug are incorporated into agar plates. In another technique, broth tubes contain the drug dilutions, and the turbidity of the subsequent culture reflects the amount of bacterial multiplication. As with the single-plate disk methods, the pathogen should be in pure culture, although in the plate dilution test, the presence of more than one organism is more obvious than in broth tubes.

PRIMARY CULTURES

When speed is absolutely vital, antibiotic-containing disks are placed on the plates after primary inoculation. This is best done after Gram stain or some other procedure has indicated bacteria to be present and has given some clue about their identity. After the primary culture has grown out and the organism or organisms have been identified, these tentative sensitivity results should be confirmed. In patients with persistent or mixed infections, and those who respond poorly to seemingly appropriate therapy, repeated isolations and a variety of susceptibility tests may be indicated.

MYCOTIC INFECTIONS

Laboratory diagnosis of mycotic infections follows the same theoretical approach as bacterial diagnosis. If clinical specimens contain the organisms in viable state, cultures on artificial media yield diagnostic growth. Problems arise, however, in distinguishing in vivo saprophytes or laboratory contaminants from significant pathogens. Pathogenic fungi coexist with bacteria, which may or may not also have pathogenic significance. Some fungi, ordinarily saprophytic, may become virulent in debilitated hosts. Systemic fungal infections may mimic bacterial disease, and unless special efforts are made, their presence may go undetected.

SUPERFICIAL INFECTIONS

Fungal infections or mycoses are frequently categorized as superficial, cutaneous, subcutaneous, and systemic. Direct examination of skin scrapings or hair fragments often identifies superficial or cutaneous infections. Microscopic examination of NaOH-suspended or KOH-suspended emulsions reveals morphologically characteristic hyphae or, occasionally, budding yeast forms. Cultural identification is made from growth on Sabouraud's dextrose agar, incubated at room temperature. The organisms tend to be slow growing, so cultures are ordinarily held for 30 days. Because skin and hair often harbor saprophytic bacteria and fungi in addition to pathogens, the culture medium may include antibiotics to suppress unwanted contaminants.

SUBCUTANEOUS INFECTIONS

Subcutaneous mycoses, although they do not disseminate throughout the body, may be locally destructive and difficult to treat. Sporotrichum schenckii is one of the common agents in temperate climates, producing nodular or ulcerating lesions after superficial introduction of the spores. Most other infections are more frequent in, but not confined to, tropical or semitropical areas. Local introduction is through minor breaks in the skin, especially on bare feet, and a variety of fungal types may be involved. Nocardia, an aerobic bacterium rather than a fungus, may be isolated from lesions of this sort, and grows in a fashion resembling fungi on Sabouraud's medium.

Direct examination of pus, scrapings, or fungous granules often permits rapid presumptive diagnosis, and most of the agents grow readily on Sabouraud's dextrose agar. Antibiotics inhibit cultivation of some pathogenic species. For this reason, two sets of Saubouraud's media are often inoculated, one with added antibiotics to prevent contaminating overgrowth, and one unmodified, to give these sensitive organisms a chance to reveal themselves.

SYSTEMIC INFECTIONS

Systemic mycoses are becoming increasingly familiar to clinicians. These infections can usefully be divided into two groups, so-called primary disease and secondary, or opportunistic, invasion.[31] In the first group are histoplasmosis, coccidioidomycosis, blastomycosis, paracoccidioidomycosis (South American blastomycosis), and systemic sporotrichosis. Nocardiosis and actinomycosis are often included in this group because the clinical findings are comparable, but the organisms are bacteria rather than fungi. These illnesses, which afflict previously healthy individuals, must be recognized and treated on their own merits. The opportunistic infections attack patients with other diseases, who cannot mount effective defenses against agents which might not otherwise produce disease. This group includes systemic manifestations of infections with candida, aspergillus, cryptococcus, and members of the class phycomycetes, which produce mucormycosis.

Primary Infection

Primary infections tend to present initially with pulmonary symptoms, although the respiratory tract cannot always be implicated as the portal of entry, and other organs are sometimes involved. Tissue sections and smears of pus contain yeast forms of the fungi. As with bacterial infections, definitive diagnosis requires cultivation for identification, although clinical data, skin testing, and the morphology of the tissue forms may suggest the diagnosis.

Secondary Infection

Opportunistic fungus infections occur when fungi normally present in the individual or his environment produce local or systemic damage. Aspergillus and the phycomycetes are ubiquitous in the environment, and candida is a normal commensal. These fungi grow frequently in cultured specimens, without pathogenic significance. When large numbers of a single organism grow from repeated cultures of carefully obtained specimens, promptly processed, then pathogenic significance may be inferred.[21] Cryptococcus is not a normal inhabitant of central nervous system, lung, or urinary tract, so its presence in specimens, especially from debilitated or immunologically compromised patients, deserves prompt attention. Cryptococcal meningitis may develop as a primary disease, in which the organisms tend to be few and hard to demonstrate. The immunologic test for cryptococcal antigen sometimes helps in identifying these cases of seemingly aseptic, persisting meningitis.[15]

The opportunistic fungi and comparable bacteria have favorite portals of entry, although rapidly fatal dissemination frequently follows. Nocardia often causes severe pulmonary involvement, and later central nervous system disease, notably brain abscesses. Aspergillus nearly always involves the lung, where it may cause suppurative or granulomatous inflammation or a type of hypersensitivity reaction.[21] Mucormycosis classically presents as fulminating rhinocerebral infection, but hematogenous spread with arteritis and thrombosis often follows. Candida albicans spreads initially on surfaces—the skin, the mucosa of the respiratory or gastrointestinal tract, and sometimes the mucosa of the urinary tract—but the mycelia penetrate into the underlying tissue, and generalized sepsis, meningitis, or endocarditis may be the terminal event.

The cultivation of viruses and mycoplasmas is a topic beyond our scope. Serologic approaches to these organisms are discussed in Chapter 2.

BIBLIOGRAPHY

1. BAILEY, W.R., AND SCOTT, E.G.: Diagnostic Microbiology, ed.3. C. V. Mosby Co., St. Louis, 1970.
2. BARRY, A.L., GARCIA, F., AND THRUPP, L.D.: An improved single-disk method for testing the antibiotic susceptibility of rapidly growing pathogens. Am. J. Clin. Pathol. 53:149, 1970.
3. BAUER, A.W., KIRBY, W.M.M., SHERRIS, J.C., AND TURCK, M.: Antibiotic susceptibility testing by a standardized single disk method. Am. J. Clin. Pathol. 45:493, 1966.
4. BLAIR, T.E., LENNETTE, E.H., AND TRUANT, J.P. (EDS.): Manual of Clinical Microbiology. American Society for Microbiology, Bethesda, Md., 1970.
5. DATTA, N.: The vectors of antibiotic resistance in bacteria. Sci. Basis Med. Annu. Rev. 1969, p. 267.
6. DAVIES, J.: Bacterial resistance to aminoglycoside antibiotics. J. Infect. Dis. 124:Suppl. 7, 1971.
7. DAVIES, J.E., AND ROWND, R.: Transmissible multiple drug resistance in Enterobacteriaceae. Science 176:758, 1972.
8. DIAGNOSTIC STANDARDS AND CLASSIFICATION OF TUBERCULOSIS. National Tuberculosis and Respiratory Disease Association, New York, 1969.
9. DUBOS, R.J., AND HIRSCH, J.G. (EDS.): Bacterial and Mycotic Infections of Man, ed. 4 J.B. Lippincott Co., Philadelphia, 1965.
10. DUPONT, H.L., FORMAL, S.B., HORNICK, R.B. ET AL.: Pathogenesis of Escherichia coli diarrhea. N. Engl. J. Med. 285:1, 1971.
11. ETKINS, S., AND GORBACH, S.L.: Studies on enterotoxin from Escherichia coli associated with acute diarrhea in man. J. Lab. Clin. Med. 78:81, 1971.

12. EWING, W.H.: Isolation and identification of *Escherichia coli* serotypes associated with diarrheal disease. National Communicable Disease Center, Atlanta, Jan., 1963.
13. EWING, W.H.: Revised definitions for the family Enterobacteriaceae, its tribes and genera. National Communicable Disease Center, Atlanta, 1967.
14. FARRAR, W.E., JR., AND EIDSON, M.: Antibiotic resistance in Shigella mediated by R factors. J. Infect. Dis. 123:477,1971.
15. GOODMAN, J.S., KAUFMAN, L., AND KOENIG, M.G.: Diagnosis of cryptococcal meningitis: Value of immunologic detection of cryptococcal antigen. N. Engl. J. Med. 285:434, 1971.
16. GRADY, G.F., AND KEUSCH, G.T.: Pathogenesis of bacterial diarrheas. N. Engl. J. Med. 285:831, 1971.
17. JACOBY, G.A.: An R factor defects to our side. N. Engl. J. Med. 286:602, 1972.
18. JAROLMEN, H., AND KEMP, G.: R factor transmission in vivo. J. Bacteriol. 99:487, 1969.
19. KASS, E.H.: Pyelonephritis and bacteriuria; a major problem in preventive medicine. Ann. Intern. Med. 56:46, 1962.
20. KISER, J.S., GALE, G.O., AND KEMP, G.A.: Resistance to antimicrobial agents. Adv. Appl. Microbiol. 11:77, 1969.
21. KLAINER, A.S., AND BEISEL, W.R.: Opportunistic infection: A review. Am. J. Med. Sci. 258:431, 1969.
22. LYNCH, M.J., RAPHAEL, S.S., MELLOR, L.D. ET AL.: Medical Laboratory Technology, ed. 2. W.B. Saunders Co., Philadelphia, 1969.
23. MARTIN, W.J.: "Enterobacteriaceae," *In* Blair, J.E., Lennette, E.H., and Truant, J.P. (eds.): Manual of Clinical Microbiology. American Society for Microbiology, Bethesda, Md., 1970.
24. MOU, T.W., AND FELDMAN, H.A.: The enumeration and preservation of bacteria in urine. Am. J. Clin. Pathol. 35:572, 1961.
25. RESNICK, B., CELLA, R.L., SOGHIKIAN, K. ET AL.: Mass detection of significant bacteriuria. Arch. Intern. Med. 124:165, 1968.
26. RUDOLPH, A.H.: Control of gonorrhea. J.A.M.A. 220:1587, 1972.
27. SMITH, D.H.: R factor infection of Escherichia coli lyophilized in 1946. J. Bacteriol. 94:2071, 1967.
28. TERAWAKI, Y., TAKAYSAU, H., AND AKIBA, T.: Thermosensitive replication of a kanamycin resistance factor. J. Bacteriol. 94:687, 1967.
29. TILLOTSON, J. R., AND LERNER, A.M.: Hemophilus influenzae bronchopneumonia in adults. Arch. Intern. Med. 121:428, 1968.
30. TRUANT, J.P., BRETT, W.A., AND THOMAS, W., JR.: Fluorescence microscopy of tubercle bacilli stained with auramine and rhodamine. Henry Ford Hosp. Med. J. 10:287, 1962.
31. UTZ, J.P.: Pulmonary infection due to opportunistic fungi. Adv. Intern. Med. 16:427, 1970.
32. WATANABE, T.: Infectious drug resistance in enteric bacteria. N. Engl. J. Med. 275:888, 1966.
33. WEINSTEIN, L., AND DALTON, A. C.: Host determinants of response to antimicrobial agents. N. Engl. J. Med. 279:467, 1968.

CHAPTER **8**

Urine

PHYSIOLOGY

THE NEPHRON

The kidneys, which together constitute 0.5 per cent of total body weight, receive 20 per cent of cardiac output, a testimonial to the complexity and importance of renal function. Approximately 1500 L of blood pass through the kidneys each day; approximately 150 L of fluid per day enter the proximal convoluted tubules as potential urine; approximately 1.5 L per day is the usual output for a metabolically stable adult. The magnitude of renal activity is obvious! The functional unit of renal activity is the nephron, of which each kidney contains approximately 1.5 million. Comprising the nephron are the glomerular capillary loop, the proximal convoluted tubule, the loop of Henle, the distal convoluted tubule, and the collecting duct, which unites with other ducts to connect, ultimately, with the renal pelvis.

Glomerular Function

Glomerular blood flow is regulated by the afferent (preglomerular) and efferent (postglomerular) arterioles. The principal function of the glomerular capillary loop is filtration, whereby fluid and associated solutes leave the blood stream for processing into urine. Filtration pressure, the *push* that expels fluid from the capillary lumen, is the net sum of outward-directed hydrostatic pressure and in-pulling colloid osmotic pressure. Serum protein

216

levels principally determine osmotic pressure, while changes in arteriolar constriction regulate the intracapillary hydrostatic pressure.

After leaving the capillary lumen, the filtrate traverses a maze of cellular and acellular elements which permit plasma solutes to pass, but restrict larger molecules, notably proteins. Small amounts of the smallest plasma proteins normally enter the filtrate. Hemoglobin, a compact, spherical molecule,[23] can readily pass the filter, but its presence in plasma is highly abnormal. Abnormal quantities of protein may enter the filtrate if hydrostatic pressure is exceptionally high, if there is damage to the endothelial, basement membrane or epithelial structures comprising the physical barrier, or if exceptionally small protein molecules are present in plasma for any reason.

The Proximal Tubule

The 150 L of filtrate that enter the convoluted tubule contain more than a kilogram of sodium chloride and innumerable other constituents. While traversing the proximal convoluted tubule, the urine-to-be loses 80 to 85 per cent of its water and salt, and virtually all its sugar, amino acids, and proteins. The epithelial cells lining this segment expend energy in the reabsorption of sodium; water and chloride passively accompany the reabsorbed sodium back into the general circulation. This portion of salt and water regulation does not respond to changing physiologic stimuli, and final regulation occurs more distally.

Secretion and Absorption. The proximal tubular cells transport a multitude of other substances, most of them from the tubular lumen into capillary blood, but some secreted in the reverse direction, so that urinary concentration exceeds the filtered level. These transport mechanisms depend upon the coupling of transported substance with an intracellular carrier, and their capacity is finite. The exact nature of these carriers is unknown, although certain common reabsorptive pathways are known to exist. Glucose, fructose, xylose, and galactose share one system; different classes of amino acids share several different systems. Secretion, which is net transport from blood or interstitial fluid into tubular urine, employs comparable carrier systems. One well-defined common secretory pathway is shared by such organic ions as penicillin, para-aminohippuric acid (PAH), and phenolsulfonphthalein (PSP). The tubules can clear a small amount of protein from the filtrate by a carrier system involving lipoprotein complexes, but the maximum capacity is quite low.

Measurement of absorptive or secretory capacity for a given substance provides a functional estimate of tubular epithelial capacity; the descriptive term for maximum rate of tubular transport is T_m, the substance being specified by a subscript, as $T_{m(PAH)}$ or $T_{m(glucose)}$. If the tubular fluid contains more glucose, for example, than the reabsorptive mechanism can handle, the T_m is exceeded and the excess material remains in the urine.

The Loop of Henle

Fluid and electrolyte recovery in the proximal tubule reduces the minute volume of tubular content from 120 ml to 20 ml, but excretion at this rate would still produce 29 L of urine per day. Entering the loop of Henle, the tubular fluid is isosmotic with plasma, i.e., approximately 300 mOsm/L. The loop descends into the renal medulla, where the interstitial fluid is highly hypertonic. Water and electrolytes move between tubular lumen and interstitial fluid in a complex series of relationships known as *countercurrent multiplication of concentration.* [29] Following its passage through Henle's loop, the fluid entering the distal convoluted tubule is hypotonic to the concentrated interstitial fluid just outside the tubule.

The Distal Tubule

In the distal convoluted tubule and collecting ducts, the day-to-day, minute-to-minute adjustments of volume and electrolyte composition occur. Antidiuretic hormone (ADH) controls volume excretion by varying the interaction between dilute tubular contents and concentrated interstitial fluid. When ADH is present, the wall of these segments becomes permeable to solute-free water. From the interstitial fluid, this water returns to the circulation, thus conserving body water and leaving urine fairly concentrated. Without ADH, the walls resist water movement, the tubular fluid remains hypotonic, and large volumes of dilute urine are excreted.

Both proximal and distal convoluted tubules participate in acid-base and potassium ion regulation. In the proximal tubule, potassium and bicarbonate are removed from the filtrate, while hydrogen ion content of the tubular fluid increases. The proximal tubular epithelium regenerates bicarbonate ions and restores them to the circulation along with sodium ions. In the distal tubule, the epithelium adjusts the excretion of hydrogen and potassium ions; as long as the organism maintains approximate metabolic equilibrium, these ions are excreted in a roughly reciprocal fashion. Excess hydrogen ions are excreted by combination with ammonia (to form ammonium ions) or with filtered buffers like $HPO_3^=$. When H^+ excretion is increased, urinary K^+ concentration diminishes. If whole-body potassium stores are low, K^+ will be conserved and H^+ excreted. This may occur even if the stimulus to K^+ depletion is one which leads to overall alkalosis, so the urine may be paradoxically acid in the face of whole-body alkalosis.

PHYSIOLOGIC DERANGEMENTS

Renal function is so intimately dependent upon the interrelations of blood vessels and epithelial elements that distinct separation of disease states is very difficult. It is useful to consider vascular disease, glomerular disease, and tubular disorders in separate categories, but the glomerulus is, after all, a tuft of blood vessels, and tubular function at all levels in the nephron requires interchange with interstitial fluid and the capillaries of the interstitium.

Acute drop in renal perfusion reduces urine flow because of decreased filtration and, if severe, because of hypoxic damage to the metabolically active and highly vulnerable tubular epithelial cells. Marked increase in arterial or arteriolar pressure leads to structural changes in the blood vessels, originally to protect against damage but leading to irreversible changes if prolonged.

Sites of Damage

If the glomerulus sustains damage either from inflammatory conditions or vascular disease, its filtration functions suffer, so large molecules like serum proteins or even intact erythrocytes or leukocytes can enter the tubular contents. Damage to the tubular cells impairs their secretory and reabsorptive capacities, and interferes with the regulatory mechanisms for electrolyte and acid-base control, as well as control of volume and concentration. If the interstitium of cortex or medulla is altered by inflammation, scarring, or deposition of abnormal elements, then concentrating power and metabolic exchange will be affected.

Abnormal Urinary Constituents

Red or white blood cells may enter the urine from any level in the urinary tract. If these cellular elements or other constituents originate in the kidney and spend sufficient time in the tubules, they may become packed together and assume the shape of the tubular lumen. These are called casts, and, when seen in the urine, are incontrovertible evidence of intrarenal disease. Red or white cells of renal origin may sometimes appear loose in the urine, and desquamated tubular epithelial cells sometimes are found in urinary sediment. More often, however, the inciting abnormality sets up conditions conducive to cast formation.

Cast Formation. Casts consist of inspissated tubular contents passed directly into urine and therefore fairly accurately reflect renal parenchymal disease. Hyaline casts, composed largely of the Tamm-Horsfall mucoprotein which is a product of the normal nephron,[43] are present in small numbers in normal urine, but increase when urinary protein is increased and urine is highly concentrated. Increased acidity and electrolyte concentration enhance precipitation of Tamm-Horsfall mucoprotein.[38] The sticky protein casts attract white cells or tubular cells to their surface, and cellular inclusions in hyaline casts are fairly common. Bilirubin or hemoglobin, if present in the urine, may lend color to these normally colorless cylinders. Mucous threads, fibers, and other artefacts may occasionally be mistaken for hyaline casts, which are difficult to see against a brightly lighted background. Other kinds of casts include cellular elements or debris from blood or epithelial cells and appear granular or overtly cellular. These are more obvious on microscopic examination, and often accompany more destructive renal processes.

Chemical Abnormalities. The chemical composition of urine depends on what enters the tubular filtrate, that is, the composition of blood as it reflects systemic metabolism and the activity of the nephron in modifying the filtrate. For some substances, comparison of blood and urine levels provides some idea of the site of abnormality. For others, urinary composition may be an important clue to systemic disease. The urinary levels of sodium, potassium, calcium, phosphates, and bicarbonate reflect both renal and systemic problems, and must be evaluated with many variables in mind. Routine urinalysis ordinarily includes qualitative search for such common pathologically significant elements as glucose, ketone bodies, protein, blood, and bile pigments. When specific diseases are under consideration, a host of other qualitative or quantitative procedures may be indicated. Table 14 shows values of the constituents of normal urine.

RENAL FUNCTION TESTS

GLOMERULAR BLOOD FLOW

Urine constitutes an end-point of renal function, but a single specimen, or even a timed collection, often cannot provide information about the dynamics of the functioning kidney. Several well-established procedures are available to investigate glomerular flow rate and tubular excretory capacity. The volume of blood going through the glomerulus cannot, of course, be partitioned and measured separately from the total renal

Table 14. Normal Values for Urine

Test	Normal Values	Remarks
Addis count	WBC 1,800,000; RBC 500,000; casts (hyaline) 0–5000	Rinse bottle with 10% neutral formalin and discard excess 12-hr specimen
Albumin Qualitative Quantitative	Negative 10–100 mg/24 hr	Single specimen 24-hr specimen
Aldosterone	2–23 μg/24 hr	24-hr specimen; keep refrigerated.
Amino acid nitrogen	100–290 mg/24 hr	24-hr specimen; collect in thymol; refrigerate
Ammonia	700 mg/24 hr	24-hr specimen
Amylase	2–50 Wohlgemuth u/ml	Single specimen
Amylase, total in 24 hr	6–30 Wohlgemuth u/ml Up to 5000 Somogyi u/24 hr	24-hr specimen
Bence-Jones protein	Negative	First morning specimen
Bilirubin	Negative	Single specimen
Blood, occult	Negative	Single specimen
Calcium Sulkowitch Quantitative	Positive 1+ 30–150 mg/24 hr 100–250 mg/24 hr	Single specimen Average diet High-calcium diet; 24-hr specimen
Catecholamines	Less than 230 μg in 24 hr	24-hr specimen; use 1 ml conc. H_2SO_4 for preservative
Chloride	110–250 mEq/24 hr	24-hr specimen
Coproporphyrin	50–200 μg/24 hr. Children: 0–80 μg/24 hr	24-hr specimen in 5 Gm of Na_2CO_3
Creatine	Less than 100 mg in 24 hr, or less than 6% of creatinine. Pregnancy: up to 12% of creatinine. Children under 1 yr: may equal creatinine. Children over 1 yr: up to 30% of creatinine	24-hr specimen
Creatinine	Females: 0.8–1.7 Gm/24 hr Males: 1–1.9 Gm/24 hr	24-hr specimen

Table 14.   (Continued)

Test	Normal Values	Remarks
Estrogens	Females: 4–60 μg/24 hr Males: 4–25 μg/24 hr	24-hr specimen; refrigerate
Fishberg concentration test	Specific gravity: 1.022 to 1.032	Collect specimens at 7,8 and 10 A.M.
Fishberg dilution test	Volume of 40 ml in first hour with specific gravity 1.001 to 1.003	Collect 4 hourly specimens after drinking 1200 ml of water
Glucose Qualitative	Negative	Single specimen
Quantitative	Less than 100 mg/100 ml	24-hr specimen
Gonadotropic hormone, pituitary	10 to 15 mouse uterine u/24 hr	24-hr specimen; collect with toluene
17-Hydroxycortico-steriods	Females: 2–8 mg/24 hr Males: 3–10 mg/24 hr	24-hr specimen; tranquilizers interfere
5-Hydroxyindoleacetic acid	2–9 mg/24 hr	24-hr specimen; tranquilizers interfere
Indican	4–20 mg/24 hr	24-hr specimen
17-Ketosteriods	24-hr excretion:	24-hr specimen
Lead	0.021–0.038 mg/liter	24-hr specimen
pH	4.8 to 7.8	Single specimen
Phenylpyruvic acid	Negative	Single specimen
Phosphorus	0.9–1.3 Gm/24 hr	24-hr specimen
Porphobilinogen	Negative	Single specimen
Potassium	25–100 mEq/24 hr	24-hr specimen
Pregnanediol	Children: negative. Females: 1–8 mg/24 hr. Males: 0–1 mg/24 hr	24-hr specimen; refrigerate
Pregnanetriol	Children: Less than 0.5 mg/ 24 hr. Females: 0.5–2 mg/ 24 hr. Males: 1.0–2.0 mg/ 24 hr	24-hr specimen; refrigerate
Protein Bence-Jones	Negative	First morning specimen
Qualitative	Negative	Single specimen
Quantitative	10–100 mg/24 hr	24-hr specimen

17-Ketosteriods, 24-hr excretion:

Age	Females	Males
10	1–4 mg	1–4 mg
20–30	4–16 mg	6–26 mg
50	3–9 mg	5–18 mg
70	1–7 mg	2–10 mg

Table 14. (Continued)

Test	Normal Values	Remarks
Serotonin	*See* 5-Hydroxyindoleacetic acid	
Sodium	About 110 mEq/24 hr	24-hr specimen
Specific gravity	1.002–1.030 1.015–1.025	Single specimen 24-hr specimen
Sugars	Negative	Single specimen
Urea clearance	Maximum: 75 ml Standard: 54 ml	Serum and urine
Uric acid	0.5–1.0 Gm/24 hr	24-hr specimen
Urobilinogen Semiquantitative	Up to 1 Ehrlich u/2 hr	2-hr specimen; collect between 1 and 3 P.M.
Quantitative	1.0–4.0 mg/24 hr	24-hr specimen; collect in dark container with 5 Gm of Na_2CO_3
Vanilmandelic acid	0.7–6.8 mg/24 hr	24-hr specimen in 3 ml 25% H_2SO_4; omit fruit and coffee 2 days before test
Volume	Adults: 1000-1500 ml/24 hr (about 15–21 ml/kg body wt) Children: 3 to 4 times as much as adults per kg of body wt	

blood flow. Instead, the glomerular flow is inferred from the rate at which certain materials leave the circulation and enter the filtrate, resulting in a figure called the glomerular filtration rate.

Inulin Clearance

Glomerular filtration rate (GFR) is usually expressed in terms of clearance, a figure representing the amount of plasma from which some substance is totally cleared in one minute. Such clearing does not actually occur, nor could it be precisely measured if it did. Clearance is calculated from the ratio of substance excreted to the concentration of that substance in the plasma, that is, the amount available to the kidney for excretion. The amount excreted is readily measured; it is the concentration of the substance in the urine (U) multiplied by the volume of urine excreted in the selected time (V). Dividing the amount excreted by the concentration in plasma (P) tells how many milliliters of plasma yielded that amount of material, assuming that each milliliter of plasma flowing through the glomerulus released all its substance into the urine. The clearance formula, then, is $(U \times V)/P$.

Measurement. Accurate measurement of clearance requires that the substance be one that can accurately be measured at both plasma and urine levels. It also requires that the proportion of urinary concentration to plasma concentration [U]/[P] be constant over a wide range of plasma levels, and that the substance not be secreted, absorbed, or metabolized. The substance that best fulfills these requirements is inulin, a metabolically inert polysaccharide of fructose.

The rate of plasma flow through the glomerulus can be measured very accurately if inulin is infused at such a rate that a constant plasma level is maintained and complete, meticulous urine collection is achieved. The glomerular filtration rate, as so determined, is 124 ± 15 ml of plasma/min/ 1.73 m² of body surface in healthy young men and 110 ± 15 ml/min/1.73 m² for healthy young women.[40] These values diminish slightly with aging, even when no demonstrable renal disease coexists.

Abnormalities. Diseases that affect the glomerular tuft and renal vascular disease have the most immediate effect on GFR, but any significant degree of renal disease can diminish the filtration rate. Nonrenal conditions which impair small vessel circulation may also decrease glomerular plasma flow, such as congestive heart failure, cirrhosis with ascitic accumulation, shock from any cause, or dehydration.

Endogenous Clearance Tests

Inulin clearance is not suitable for routine laboratory use because the plasma levels must be monitored by frequent and very accurate measurement, and urine collection must be extremely careful. From research studies using inulin clearance, however, has come knowledge of the relative accuracies and shortcomings of other clearance techniques. In clinical situations, glomerular filtration rate is usually estimated from values for urea clearance or creatinine clearance. Both procedures have shortcomings, but creatinine clearance is perhaps more widely used. Both are endogenous clearance tests, meaning that the substance measured is already present in the circulation. This makes it unnecessary to achieve and maintain a constant plasma level of the material during the test period, since the assumption is made that the plasma level remains stable for this period. A highly unstable metabolite, like glucose, could not be used.

Creatinine Clearance. One problem, affecting both creatinine and urea, is that excretory levels reflect more than just filtration. The tubules normally secrete a small amount of creatinine into the urine, and reabsorb a moderate amount of urea. When plasma creatinine is high, secretion is enhanced. Since patients with impaired renal function have increased plasma creatinine, the degree of inaccuracy is cumulative. For this reason, creatinine clearance rates in seriously ill patients cannot usefully be referred to absolute normal values. A better approach is to follow sequential values in an individual patient who then serves as his own control.

For creatinine clearance, a 12- or 24-hour urine specimen is collected. The sample for plasma determination should be drawn some time during this period. Plasma levels are normally so low (0.7 to 1.5 mg/100 ml) that strictly accurate determinations are difficult. In addition, plasma contains noncreatinine reactants which are chromogenic in the alkaline picrate procedure usually employed. This small degree of error is probably balanced in calculation, however, by the inaccuracy that results from tubular secretion.

Urea Clearance. Tubular reabsorption of urea presents a more serious problem, because the rate of absorption varies with the rate of urine flow. When flow is slow, quite a lot of filtered urea is removed. For reasonably reliable results, urine flow must be 2 ml/min or greater. Plasma urea concentrations are somewhat more variable than creatinine levels, one reason for using a shorter collection period for urea than for creatinine clearance. If urea clearance is measured during two consecutive one hour collections, sufficient hydration can be achieved that urine flow remains above 2 ml/min and plasma fluctuations are unlikely to be serious. The short collection periods may, however, introduce serious artefacts if bladder emptying is incomplete.

Normal Values. The values for creatinine clearance, properly done, bear a close relationship to those measured by inulin clearance. Normal creatinine clearance values are approximately 125 ml/min for men and 110 ml/min for women. Urea clearance is often expressed in terms of per cent of normal function instead of in absolute terms. The normal or 100 per cent level is taken as 75 ml/min if urine flow has been 2 ml/min or greater, and 54 ml/min (calculated with the square root of the urine volume) if flow was less than 2 ml/min. Values between 75 and 125 per cent of normal indicate adequate filtration function.

TUBULAR TRANSPORT MECHANISMS

Inulin does not undergo tubular transport, but certain other materials enter the urine both by glomerular filtration and tubular secretion. Comparing this excretion against purely glomerular excretion permits estimation of tubular transport capacity. A single transport path is known to secrete phenolsulfonphthalein (PSP) and para-aminohippuric acid (PAH) into the urine, and also to transport penicillin, glucuronides, and such x-ray contrast media as Diodrast. That portion of PSP or PAH which is bound to plasma proteins does not pass the glomerular filter, but reaches the tubules from the postglomerular interstitial circulation. At fairly low plasma levels, virtually all the PAH in a volume of blood can be removed by one passage through the kidney; one passage removes about 50 per cent of the PSP.[41] The excretory rate of these substances varies with the renal blood flow and the degree of tubular function.

PAH Excretion

Since PAH is excreted both by tubular secretion and glomerular filtration, tubular transport capacity (T_m) can be measured by comparing PAH excretion with the values for glomerular filtration rate obtained by inulin clearance. The increment of PAH over inulin values represents the tubular capacity. Both technical and clinical problems limit wide-spread employment of this approach.

PSP Excretion

Simpler than measuring PAH excretion but still a useful measure of tubular transport is measuring PSP excretion. In this test, urinary content of PSP is measured at 15, 30, 60, and 120 minutes after intravenous injection. With normal renal blood flow, normal tubular function, and unobstructed urine flow, at least 25 per cent of the total dose should appear in urine at 15 minutes, and 60 to 70 per cent should have been excreted within an hour.

The plasma PSP level achieved with the usual dose does not reach the maximum capacity of normally functioning tubules, so the amount of dye excreted relates more closely to the amount of blood coming in contact with the tubules than to the functional capacity of the tubular epithelium. If obstruction and oliguria are ruled out, reduced early (15 minutes) PSP excretion is more likely to indicate impaired renal perfusion than diminished tubular function. Congestive heart failure or isolated renal vascular disease produce abnormal PSP results before the degree of circulatory impairment reduces tubular function. Depressed tubular function rarely occurs without impaired perfusion. Markedly abnormal PSP results indicate extensive damage, and the one hour total excretion will be reduced.

Problems in Interpretation. Since injected contrast media, chlorothiazide, penicillin G, and PSP all share a common tubular mechanism, the test should not be performed if these drugs are in use. Patients with severe hypoproteinemia may excrete unexpectedly large amounts of PSP because more dye is unbound and filterable, thus by-passing tubular transport. The dose of PSP must be accurately measured and injected, and, because the collecting periods are so short, the patient must be thoroughly hydrated.

Concentrating Ability

The complex functions of concentrating and diluting urine require interaction among the distal nephron, the interstitium of the medulla, the pituitary hormone ADH, and other whole-body volume regulators. Intact functioning requires not only anatomic integrity but a high level of subtle regulatory capacity. Impaired concentrating ability may be an early sign of renal damage, apparent before measurable change occurs in the GFR or the renal perfusion rate, and long before gross signs of damage become obvious.

Specific Gravity

Several different means are available to measure urine concentration, that is, the relative amounts of solute and water. The oldest is measurement of specific gravity, using a float or urinometer which has been calibrated against distilled water. The specific gravity of urine from normal individuals can vary between 1.000 and 1.035. The procedure requires a large volume of urine and careful technique to avoid contaminating the specimen, or misusing or misreading the urinometer. Other technical problems include the need to correct for temperature changes and the necessity for frequent instrument calibration. Simpler, but employing the same basic principles, is measurement cf urinary solute load by its refractive effect on transmitted light. This can easily be measured on a few drops of urine without temperature interference. Urine refractometers are calibrated to translate refractive index directly to specific gravity.

Significant Alterations. Specific gravity and refraction are influenced by the number and the nature of the solute particles. Large molecules in the urine, particularly proteins, glucose, and radiopaque dyes, exert a disproportionate effect on specific gravity. Artefact introduced by these substances may obscure small but significant changes in true concentration. The specific gravity of plasma, which contains proteins, glucose, lipids, and other macromolecules, is approximately 1.010. When the kidneys lose their ability to concentrate or dilute, excreted urine cannot reflect responses to physiologic stimuli, and urine specific gravity becomes fixed at 1.010, the plasma level.

Osmolality

An index of renal function more sensitive than specific gravity is urine osmolality. Osmolality reflects only the number of solute particles in a fluid, regardless of their size or composition. Osmolality is measured by the effect of solute particles on the freezing point of a fluid. Pure water freezes at 0°C. One osmole, which is one gram-molecular weight of an undissociated solute, dissolved in one kilogram of water depresses the freezing point to −1.86°C. Osmolality is expressed as osmoles (Osm) or milliosmoles (mOsm) per kilogram of water.

Normal plasma has an osmolality of 285 mOsm/kg. More than 90 per cent of this value derives from sodium ions and complementary chloride and bicarbonate. In health, glucose, urea, plasma proteins, potassium, and so forth contribute very little to this value. Urine osmolality can vary between 50 and 1400 mOsm/kg, depending upon fluid volume, solute load, and renal function. Urine specific gravity of 1.022 corresponds to an osmolality of 800 mOsm/kg. Since urine osmolality can be measured to accuracies of ±2 mOsm/kg,[6] osmolality provides a far wider range and more sensitive index of renal concentrating ability than does specific gravity measurement. More important, the presence in urine of glucose, protein, or radio-contrast material does not affect osmolality determinations. These materials can be demonstrated in other fashions, without distorting the evaluation of renal concentrating ability.

Significant Alterations. Serum osmolality rises with hyperglycemia, uremia, hemoconcentration from most causes, and the presence of circulating abnormal solutes, as in certain kinds of acidosis and shock. Under these conditions, urine osmolality should also be elevated. One effect of antidiuretic hormone (ADH) is to lower serum osmolality, producing relative urinary hyperosmolality until physiologic or pharmacologic measures achieve metabolic stabilization. Persistently high urine osmolality in the face of serum hypo-osmolality and hyponatremia suggests "inappropriate" ADH secretion. Urine is hypo-osmolal to serum in most types of physiologic or induced diuresis. Osmotic diuresis, which can occur with uremia and hyperglycemia as well as after infusion of mannitol or other substances, leads to urine isosmolal with serum.

Value of Random Specimens. Determining the specific gravity or osmolality of a random urine specimen provides a spot check of renal concentrating ability, but in an uncontrolled fashion. A standard of adequate concentrating ability is achievement, under appropriate stimulus, of urinary specific gravity of 1.025, or osmolality of 900 mOsm/kg. If a random specimen, often the first or second voided morning specimen, attains these or higher levels, then adequate concentrating function can be inferred and further testing is unnecessary. Care must be taken that none of the above-mentioned artefacts has spuriously raised the specific gravity. If concentrating ability requires further study, the patient can be subjected to controlled water deprivation, and subsequent concentration observed.

Concentration Tests

The Mosenthal Test. The classical concentration test is that of Mosenthal, requiring a 24-hour period of water deprivation, although relatively normal food intake is permitted. Following a day and a night of fluid restriction, the patient saves the first voided morning specimen, but remains recumbent. After one hour recumbent, he voids again, and then after one hour of upright activity, saves the third specimen voided. Of these three specimens, at least one should have a specific gravity of 1.025. The first specimen is usually the most concentrated, but patients with congestive heart failure or mobilizing edema fluid for any reason may have a relatively dilute overnight specimen, so the second or third specimen would become more concentrated. Comparing the second and third specimen also permits detection of orthostatic proteinuria.

Fourteen-Hour Deprivation. A shorter period of fluid restriction is easier to control, and gives similarly useful results.[19] If the patient eats his evening meal before 6 P.M. and takes no fluids thereafter, the morning specimens will reflect 14 hours without intake. Jacobson[19] recommends that the first voided morning specimen not be used, since the overnight accumulation may include dilute urine from the early evening. Sampling the second voided specimen measures concentrating ability during a short period of known fluid restriction. The second morning sample should achieve either a minimum osmolality of 850 mOsm/kg or specific gravity of 1.026. If this concentration is not achieved, additional samples can be measured by prolonging the fluid restriction for another six hours. In some physiologically normal individuals, water deprivation for 22 hours may be necessary before maximum concentrating ability is induced.[32]

Significance. Failure to concentrate normally indicates renal damage, which may be localized to medulla or may involve the entire nephron. Impaired concentrating ability may be the first sign of subtle damage or an early indicator of unsuspected infection. Patient cooperation, naturally, is essential. Before diagnosing impaired concentrating ability, the physician must be sure the patient has not taken nocturnal fluids, either accidentally or deliberately. Diminished concentrating ability usually means damaged kidneys, but rare etiologies may include pituitary dysfunction, with reduced antidiuretic hormone (ADH) production or renal insensitivity to

ADH. Both these possibilities can be investigated by noting the response to exogenous ADH.

Concentration tests are meaningless in patients taking diuretic drugs. Metabolically-induced conditions of osmotic diuresis or increased solute load also invalidate the results, since renal concentrating ability is inversely proportional to the solute load. The patient should be in a state of adequate diet and normal hydration. Protein deficiency impairs renal concentrating ability, and patients who have been markedly overhydrated for several days may have impaired concentration if dehydration is then imposed.[32]

Renal damage can also impair diluting ability, but this is less readily demonstrated than impairment of maximum concentration and gives no more information than concentration testing.

THE ROUTINE URINALYSIS

Routine urinalysis includes the observation of color, concentration, and pH of the urine, along with microscopic examination of formed elements and a search for pathologically significant elements not normally present, such as glucose, protein, blood, ketones, and bile pigments. The technology of routine urinalysis has changed from manual tests for individual constituents to use of chemical-impregnated paper strips and reagent tablets. The results offer equal or greater accuracy, as long as the limitations are appreciated, and much greater speed and convenience. The strips should be protected from moisture or volatile fumes, and should not be used if discolored. Personnel using the strips should avoid touching the test areas with their fingers. In reading the results, recommended time intervals are important, and a good light is indispensable.

Urine pH

Urinary pH is measured only roughly. The normal pH is slightly acid, approximately 6 when the usual acid-residue diet is consumed. The limits of pH variation are from 4.5 to nearly 9. The combination of bromthymol blue and methyl red used in the testing strips permits discrimination to approximately one half pH unit within this range.

Urine acidification requires metabolic work by the kidney, including reabsorption and reconstitution of bicarbonate ion, ammonium ion excretion, and excretion of free hydrogen ions. With good renal function, urine pH tends to reflect plasma pH, permitting compensation when acid-base derangements are present, but there are several notable exceptions.

Significant Alterations. If tubular function is deficient, the kidney may be unable to produce an appropriate gradient between urine and plasma pH. This syndrome of renal tubular acidosis may be primary, due to congenital or acquired renal disease and resulting in subsequent metabolic abnormalities if uncorrected, or it may be secondary to other conditions which produce acidosis and also impair renal reactivity. Urine may be inappropriately acid during metabolic alkalosis, because of obligatory hydrogen ion excretion if potassium is severely depleted. With the kind of severe dehydration and salt loss that tends to produce this picture, ketones and organic acids frequently accumulate, enhancing urinary acidity and ultimately producing a picture of mixed alkalosis and acidosis

Alkalinity. Significantly alkaline urines are relatively rare. They may result from a diet disproportionately high in fruits and vegetables and low in meat protein, or from alkalinizing drugs given to prevent precipitation of urate or other stones. Ammonia-splitting bacteria convert urine from acid to alkaline, so a strongly alkaline reaction may mean that the specimen has been sitting around too long. If a freshly voided specimen is alkaline, urinary tract infection should be investigated.

Acidity. Strongly acid reactions accompany nearly all forms of acidosis except, as mentioned above, when there is intrinsic or acquired renal damage. A test of acidifying capacity is the administration of large doses of ammonium chloride (12 Gm daily for 3 days), which should result in urine acidification to pH 4.5 to 5.5. In renal tubular failure, pH fails to go below 6 or 6.5. High meat diets and acidifying drugs produce persistently acid urine.

COLOR

Normal urine ranges in color from pale yellow to deep gold, depending on the concentration of solutes. Although usually clear, urine may turn cloudy on standing if urates precipitate in acid urine, or phosphates precipitate at alkaline pH. The most common pathologically significant color changes result from the presence of blood, hemoglobin degradation products, or bilirubin and its metabolites. Fresh blood imparts a cloudy red-pink or reddish-brown appearance; deeper brown or brownish-grey shades develop if urinary acidity converts hemoglobin to acid hematin or methemoglobin. Myoglobin also produces a red-brown appearance. Closely related chemically to hemoglobin, myoglobin may enter urine after severe destruction of muscle, the only tissue that contains myoglobin.

Hemoglobin Testing

Virtually all tests for hemoglobin, in urine, feces, and other materials, exploit the peroxidase properties of the molecule, whereby oxygen catalytically released from hydrogen peroxide affects an indicator color. For urine, orthotoluidine is used as indicator, and it is sensitive to hemoglobin in extremely low concentrations. Myoglobin, when present, also produces a positive test. Since the test detects hemoglobin free in solution, it sometimes fails to reveal that intact red cells are present. Microscopic examination of the centrifuged sediment is the best way to demonstrate red blood cells in the urine, while orthotoluidine testing is valuable if hemoglobinuria is of other origin, or if red cells originally present have lysed. Both chemical and microscopic examinations should be applied to all specimens, since neither test will reliably detect all significant abnormalities.

Blood can enter the urine from trauma, hemorrhage, infarction, or infection at any level in the urinary system. Cell-free hemoglobinuria, if not the result of red cell lysis after the urine is voided, indicates intravascular hemolysis, usually due to acquired hemolytic anemia of the cold agglutinin type, paroxysmal nocturnal hemoglobinuria, drug-induced hemolysis, or transfusion reactions.

Free Hemoglobin. Extracellular hemoglobin enters urine only after the hemoglobin-binding capacity of plasma haptoglobin is exceeded. Normal haptoglobin levels can bind as much as 3 Gm of hemoglobin, the amount released from approximately 20 ml of blood. Hemoglobinuria begins within one or two hours of an acute hemolytic event, and does not usually persist beyond 24 hours, although hemosiderin may be excreted for 3 to 5 days thereafter. In paroxysmal nocturnal hemoglobinuria, as in other states of persistent or repeated hemolysis, the sediment may contain hemosiderin granules in casts or in the cytoplasm of epithelial cells. Its presence is detected by treating the sediment with ammonium sulfide, which highlights the hemosiderin as distinct black granules.

Other Significant Colors

Bilirubin and related pigments produce shades ranging from orange through yellow to greenish-brown. Chemical tests for these products are described later in the chapter. Uncommon, but diagnostically significant, causes for peculiar coloration include the following: clear urine which turns dark red on standing suggests porphobilinogen excretion, found in acute intermittent porphyria; clear urine which turns brown or black on standing suggests homogentisic acid, excreted in the amino acid disorder alkaptonuria; or melanogen, excreted in disseminated malignant melanoma.

Artefactual Changes

A number of drugs or dietary items affect urine color, but in themselves have little pathologic importance. Pyridium, used to relieve the pain of bladder and other urinary tract diseases, imparts a lurid orange hue. The vitamin riboflavin, in large doses, turns urine bright orange. Certain dye-stuffs in candies or drugs may sometimes produce red or yellow urine. Alkaline urine turns red in the presence of several related substances including excreted phenolphthalein, sometimes used as a laxative, phenol-sulfonphthalein (PSP) which has laxative effect but is usually administered for a renal function test, and Bromsulphalein (BSP) which is used in liver function testing. Large quantities of phenacetin, used in innumerable pro-prietary pain-relieving preparations, may turn urine brownish-grey or black.[27] The anticonvulsant drug Dilantin and psychoactive drugs of the phenothiazine group may cause pink, red, or reddish-brown urine.

SUGAR

Normal urine contains virtually no sugar. Although approximately 250 Gm of glucose pass through the kidneys daily, no more than 100 mg is excreted in 24 hours.[4] Glucose may occur in urine (glycosuria) if high blood glucose levels produce a glucose load in the filtrate which exceeds the kidneys' reabsorptive capacity, or if the proximal tubules perform this reabsorptive function imperfectly. Sugar in urine was known by the an-cients to be abnormal, and perhaps the earliest form of urinalysis was tasting the urine; the name diabetes mellitus means "flow of sweet urine."

Copper Reduction Tests

The classic present-day test for glucose is Benedict's test, in which the sugar reduces blue alkaline cupric sulphate to red cuprous oxide. This measures reducing activity, not glucose specifically and not even carbohy-drates specifically. In addition to such sugars as fructose and galactose, other urinary constituents which may reduce copper sulfate are creatinine, uric acid, salicylates, and homogentisic acid. In addition, drugs, or contam-inants, such as ascorbic acid or some antibiotics, may cause spurious positives.

Benedict's test is sensitive to concentrations of 50 to 80 mg glucose per 100 ml urine and can be roughly quantitated according to the color and quantity of the precipitate. The single-tablet copper reduction test (Clini-test) employs the same reagents and is slightly less sensitive but far easier than Benedict's test, which requires boiling.

Glucose Oxidase Tests

Reagent-impregnated paper strips and several automated procedures employ a different, highly sensitive and highly specific test for glucose. The strips contain glucose oxidase which reacts with glucose to produce gluconic acid and hydrogen peroxide. The hydrogen peroxide induces color change in orthotoluidine or some other colored indicator, to a degree proportional to the glucose concentration. Adventitious hydrogen peroxide or bleach in the urine container will, of course, produce a false positive, while large quantities of ascorbic acid in the urine delay or abolish the color development. Other reducing substances have no effect on the glucose oxidase methods.

Nonglucose Sugars

Under some conditions, demonstration of other sugars than glucose is highly significant, and the specificity of glucose oxidase is a liability, not an advantage. This is especially true in the urine of young infants, when galactosuria is a more significant finding than glycosuria. Galactose in urine may signal the presence of the potentially disastrous hereditary condition galactosemia (see Chap. 18); infants' urines should be screened with a copper-reduction, not a glucose-oxidase, technique. Galactose will be excreted only if the child is ingesting milk in moderate quantities, so during the immediate newborn period, galactosemia cannot be diagnosed by urine testing.

Other sugars which reduce copper and may be found in urine include lactose, fructose, and five-carbon sugars. Their presence may signify dietary peculiarities or congenital metabolic abnormalities, usually fairly benign except for galactosemia. Pregnant and lactating women may excrete lactose; since glycosuria is very common in pregnancy, the presence of lactose or other sugars will not be noted unless specific tests are done. Both chemical and chromatographic tests are used to identify specific sugars.

KETONES

If tissue needs outstrip the body's available glucose supplies, fat combustion substitutes as an energy supply. Since fat metabolism is less efficient, metabolic end products accumulate and these ketone bodies are excreted in the urine. The three ketone bodies found in urine are betahydroxybutyric acid which accounts for nearly 80 per cent of the ketones present, acetoacetic acid (just under 20 per cent), and acetone which comprises no more than a few per cent.[13] The nitroprusside test generally used for screening ketonuria identifies only acetoacetic acid and acetone, but all three are excreted in parallel proportions, and there is no particular virtue in partitioning the ketones present.

Significance. Any condition of acute metabolic demand with reduced intake, often exacerbated by loss through diarrhea or vomiting or both, can produce ketonuria. In children, stress which might not outstrip an adult's glucose metabolism will produce ketonuria. In adults, significant ketonuria most frequently accompanies uncontrolled episodes of diabetes, when glucose is present but not functionally available for metabolism. The degree of ketonuria roughly reflects the severity of metabolic stress, but accurate quantitation is unnecessary. Reporting excretion as trace, slight, moderate, and severe ketonuria is usually sufficient.

Reagent strips impregnated with nitroprusside and glycine discriminate the level of ketonuria with definite color differences over the range from 5 to 10 mg/100 ml (trace-to-slight), 20 to 30 mg/100 ml (moderate), and 60 mg/100 ml or above (severe). Symptomatic ketosis occurs at levels of 50 mg/100 ml or above,[21] while levels of 20 to 30 mg/100 ml signal moderately serious metabolic imbalance, so these gradations correlate well with clinical usefulness.

PROTEIN

The classic tests for urine protein involve precipitating the proteins, either chemically or by heating. The precipitate includes all types of protein, at a minimum sensitivity of 1 to 10 mg per 100 ml, the quantity of precipitate being roughly proportional to the amount of protein present.

Reagent Strip Methods

Reagent-impregnated strips detect proteinuria with a buffered color indicator (tetrabromphenol blue) which, at pH 3, is yellow when protein is absent and green when protein is present. The advantages of this procedure, besides rapidity, is that turbidity of the specimen or the presence of radio-contrast media or other macromolecules do not affect the results. On the other hand, it detects primarily albumin, and does not indicate the presence of globulins, Bence-Jones protein, other globulin fragments, or myoglobin.

Protein Quantitation

Reagent strips permit modest quantitation of protein present in random specimens, but other techniques are used for total urinary protein excretion. The turbidity produced with sulfosalicylic acid precipitation can be quantitated fairly accurately, giving a specific figure for protein in all or part of a collected specimen. Either a total 24-hour collection or smaller timed aliquot can be used. Normal excretion is no more than 150 mg in 24 hours.

The standard curve used for quantitation goes up to concentrations of 100 mg protein in 100 ml urine. If the patient's urine has more protein than this, it can be diluted to fall within the range, and appropriate calculations made for actual concentration. Sulfosalicylic acid precipitates polypeptides, Bence-Jones protein, and proteoses (heat soluble glycoproteins) as well as albumin and normal globulins, so a variety of abnormal constituents may be included in the total figure.

Significance. Protein excretion above 150 mg per day is nearly always significant. Most often the protein is albumin. Albuminuria frequently indicates abnormal glomerular permeability, due either to intrinsic glomerular disease or to changes in blood pressure, as in hypertension, pre-eclampsia, or abnormalities of the renal veins. The list of all conditions causing proteinuria of any degree would simply be a list of all possible urinary tract diseases. Massive proteinuria, greater than 4 Gm per day, is the hallmark of the nephrotic syndrome, which can be "idiopathic," or due to lupus erythematosus, amyloid disease, or other conditions. The proteinuria in glomerulonephritis is inconstantly related to the severity or the phase of the process. When glomerular function is severely reduced, as in acute proliferative glomerulonephritis or chronic glomerulonephritis approaching "end-stage" disease, proteinuria may be minimal.

Inflammatory Signs. Large numbers of white cells accompanying proteinuria usually signal infection at some level in the urinary tract, the protein originating from the white cells, the bacteria, or the increased capillary permeability that inflammation induces. Noninfectious inflammatory diseases of the glomeruli tend to contribute both red and white blood cells accompanying proteinuria, notably in glomerulonephritis and the nephritis of lupus erythematosus. Proteinuria does not inevitably accompany renal disease. Pyelonephritis, obstructions, nephrolithiasis, tumors, and metabolic nephropathies may cause severe illness without telltale protein leakage.

Orthostatic Proteinuria. Somewhat perplexing is the significance of postural (orthostatic) proteinuria, found in up to 5 per cent of healthy adolescents and young adults, usually male. There is evidence[33] that consistent protein leakage, occurring only in the upright position and without other urinary abnormalities, is unlikely to develop into more severe disease later. Persistent proteinuria unrelated to posture, or intermittent proteinuria occurring with no predictable physiologic concomitant, carry greater likelihood of unfavorable prognosis and existing renal biopsy changes.

PROTEINS OTHER THAN ALBUMIN

Of increasing significance are the proteinurias not due to albumin. These include the classic example, Bence-Jones protein of multiple myeloma, as well as the proteins or protein components in heavy chain disease, macroglobulinemia and various tubular defects. These will be detected by heat precipitation or sulfosalicylic acid, whereupon specific immunologic, electrophoretic, or chromatographic identification should be undertaken. Reagent-strip testing does not screen adequately for these conditions. The urine found to be negative with strip testing and positive with sulfosalicylic acid signals a need for more detailed investigation.

Bence-Jones Protein

Bence-Jones protein is the most commonly sought nonalbumin protein in urine. These low molecular weight polypeptides (molecular weight 22,000 to 44,000) are immunoglobulin light chains which circulate and enter the urine as monomers, dimers, and trimers or tetramers. Approximately 60 per cent of patients with multiple myeloma have this distinctive form of proteinuria. The Bence-Jones protein precipitates reversibly at temperatures between 45° and 60°C, re-entering suspension at higher or lower temperatures.

Heat Testing. The classic test consists of placing the slightly acidified urine sample in a water bath and raising the temperature gradually to the boiling point. If turbidity develops at the mid-range, disappears as the boiling point approaches, reappears as the urine cools, and then disappears on return to room temperature, the demonstration is virtually conclusive. Turbidity may fail to clear when the urine cools if other proteins have been precipitated by the heat, or if the urine has been excessively acidified. Filtering the turbid specimen at high temperatures may remove precipitated protein and permit demonstration of the appropriately reacting Bence-Jones material, but some Bence-Jones proteins do not completely disperse at high temperature.

Electrophoresis. Heat testing may miss as many as one third of Bence-Jones proteinurias.[16] It is preferable, in patients with suspected myeloma or other dysproteinemias, to perform electrophoresis of the urine proteins. It is usually necessary to concentrate the urine sample, since electrophoresis is unsatisfactory at protein concentrations below 0.5 to 1 Gm per 100 ml. Bence-Jones protein appears as a peak at the α_2-globulin location. Serum electrophoresis usually does not reveal circulating Bence-Jones protein, since the small molecules pass rapidly through the glomerular filter and are, in addition, rapidly destroyed by bodily metabolism.[17] Most myeloma patients also produce whole immunoglobulin in a diagnostically significant monoclonal pattern, although in perhaps 20 per cent of patients the isolated light chains may be the only detectable abnormal secretory product.[17] Bence-Jones proteinuria may occasionally accompany macroglobulinemia and, rarer still, some leukemias.[47]

Electrophoretic Patterns

Electrophoresis of urine proteins may demonstrate that abnormal serum constituents, potentially damaging to the kidney, have entered the urine for excretion. Albumin is the prominent urinary protein when glomerular permeability is increased, but with normal glomerular permeability and various prerenal abnormalities, circulating globulins may appear in the urine. Bence-Jones protein is especially important because it does not appear on serum electrophoretograms. Hemoglobins, following intravascular hemolysis, and myoglobin, following extensive muscle damage, appear on urine electrophoretograms at the α_1-globulin band. In conditions of catabolic stress and "inflammatory syndrome," there may be α_1-globulin elevations without increased albumin.[2] If the stress or systemic damage alters glomerular permeability in addition, a high albumin peak accompanies the α_1 peak. Cawley[2] describes a pattern of increased α_2 and β_2 globulins with decreased albumin as indicating tubular damage of various etiologies, including phenacetin intoxication, severe chronic hypokalemia, chronic pyelonephritis, and the hereditary disorders of tubular function.

MICROSCOPIC EXAMINATION OF SEDIMENT

The urine sediment, containing cells and other formed elements, constitutes a direct sampling of urinary tract morphology. For best results, urine should be examined within an hour or two of voiding, and a concentrated urine will contain proportionally more formed elements than a dilute specimen. The first or second voided morning specimen usually gives best results, and the number of organized elements can be roughly quantitated from their number in a centrifuged aliquot. More accurate quantitation is sometimes obtained by the Addis count on a 12-hour timed collection, but more often qualitative judgments provide sufficient information. Significant elements to be sought in all specimens are red blood cells, white blood cells, epithelial cells, casts, trichomonads, bacteria, and yeasts.

Collection Technique

Sediment of normal urine may contain occasional white blood cells and squamous epithelial cells, but should be virtually free of red blood cells. Cleansing and collection procedures are critical, for urine voided through an inadequately cleansed meatus may contain leukocytes, epithelial cells, bacteria, and, especially from menstruating women, red blood cells. Over-enthusiastic cleansing, combined with poor collection technique, may introduce red cells, extraneous fibers, epithelial cells, and starch or powder granules. If technique has been satisfactory and the voided urine is examined within two or three hours, the sediment can be considered representative of the bladder contents. Urine specimens refrigerated for 12 to 24 hours can still provide valid bacteriologic information, but in the absence of preservative, casts and cells begin to deteriorate after about three hours.

Inflammation

The usual cause of urinary leukocytosis is acute infection somewhere in the urinary tract. If the infection is in the kidney, the white cells tend to be associated with cellular and granular casts, bacteria, renal epithelial cells, and relatively few red cells. The degree of pyuria need not reflect the severity of the inflammatory process, but rather the proximity of the infection to functioning nephrons, collecting ducts, and the pelvis.

Bladder infections will not produce casts, since the process occurs below the level of renal tubules, the only site where casts are formed. Cystitis frequently produces red cells in the sediment, as well as leukocytes and, often, large epithelial cells of bladder origin. Cystitis may be bacterial or nonbacterial, with little distinction in the sediment, although the cultures will provide necessary differentiation. In acute glomerulonephritis there may be significant urinary leukocytosis, although red cells usually predominate. Various noninfectious inflammatory diseases of the kidney, ureters, and bladder may contribute moderate numbers of white cells to the sediment.

Red Blood Cells

Red cells greatly in excess of leukocytes indicate bleeding into the urinary tract. Among other causes, this may be due to trauma, which can usually be elicited by history; tumor, in which case cytologic examination of the urinary sediment may permit positive diagnosis; or systemic bleeding disorders, such as thrombocytopenia, acquired hemorrhagic diatheses, congenital deficiencies, aspirin ingestion, or anticoagulant therapy. In acute glomerulonephritis, red cells enter the urine because of glomerular capillary damage, and in necrotizing arteriolarsclerosis, there may be intermittent mild hematuria because of small vessel hemorrhage.

Casts

Casts composed largely or exclusively of cells indicate exudative, hemorrhagic, or desquamative conditions of the nephron. Red cell casts suggest destructive lesions of the glomerulus, and are fairly common in acute glomerulonephritis; they are less conspicuous in severe lupus nephritis, arteritis of any cause, or necrotizing arteriolarsclerosis. White cell casts may be difficult to distinguish from epithelial cell casts, and both kinds of cells may be intermixed. During recovery from acute tubular damage, desquamated epithelial cells may aggregate as casts, but in inflammatory states, leukocytes and epithelial cells tend to be present together. So-called granular casts probably represent degenerated cellular elements embedded in the protein matrix. The nature of *waxy* casts, which are homogeneous, sharply defined, and highly refractile, is uncertain.

Cast Formation. Most casts derive from the distal convoluted tubules, where hydrogen ion and electrolyte concentrations are high, and have the narrow caliber of this segment. Occasionally casts are seen which are wide-bore and originate from the collecting tubules. Urine flow in these ducts is normally too swift for casts to form, so development of broad casts indicates severe slowing of the urinary stream and pronounced renal malfunction. The ducts where this occurs tend to be those whose contributing nephrons have been damaged or destroyed, so these wide casts reflect severe kidney damage and are sometimes called *renal failure* casts.

CRYSTALS

Most crystals or amorphous material have little clinical significance, but may obscure other elements in the sediment. Crystalluria becomes important in some disorders of amino acid metabolism, notably cystine, leucine, or tyrosine, or in patients taking poorly soluble sulfa drugs or other medications. The clinician should alert the laboratory that these elements may be present, to facilitate special examination and identification. Far more common findings in urinary sediment are crystalline or amorphous urates, calcium oxalate, and crystalline or amorphous phosphates. Bilirubin and cholesterol may occasionally be present as urinary crystals.

OTHER FINDINGS

Motile trichomonads are sometimes present in urine specimens from women with vaginitis, if collecting technique has been poor. In men, trichomonads can produce urethritis and occasionally the organisms may be seen in the urine. When fungi or bacteria are present in urine sediment, the cause may be significant infection or multiplication of a few organisms in a specimen that has been standing for too long. Globules of cholesterol and other lipids are sometimes seen in urine from patients with intense proteinuria. Since lipid vacuoles occur in tubular epithelial cells when proteinuria is severe, these globules may derive from coalesced epithelial vacuoles or degenerated cells, or they may result in some way from the high serum lipid levels usually present in these patients.

SPECIAL TESTS

BILIRUBIN AND UROBILINOGEN

Tests are available for many other substances which may appear in urine under various clinical conditions. The abnormal constituent most often sought, and found, is bilirubin. Since bilirubin is water soluble only when conjugated, it is posthepatic, direct-reacting bilirubin that appears in urine. This form, normally excreted in the bile, enters urine when blood levels are high, so jaundice of some degree always accompanies bilirubinuria. With severe jaundice, the renal excretory pathway achieves metabolic significance, and serum bilirubin levels may increase if renal function deteriorates.[8]

The classic cause for bilirubinuria is extrahepatic biliary tract obstruction, but conjugated bilirubin may enter the urine when there is portal inflammation or hepatocellular damage. In viral or toxic hepatitis, bilirubinuria may be conspicuous. Urine color may range from yellow-orange through brown, depending on the concentration, and shaking the specimen produces a yellow foam. Urine pigmented from urobilin and urobilinogen does not have yellow foam when shaken; this permits differentiation of a sort, but there are better tests available for both substances than the "foam test."

Urobilinogen

Urobilinogen is formed in the intestine from normally excreted conjugated bilirubin. Bacterial activity produces a series of colorless substances known collectively as urobilinogen (also called stercobilinogen) which, upon oxidation, form orange-brown urobilin (stercobilin) which gives normal feces their color. Some urobilinogen is absorbed from the colon into the blood stream, whence it returns to the liver, for re-excretion in bile. This enterohepatic circulation appears to serve no useful function, but the water-soluble urobilinogen enters the urinary filtrate as blood goes through the kidney.

Increased Urine Levels. Normally, urine contains small quantities of urobilinogen, but pathologic amounts appear if abnormally large amounts are present in the intestine, or if the liver cannot re-excrete the absorbed urobilinogen. With increased hemoglobin breakdown, intestinal urobilinogen increases and urinary urobilinogen rises. Urine urobilinogen levels can be a sensitive indicator of hepatic damage, since hepatic urobilinogen excretion is more vulnerable to mild parenchymal damage than is bilirubin excretion. Early hepatitis or mild toxic injury may cause elevated circulating urobilinogen because of decreased biliary-tract excretion, despite unchanged serum bilirubin levels. In such cases, elevated urine urobilinogen points to incipient liver disease. Obviously if no bilirubin enters the bile, no urobilinogen will be produced. With severe liver damage or obstruction, both urinary and fecal urobilinogen will decline. The classic association of pale stools and dark urine in obstructive jaundice results from diminished intestinal bilirubin being converted to the chromogen, while increased plasma bilirubin enters the urine.

Urine Tests

Bilirubin. Tests for urinary bilirubin employ either a diazo reaction or the oxidation of bilirubin to biliverdin. Fouchet's test employs the oxidation principle, with trichloracetic acid and ferric chloride added to whatever bilirubin remains when filtered urine is adsorbed onto barium chloride. A positive result is appearance of a green spot. Even if exposure to air has oxidized some bilirubin, this test may be positive. The diazo test, available in tablet form, reacts only with the somewhat labile nonoxidized form, so the age of the specimen may affect the results of tablet testing. Positive tests result in purple or blue-purple coloration.

Since urine contains only conjugated bilirubin, there is no need to worry about "direct" and "indirect" reactions. Urobilin, the oxidation product of urobilinogen, may produce a red spot with this test, or a muddy purple color on Fouchet's test, but both constitute negative results for bilirubin. Salicylates may also give false positives, and large amounts of ascorbic acid can interfere with both tests.

Urobilinogen. Urobilinogen testing uses Ehrlich's aldehyde reagent. Urobilin will not react, so the specimen must be protected from oxidation. Besides urobilinogen, porphobilinogen, sulfonamides, and 5-hydroxyin- loleacetic acid (5-HIAA) all react with Ehrlich's aldehyde reagent, but urobilinogen can be separated by chloroform extraction for identification if necessary. Small amounts of urobilinogen are normal, so results must be quantitated.

The Watson-Schwartz method measures the amount of urobilinogen excreted in a carefully timed two-hour collection period between the hours of 1 and 3 in the afternoon, and the results are given in Ehrlich units. The classic technique uses spectrophotometric reading for accurate quantita- tion. A reagent strip method permits semiquantitation by comparing devel- oped color against reference blocks. The normal concentration range is one tenth to one Ehrlich unit per 100 ml urine, or less than one Ehrlich unit in a two-hour collection. Patients with biliary obstruction or diminished bacte- rial flora will excrete little or no urobilinogen, but there is no reliable way of documenting abnormally low urinary urobilinogen. Strongly acid urine may give a falsely low test result. Porphobilinogen (see below) also gives positive results with Ehrlich's aldehyde reagent.

HEMOGLOBIN PRECURSORS

Porphobilinogen is a hemoglobin precursor rather than a breakdown product. It is a single-ringed structure which develops from the straight- chain molecule delta-aminolevulinic acid. Heme synthesis progresses from delta-aminolevulinic acid (ALA), through porphobilinogen to the four- ringed precursors uroporphyrinogen, coproporphyrinogen, protoporphyri- nogen, and protoporphyrin which finally combines with iron to become heme. The porphyrinogen forms are hematologically active and remain in the marrow. The inactive end products uroporphyrin and coproporphyrin are excreted in urine and feces.

Secondary Porphyrias

A group of heritable metabolic diseases, the porphyrias, produce ab- normal porphyrin values in both urine and feces. With impaired hemato- poiesis or decreased liver function[45] porphyrin excretion may also rise. Rare cases of liver disease and severe lead poisoning may elevate urinary levels of uroporphyrin, but the more frequent urinary metabolite in secondary porphyria is coproporphyrin. Mild coproporphyrinuria may accompany heavy metal poisoning; carbon tetrachloride or benzene toxicity; Hodg- kin's disease; some cases of hemolytic, aplastic, or megaloblastic anemia;

and, in an unpredictable fashion, liver disease of various kinds. Substantial porphyrinuria, however, usually signifies a primary metabolic disorder.

Primary Porphyrias

Erythropoietic Porphyria. The porphyrias are divided into two different groups, classified as erythropoietic and hepatic. In the erythropoietic forms, the major accumulation of porphyrins is in the erythrocytes. Up to 50 mg of urinary uroporphyrin per day may be excreted in the least rare of these conditions; in the other forms, fecal and urinary uroporphyrin, coproporphyrin, and protoporphyrin levels are not significant. Urinary levels of ALA and porphobilinogen are normal in all the erythropoietic conditions, and definitive diagnosis rests on red cell studies.

Hepatic Porphyrias. In the hepatic porphyrias, red cell levels of heme precursors are normal, and diagnosis rests on urinary and fecal determinations. The three major forms of hepatic porphyria are: acute intermittent porphyria, characterized by markedly increased urinary ALA and porphobilinogen, moderate urinary uroporphyrin, and mildly elevated urinary coproporphyrin; porphyria cutanea tarda, in which ALA and porphobilinogen are normal, but urinary uroporphyrin and coproporphyrin are both markedly elevated; and variegate porphyria, a disease chiefly associated with South Africa, in which porphobilinogen and ALA appear in urine during acute attacks, along with both coproporphyrin and uroporphyrin. Fecal levels of protoporphyrin are markedly elevated in variegate porphyria, a finding distinctive for this condition.

Porphobilinogen Determination. Normal porphobilinogen excretion is 1 to 1.5 mg per day. During active episodes of acute intermittent porphyria, porphobilinogen excretion increases enormously. When the disease is latent, the substance may or may not be present in diagnostic amounts. Porphobilinogen converts to dark red porphobilin and colorless porphyrins on standing. Since these do not react with the aldehyde reagent, fresh specimens should be used for testing. On the other hand, the observation that a specimen turns wine-colored on standing may indicate that porphyria should be considered in a patient's differential diagnosis.

If the Ehrlich's aldehyde test is positive on whole urine, chloroform extraction can be used to remove most extraneous Ehrlich-reactive materials. The aqueous phase remains Ehrlich-reactive if porphobilinogen is present. Subsequent butanol extraction gives even better identification, since butanol removes all the Ehrlich-reactive material except porphobilinogen, which steadfastly remains in the aqueous phase. In porphyria cutanea tarda, another hepatic porphyria, porphobilinogen may occasionally be increased.

Screening with Ultra-violet Light. The simplest screening test for urinary porphyrins is to view the specimen with ultraviolet light. The porphyrins exhibit orange fluorescence in highly acid urine, and orange-red to red fluorescence as the pH rises. Coproporphyrin is extracted from the aqueous urine with ethyl acetate or ether at lower pH, in the range of 3 to 3.5,[7] or by absorption onto alumina or column chromatography. Quantitation is possible by spectrophotometric or fluorometric measurement, but the degree and shade of fluorescence may permit sufficient estimation for diagnostic purposes.

Delta-Aminolevulinic Acid. In acute intermittent porphyria, delta-aminolevulinic acid (ALA) is markedly increased, as well as porphobilinogen. At least a part of the metabolic defect in this disease is an increase in the hepatic enzyme ALA-synthetase, leading to build-up of both substances.[44] Screening batteries to diagnose porphyria do not usually include testing for urinary ALA, because porphobilinogen testing is more productive. Urinary ALA levels are, however, used in screening for lead poisoning, since lead toxicity very early impairs hemoglobin synthesis at the stage where ALA is converted to porphobilinogen. Thus ALA builds up to be excreted in the urine, where it can be detected and quantified. Normal urine ALA levels should be below 0.5 mg/100 ml; values above that, in populations at risk, suggest toxic damage.

Industrial exposure, either acute or chronic, is a hazard in adults. Childhood plumbism tends to be insidious and associated with pica and with deteriorated housing conditions. Urinary ALA levels may occasionally be within normal limits despite significant levels of blood lead, so the screening test is not ideal. Measuring blood lead is difficult and expensive, so the search continues for a better screening test for early plumbism. One very promising approach is measurement of blood ALA-dehydratase, the enzyme whose reduced activity leads to ALA accumulation,[14] but urinary ALA determination remains, at present, an important tool for evaluating possible lead toxicity.

CALCIUM

Urinary calcium excretion is largely determined by serum calcium levels and the equilibrium between calcium and phosphates. A normal individual excretes as much as 200 to 400 mg calcium daily on diets containing between 500 mg to 1 Gm of calcium.[30] Marked changes in dietary intake produce only slight variation in urinary calcium excretion. The serum calcium level is far more important than calcium intake in determining excretion. Normally, up to 99 per cent of filtered calcium is reabsorbed. When serum calcium levels fall to 7.5 mg per 100 ml or below, virtually all the filtered calcium is salvaged, leaving practically none in the excreted urine. Calcium excretion rises with high sodium and magnesium intakes, while increasing dietary phosphate reduces calcium excretion. Metabolic acidosis and glucocorticoid excess also increase calciuria.

Hypercalciuria

Increased calcium excretion almost always accompanies elevated serum calcium levels. Hyperparathyroidism produces the most striking hypercalciuria, but increased excretion occurs whenever calcium is mobilized from bone, as in metastatic malignancies, Paget's disease of bone, and prolonged skeletal immobilization. Hypercalciuria may also accompany multiple myeloma, sarcoid, vitamin D intoxication, and some cases of thyrotoxicosis. Calcium excretion fluctuates throughout the day, being heaviest just after meals and lowest at night, so accurate evaluation of total calcium excretion requires 24-hour determination. The specimen should be collected with 10 ml of concentrated hydrochloric acid so calcium salts will not precipitate. Calcium excretion greater than intake is always excessive, and excretion above 400 to 500 mg in 24 hours is reliably abnormal.

The Sulkowitch Test

The quantitative methods used for serum calcium can also be used for urine determinations. The Sulkowitch test is a simple, time-honored means for qualitative evaluation. Although the results cover a wide range of quantitative equivalents, the test remains useful. In the Sulkowitch test, a calcium oxalate precipitate forms in the presence of acetic acid and oxalates, the amount of precipitate roughly proportional to the amount of calcium present.

Range of Results. The traditional interpretation is that normal urine produces a fine white cloud, neither a clear solution which indicates no calcium at all, nor a heavy precipitate reflecting excessive excretion. If normal excretion is taken as 150 mg in 24 hours, and normal urine volume as 1500 ml, then an average normal specimen should contain roughly 10 mg per 100 ml. Ritter and his colleagues[35] found that a 2+ Sulkowitch reading corresponded to a mean of 9 mg/100 ml, but 2+ readings could be found in urine specimens ranging from 3 to 23 mg/100 ml. Negative results clearly indicate decreased calcium excretion, covering a range from 1 to 3.45 mg/100 ml, and 4+ is clearly increased (30 to 43 mg/100 ml) but between these extremes, the range of scatter is wide.

The Sulkowitch test is used primarily on random specimens, to identify the reduced calcium excretion that accompanies decreased serum levels or to document excessive excretion if other signs and symptoms point to hyperparathyroidism. Specimens should be selected with diurnal variation in mind. To rule out hypercalciuria, an early morning specimen should be examined, since excretion is lowest then. If hypocalcemia is suspected, the sample should be taken after a meal, when excretion is maximal. The test is sufficiently simple that repeated determinations are feasible, at home by the patient himself, if necessary.

AMINO ACID ABNORMALITIES

Amino acids appear in urine either when metabolic dysfunction presents abnormal amino acid loads to a normal kidney, or when an abnormal kidney is unable to process the normally constituted glomerular filtrate. Most of the abnormal filtered loads result from inborn errors of metabolism, although occasional acquired conditions, such as severe liver disease or intravenous alimentation with protein hydrolysates, may produce generalized aminoaciduria. Inborn renal tubular disorders usually involve specific transport mechanisms, whose malfunction results in excretion of predictable amino acids. With acquired renal damage, the degree of aminoaciduria reflects the severity of the damage. Chromatography of urine and plasma is essential for accurate diagnosis, although screening procedures are available for several particularly significant conditions.

Phenylketonuria

More urine amino acid tests are done for phenylketonuria, the clinical syndrome arising from phenylalanine hydroxylase deficiency, than for any other amino acid disorder. This is partly because it is less rare than most (an autosomally recessive condition estimated to occur once every 20,000 live births),[22a] and also because prompt recognition and treatment can avert the disastrous consequences of the metabolic abnormality. The enzyme deficiency prevents conversion of phenylpyruvic acid to tyrosine. The accumulating phenylalanine is converted into phenylpyruvic acid and thence to phenyllactic and phenylacetic acids, all of which appear in the urine.

Urinary screening uses ferric chloride, which produces a blue-gray appearance in the presence of phenylpyruvic acid. Blood phenylalanine level is a more distinctive indicator of phenylketonuria than urinary screening. This is most often evaluated by Guthrie's technique of measuring the growth-enhancing effect that phenylalanine has on cultures of B. subtilis. In the test procedure, an inhibiting agent is introduced into the growth medium. Phenylalanine, at levels above 4 mg/100 ml, overcomes the inhibition; the higher the phenylalanine concentration, the greater the bacterial growth.

Ferric Chloride Testing. Ferric chloride-impregnated strips are available for simple, rapid screening. Ferric chloride also signals urinary abnormalities in patients with tyrosinosis, alcaptonuria, "maple-syrup urine disease" (branched chain ketoaciduria), histidinemia, and "oasthouse urine disease" (excretion of β-hydroxybutyric acid, tyrosine, and methionine as well as phenylalanine), so the screening strips are useful for many of these rare conditions. In most amino acid disorders, abnormal metabolites reliably appear in urine only when postnatal diet and metabolism are stabilized. For best results, screening should be done at several weeks of age, rather than in the immediate newborn period. More detailed study is required of infants with positive or suggestive results.

Alkaptonuria

Alkaptonuria, the syndrome accompanying homogentisic acid oxidase deficiency, can be detected by observing that the urine turns black on standing or if alkalinized. The urinary metabolite is homogentisic acid, a fairly late-stage product of phenylalanine metabolism. In affected individuals, this substance is present in urine, but not in serum, shortly after birth and throughout life. The symptoms of connective tissue and joint degeneration do not appear until late in adult life. Homogentisic acid reduces Benedict's reagent, gives a purple-black color with ferric chloride, and blackens a saturated solution of silver nitrate.

Cystinuria

In cystinuria, the dibasic amino acids cystine, lysine, arginine, and ornithine are excreted excessively, with cystine predominating. Cystine is poorly soluble, and its lifelong presence at high concentration often leads to urinary tract calculi and renal damage. The screening test is not difficult. Sodium nitroprusside added to alkalinized urine treated with sodium cyanide produces a magenta color proportional to the amount of amino acid present. The flat, hexagonal, cystine crystals can also be recognized on microscopic examination of concentrated urine specimens.

The disease is transmitted as an autosomal recessive, with an incidence of at least 1:20,000. Heterozygotes also excrete excessive quantities of cystine, and mass screening has revealed an incidence of presumed heterozygotes of 1:200.[3] Therapy is directed toward maintaining a high volume of dilute urine so that crystallization does not occur. Except for the renal damage induced by cystine stones, even the homozygous condition is relatively innocuous. Positive cyanide-nitroprusside tests also occur in cystinosis (a far more damaging but less common condition) and homocystinuria. Urine and plasma chromatography readily distinguish these conditions, over and above the differences in clinical presentation.

PRODUCTS OF MELANOGENIC NEOPLASMS

Some patients with melanin-producing malignant tumors excrete in urine a colorless precursor, melanogen, which is readily identifiable and specific for the disease. Colorless initially, melanogen darkens spontaneously if left at room temperature for 24 hours. Ferric chloride, with added HCl, turns the urine brownish-black, and sodium nitroprusside (Thormählen test) produces a dark bluish-black or greenish-black reaction. Homogentisic acid behaves somewhat like melanogen, in that it darkens spontaneously on standing and blackens ferric chloride and ammoniacal silver nitrate. Melanogen, however, does not darken more rapidly when alkalinized, as does homogentisic acid. It also reacts more slowly with silver nitrate than homogentisic acid, which starts turning black even before ammonia is added.

CARCINOID TUMORS

Another urinary constituent identified with neoplasm is 5-hydroxyindoleacetic acid (5-HIAA), a denaturation product of serotonin. Serotonin is a vasoconstricting and neuroactive indoleamine produced by argentaffin cells of the gastrointestinal tract, and present in the blood bound to platelets. Argentaffin tumors, also called carcinoid tumors, elaborate great quantities of serotonin, resulting in large quantities of the metabolic end-product 5-HIAA. Determination of urinary 5-HIAA, a fairly simple test, is the diagnostic procedure for hormonally active argentaffin tumors. Normal persons excrete 2 to 10 mg of 5-HIAA daily, while patients with active carcinoid may excrete 50 to 500 mg or more. Carcinoid syndrome is the only condition causing pronounced 5-HIAA excretion, although minor elevations may occur in nontropical sprue.

Urinary testing depends upon the reaction of 5-HIAA with nitrosonaphthol to produce a purple color. Phenothiazine drugs interfere with the reaction, and false positives may result from ingestion, within 72 hours, of reserpine, acetanilid-containing preparations, or serotonin-containing foods like bananas or pineapple. Both the screening and the quantitative procedures employ the same reaction, but in the quantitative technique potentially interfering ketoacids are removed and 5-HIAA is twice extracted to enhance specificity and intensity of the reaction.

DRUG METABOLITES

Urine tests for drug metabolites may be used as guides to the blood level and possible toxicity of the drug in question, or to monitor whether or not a patient has taken certain drugs. Chromatography, either thin-layer or gas-liquid, affords the most accurate and complete information about drug metabolites. Large-scale screening programs for drugs of abuse use thin-layer chromatography, and comprehensive toxicology laboratories use these techniques along with radioimmunoassay. The older, presumptive tests for toxicology screening continue to be useful, but with limitations. Salicylates, barbiturates, phenothiazines, and the morphine derivatives are the substances most often of emergency importance. Chronic ingestion of heavy metals may also be at issue.

Barbiturates

The urine is not the best specimen for barbiturate testing. Short-acting barbiturates may be lethal before significant quantities are excreted, and with the longer-acting preparations, the urinary level correlates poorly with blood levels. Stomach contents can be tested in the same fashion as urine, often with more useful results for immediate toxicologic diagnosis. Blood levels are essential for monitoring therapy. The screening procedure involves formation of chloroform-soluble mercuric complexes, which turn purple when reacted with diphenylcarbazone. Hydantoins, certain analgesics, and glutethimide (Doriden) also react in this way. If the first chloroform extract is subjected to controlled hydrolysis, barbiturates remain measurable, but the other drugs lose reactivity.

Salicylates

Salicylates and phenothiazines both produce a purple reactant with ferric chloride. Ferric chloride-impregnated reagent strips turn purple in the presence of either group, but concentrated sulfuric acid intensifies the color produced by phenothiazines, and may diminish the purple produced by salicylates. This procedure is really too sensitive to be useful, since ingestion of as little as 300 mg (one adult tablet) of aspirin can produce a positive result. If salicylate toxicity is suspected, evaluation of acid-base status and determination of blood salicylate levels are essential, since the quantity of urinary salicylates may not reflect clinical severity.

Phenothiazines

An effective screening test for documenting phenothiazine derivatives in urine uses a mixture of perchloric acid, nitric acid, and ferric chloride (FPN reagent[10]) to produce a pink-through-violet color, which depends on the drug and its dose. Chromatography or ultraviolet spectral absorption are needed for identification of specific drugs.

Drugs of Abuse

Satisfactory identification of morphine, amphetamines, and other organic bases requires chromatographic analysis. Thin-layer techniques which are both rapid and reliable are available for this purpose.[5]

HEAVY METALS

To screen for heavy metals, the Reinsch test is simple and valuable. A shiny copper wire is heated in the acidified specimen, which may be urine, blood, or gastric fluid. If arsenic, mercury, bismuth, or antimony are present, a deposit coats the surface roughly proportionally to the concentration of the metal. Mercury produces a shiny or silvery deposit, while the others are gray to black. More specific quantitative tests are available if the screening test is positive.

URINARY CALCULI

It is often helpful to analyze stones that occur in the urinary tract, since their composition may highlight a treatable metabolic condition, but in about half the cases of nephrolithiasis no etiology can be found.[31] The incidence of urinary calculi appears to be increasing,[24] a tendency some have attributed to increasingly sedentary life styles and improper diet or hydration or both.

CALCIUM

Calcium is the most common constituent of renal stones, and hypercalcemia is often associated with stone formation. Oxalates and phosphates usually accompany calcium. Conditions to be considered with calcium stones include hyperparathyroidism, hypervitaminosis D, milk-alkali syndrome, multiple myeloma, sarcoid, and various bone diseases.

CYSTINE

Cystine stones comprise less than 1 per cent of identified stones,[15] but when found, this observation should prompt a workup for the heritable amino acid abnormality cystinuria (see p. 248). Cystine stones tend to be soft, lustrous, and white or yellowish-white. Several fairly simple chemical tests using sodium cyanide and nitroprusside or naphthoquinone reagent can identify cystine calculi, and subsequent investigation should include urine chromatography for amino acid analysis. Prevention of further cystine stones is, therapeutically, fairly straightforward. Since prevention requires lifelong awareness and cooperation from the patient, the diagnosis should be made as early and as reliably as possible.

URATES

Uric acid or urate-containing stones accounted for approximately 10 per cent of Herring's series of 10,000 analyses.[15] Patients with high serum uric acid are likely to form stones, whether the hyperuricemia results from a gouty diathesis, or from cell destruction. When urine is highly concentrated or very acid, urate precipitation is more likely. In some patients, inappropriate tubular function leads to persistently acid urine. Dehydration or chronically low fluid intake predisposes to stones of all kinds, especially urates. Therapy aims at maintaining large volumes of dilute urine with neutral or higher pH. Urate calculi are identified by the murexide test or by development of blue color when a sodium carbonate suspension of the stone is reacted with phosphotungstic acid.

PHOSPHATES

Phosphate is a common anion in renal stones, but occurred as the principal constituent in only 16 per cent of Herring's series. Stones that are predominantly phosphates tend to be friable, pale, and variable in size. "Staghorn" calculi often consist largely of phosphates, as do stones in any location associated with infection, stasis, and alkaline pH. Phosphates produce a yellow precipitate when ammonium molybdate is added to the pulverized stone, and calcium phosphate produces a dense white precipitate when sodium hydroxide reacts with an acid extract of the stone. Other cations that accompany phosphates are ammonium and magnesium, which occur together as part of so-called triple phosphate stones.

OXALATES

Calcium oxalates, in various chemical combinations, are the most common findings when stones are analyzed. These produce a fine white precipitate when sodium hydroxide is mixed with the acid extract. The oxalate constituents produce a slow bluish-green reaction with resorcinol reagent, and release gas bubbles when magnesium dioxide is added to an acid extract of pulverized stone.

Very rare stone constituents include xanthine, glycine, silica, and sulfonamide crystals.

BIBLIOGRAPHY

1. BRICKER, N.S., AND KLAHR, S.: The physiologic basis of sodium-excretion and diuresis. Adv. Intern. Med. 16:17, 1970.
2. CAWLEY, L.P.: Electrophoresis and Immunoelectrophoresis. Little, Brown, Co., Boston, 1969.
3. CRAWHALL, J.C., SCOWEN, E.F., THOMPSON, C.J., AND WATTS, R.W.E.: The renal clearance of amino acids in cystinuria. J. Clin. Invest. 46:1162, 1967.
4. DATE, J.W.: Quantitative determination of some carbohydrates in normal urine. Scand. J. Clin. Lab. Invest. 10:155, 1958.
5. DAVIDOW, B., LiPETRI, N., QUAME, B. ET AL.: A thin layer chromatographic screening test for the detection of users of morphine and heroin. Am. J. Clin. Pathol. 46:58, 1966.
6. DONAT, P. E., BARLOW, R.S., AND ALBERS, D.D.: Fourteen-hour concentrated urine osmolality as a renal function test in children. J. Urol. 104:478, 1970.
7. FERNANDEZ, A.A., AND JACOBS, S.L.: Porphyrins, porphobilinogen and aminolevulinic acid in urine. Stand. Meth. Clin. Chem. 6:57, 1970.
8. FLEISCHNER, G., AND ARIAS, I.M.: Recent advances in bilirubin formation, transport, metabolism, and excretion. Am. J. Med. 49:576, 1970.
9. FLOCKS, R.H.: Urinary tract infection. Med. Clin. North Am. 54:397, 1970.
10. FORREST, I.S., FORREST, F.M., AND KANTER, S.L.: Elimination of false negative results with the FPN Forrest test for phenothiazine derivatives in urine. Clin. Chem. 12:379, 1966.
11. GUTHRIE, R., AND SUSI, A.: A simple phenylalanine method for detecting phenylketonuria in large populations of newborn infants. Pediatrics 32:338, 1963.
12. HENDLER, E.D., KASHGARIAN, M., AND HAYSLETT, J.P.: Clinicopathological correlations of primary haematuria. Lancet 1:458, 1972.
13. HENRY, R.J.: Clinical Chemistry: Principles and Techniques. Harper & Row, New York, 1964.
14. HERNBERG, S., NIKKANEN, J., MELLIN, G. ET AL.: δ-amino levulinic acid dehydrase as a measure of lead exposure. Arch. Environ. Health (Chicago) 21:140, 1970.
15. HERRING, L.C.: Observations on the analysis of ten thousand urinary calculi. J. Urol. 88:545, 1962.
16. HOBBS, J.R.: The detection of Bence Jones proteins. Biochem. J. 99:15 P, 1966.
17. HUMPHREY, J.H., AND WHITE, R.G.: Immunology for Students of Medicine. ed.3. F.A. Davis Company, Philadelphia, 1970.
18. HUTH, E.J.: Kidney stones: a medical approach to diagnosis (with some brief comments on some treatments). Med. Clin. North Am. 47:959, 1963.
19. JACOBSON, M.H., LEVY, S.E., KAUFMAN, R.M. ET AL.: Urine osmolality. A definitive test of renal function. Arch. Intern. Med. 110:83, 1962.
20. KAITZ, A.L., AND LONDON, A.M.: Osmolar urinary concentrating ability and pyelonephritis in hospitalized patients. Am. J. Med. Sci. 248:7, 1964.

21. KILLANDER, J., SJOLIN, S., AND ZAAR, B.: Rapid tests for ketonuria. Scand. J. Clin. Lab. Invest. 14:311, 1962.

22. KING, S.E.: Postural adjustments and protein excretion by the kidney in renal diseases. Ann. Intern. Med. 46:360, 1957.

22A. KNOX, W.E.: "Phenylketonuria," In Stanbury, J.B., Wyngaarden, J.B., and Frederickson, D.S. (eds.): The Metabolic Basis of Inherited Disease, ed. 3. McGraw-Hill Book Co., New York, 1972.

23. LATHEM, W.: The renal excretion of hemoglobin: Regulatory mechanisms and the differential excretion of free and protein-bound hemoglobin. J. Clin. Invest. 38:652, 1959.

24. LONSDALE, K.: Human stones. Science 159:1199, 1968.

25. MAURICE, P.F., AND HENNEMAN, P.H.: Medical aspects of renal stones. Medicine 40:315, 1961.

26. MAUZERALL, D., AND GRANICK, S.: The occurrence and determination of δ-aminolevulinic acid and porphobilinogen in urine. J. Biol. Chem. 219:435, 1956.

27. MILLER, A.L., WORSLEY, L.R., AND CHU, P.K.: Brown urine as a clue to phenacetin intoxication. Lancet 2:1102, 1970.

28. NOBEL, S.: Toxicology in a general hospital. Stand. Meth. Clin. Chem. 6:73, 1970.

29. PITTS, R.F.: Physiology of the Kidney and Body Fluids, ed. 2. Year Book Medical Publishers, Chicago, 1968.

30. POTTS, J.T., REITA, R.E., DEFTOS, L.J. ET AL.: Secondary hyperparathyroidism in chronic renal disease. Arch. Intern. Med. 124:408, 1969.

31. REINER, M., CHEUNG, H.L., AND THOMAS, J.L.: Calculi. Stand. Meth. Clin. Chem. 6:193, 1970.

32. RELMAN, A.S., AND LEVINSKY, N.G.: "Clinical examination of renal function," In Strauss, M.B., and Welt, L.G. (eds.) Diseases of the Kidney, ed. 2. Little, Brown & Company, Boston, 1971.

33. RENNIE, I.D.B.: Proteinuria. Med. Clin. North Am. 55:213, 1971.

34. RENNIE, I.D.B., AND KEEN, H.: Evaluation of clinical methods for detecting proteinuria. Lancet 2:489, 1967.

35. RITTER, S., SPENCER, H., AND SAMACHSON, J.: The Sulkowitch test and quantitative urinary calcium excretion. J. Lab. Clin. Med. 56:314, 1960.

36. ROBINSON, R.R.: Idiopathic proteinuria. Ann. Intern. Med. 71:1019, 1969.

37. ROSENBERG, L.E., AND SCRIVER, C.R.: "Disorders of amino acid metabolism," In Bondy, P.K. (ed.): Duncan's Diseases of Metabolism, ed.6. W.B. Saunders Company, Philadelphia, 1969.

38. RUTECKI, G.J., GOLDSMITH, C., AND SCHREINER, G.E.: Characterization of proteins in urinary casts. N. Engl. J. Med. 284:1049, 1971.

39. SHERLOCK, SHEILA: Disease of the Liver and Biliary System, ed.4. F.A. Davis Co., Philadelphia, 1968.

40. SMITH, H.W.: Principles of Renal Physiology. Oxford University Press, New York, 1956.

41. SMITH, H.W., GOLDRING, W., AND CHASIS, H.: The measurement of the tubular excretory mass, effective blood flow, and filtration rate in the normal human kidney. J. Clin. Invest. 17:263, 1938.

42. STOTT, R.B., OGG, C.S., CAMERON, J.S., AND BEWICK, M.: Why the persistently high mortality in acute renal failure. Lancet 2:75, 1972.

43. TAMM, I., AND HORSFALL, F.L., JR.: A mucoprotein derived from human urine which reacts with influenza, mumps, and Newcastle disease viruses. J. Exp. Med. 95:71, 1952.

44. TSCHUDY, D.P.: "Porphyrin metabolism and the porphyrias," In Bondy, P.K. (ed.): Duncan's Diseases of Metabolism, ed.6. W.B. Saunders Co., Philadelphia, 1969.

45. TSCHUDY, D.P.: Recent progress in the hepatic porphyrias. Progr. Liver Dis. 3:13, 1970.

46. TSCHUDY, D.P., PERLROTH, M.G., MARVER, H.S. ET AL.: Acute intermittent porphyria: the first "over-production disease" localized to a specific enzyme. Proc. Natl. Acad. Sci. U.S.A. 53:841, 1965.

47. WINTROBE, M.M.: Clinical Hematology, ed.6. Lea & Febiger, Philadelphia, 1967.

48. WOODS, J.W., AND WILLIAMS, T.F.: "Hypertension due to renal vascular disease, renal infarction, renal cortical necrosis," In Strauss, M.B., and Welt, L.G. (eds.): Diseases of the Kidney, ed. 2. Little, Brown & Co., Boston, 1971.

CHAPTER 9

Feces

Examination of the feces often receives short shrift in laboratories and clinics. Unlike urine, blood, or spinal fluid, it often cannot be collected on demand and patients usually dislike collecting and delivering it for examination. Nursing and laboratory personnel tend to share the patient's aversion, and the doctor often excuses himself from contact with excreta. Yet disease of the gastrointestinal tract is widespread and examination of feces helps elucidate many common clinical dilemmas.

Various means of collecting feces are available. The physician performing a rectal examination should sample whatever fecal material is within finger range. This constitutes a random, rather small sample, chiefly important for documenting unsuspected occult bleeding or striking abnormalities of color or consistency. The specimen collected at the time of defecation, constituting a single evacuation, permits a number of tests and inferences. Conditions suggested from single specimen findings sometimes require documentation by quantitative tests on timed collections.

THE NORMAL SPECIMEN

The average, normal adult excretes 100 to 300 Gm of fecal material per day. Of this, as much as 70 per cent may be water, and of the remaining material up to half may be bacteria and their debris. Vegetable residues, small amounts of fat, desquamated epithelial cells, and other miscellany constitute the rest. The feces are what remains of approximately 10 L of fluid material entering the intestinal tract each day. Ingested food and fluid, saliva, gastric secretions, pancreatic juice, and bile all contribute to input; the output depends on a complex series of absorptive, secretory, and fermentative processes.

255

The small intestine is approximately 23 feet long, the large intestine between 4 and 5 feet.[2] The small intestine degrades ingested fats, proteins and carbohydrates to absorbable units, and then absorbs them. Pancreatic, biliary, and gastric secretions operate on the luminal contents to prepare them for active mucosal transport. Other vitally important substances absorbed in the small intestine include fat-soluble vitamins, iron, and calcium. Vitamin B_{12}, after complexing with intrinsic factor, is absorbed in the ileum. The small intestine also absorbs, for return to the blood, as much as 9.5 L of water, and associated electrolytes. The large intestine is shorter, and performs less complex functions than the small intestine. The right or proximal colon absorbs much of the remaining water. Bacteria within the colonic lumen degrade many of the end-products of metabolism, and the distal portion of the colon stores the feces until a convenient time for evacuation.

Normally evacuated feces reflect the shape and caliber of the colonic lumen. The normal consistency is somewhat plastic, neither fluid, mushy, nor hard. The usual brown color results from bacterial degradation of bile pigments into stercobilin, while the odor derives from indole and skatole, degradation products of proteins. In persons with normal gastrointestinal motility, consuming a mixed dietary intake, colonic transit time is 24 to 48 hours. Small intestinal contents (chyme) begin to enter the cecum as soon as 2 to 3 hours after a meal, but the process is not complete until 6 to 9 hours after eating.[5]

LABORATORY EXAMINATION

GROSS APPEARANCE

Stool examination should evaluate size, shape, consistency, color, odor, and the presence or absence of blood, mucus, pus, tissue fragments, food residues, or parasites. This examination should be done before the patient is exposed to barium or purges.

Alterations in size or shape indicate altered motility or abnormalities in the colonic wall. Thus, very large caliber indicates dilatation of the viscus, while excessively small, ribbon-like extrusions suggest decreased elasticity or partial obstruction. Small, round, hard masses accompany habitual, moderate constipation, but severe fecal retention can produce huge impacted masses with small volumes of pasty material excreted as overflow.

Color

Alterations in color may have diagnostic significance, but may reflect only dietary peculiarity. Diets high in milk and low in meat produce light colored stool with little odor. Excessive fat intake may produce a clay-like appearance, and large quantities of green vegetables may color stool green. Black or very dark brown feces may result from iron or bismuth ingestion, or from an unusually large proportion of meat in the diet. A good history helps distinguish these adventitious changes from significant abnormalities.

The usual cause of clay-colored stools is that reduced quantities of bile pigments enter the intestine because of intrinsic hepatobiliary disease or obstruction. The presence of excessive fat in a light-colored stool suggests malabsorption, a condition in which accurate dietary history is most important. Black feces suggest bleeding fairly high in the gastrointestinal tract, but this must be confirmed chemically. Unchanged bile pigments in feces indicate intestinal transit too rapid to allow bacterial degradation.

Other Elements

Grossly visible blood is never normal. Blood streaked on the outer surface usually suggests hemorrhoids or anal abnormalities, but can also arise from abnormalities higher in the colon. If transit time is sufficiently rapid, blood from the stomach or duodenum may appear as bright or dark red in the feces.

Mucus is also abnormal if grossly visible. Colonic mucosa secretes mucus in response to parasympathetic stimulation, so fecal mucus appears in conditions of parasympathetic excitability. The classic example is *mucous colitis* in which increased motility and mucus secretion occur without bleeding or inflammation. Mucus may signal other diffuse or localized abnormalities of the distal colon, especially the well-differentiated, mucus-producing tumors. If there is sufficient destruction of colonic mucosa, as in severe ulcerative colitis, mucus production ceases in the involved segments. Mucus incorporated within the fecal mass, rather than streaked on the surface, suggests an abnormality more proximal in the colon, and the mucus particles are usually smaller.

Recognizable pus is seldom seen in or on feces unless a draining rectal infection is present. Pus intermixed with tissue fragments and necrotic debris can, however, result from some ulcerating or fungating process. More often, acute inflammation produces excessive numbers of leukocytes which are intermixed with the feces and seen only on microscopic examination.

MICROSCOPIC EXAMINATION

Parasites

Microscopic examination of fecal material may augment the observations from gross inspection. Parasites and their ova usually require microscopic examination for diagnosis, although adult nematodes or tapeworm segments may occasionally be only too obvious in the gross material. For significant parasitologic evaluation, the stool specimen must be fresh, and the examiner must be experienced. To diagnose and identify amoebae and other motile parasites, the examiner should observe freshly passed material while it is still warm. Bloody or mucus-containing fragments give the best results, and both a saline emulsion and an iodine emulsion should be examined. Concentrating the stool sample helps in finding helminth ova; their presence in a simple emulsion indicates that large numbers are present. Zinc sulfate flotation of washed, concentrated fecal material is widely used, although various methods of concentration, fixation, or staining find favor in various laboratories.

Undigested Material

Besides demonstrating parasites, microscopic examination of feces permits rapid screening of digestive efficiency. If visibly striated meat fibers can be seen, proteolysis is inadequate. The significance of fats in a random specimen is less clear. A certain amount of fecal fat is normal, corresponding to 5 to 7 per cent of dietary intake. By no means all, or even most, of this fat comes directly from dietary input,[11] but the approximate proportion is fairly predictable. Recent dietary intake influences the fat content of random or single specimens. A patient with malabsorption problems may restrict his fat intake because of anorexia, resulting in normal excretion at the time of examination. Conversely, a metabolically normal patient with abnormally high intake may excrete more fat than the expected normal. If there is reason to suspect abnormal fat metabolism, evaluation of a random specimen should include available information about recent intake.

Cellular Elements

A certain number of epithelial cells may be present in feces, but large numbers of epithelial cells or of mucus indicate an irritated mucosa White cells are not normal constituents, so their presence indicates inflammation at some point in the lower alimentary tract or excretory organs. While large numbers of white cells suggest a fairly serious or extensive inflammatory process, the absence of leukocytes does not mean inflammation is absent. An inflammatory process deep in the wall or a surface condition which does not attract neutrophils will contribute few leukocytes to the fecal content. Unaltered red blood cells, when present, usually come from the anus or rectum. Intraluminal blood from higher in the gastrointestinal tract undergoes damage to the cells even if the hemoglobin remains undegraded.

CHEMICAL EXAMINATIONS

Chemical tests performed on feces usually seek blood, abnormal quantities of fats, or rarely, increased protein. Accurate testing for blood in the stool is one of the most significant laboratory tools available, since both positive and negative results have important implications.

Blood

Most tests for blood in biologic specimens utilize the catalytic effects of heme compounds on the oxidation of such organic substances as benzidine or guaiac. Of the hemoglobin breakdown products, only hematin retains this peroxidase activity, which is also present in myoglobin and certain plant enzymes. Since small amounts of fecal peroxidase activity may derive from dietary meat or, rarely, vegetable substances, and since small quantities of blood may not have clinical significance, tests for fecal blood must have appropriate sensitivity. Too many false positives wreak havoc with patients. False negatives may prevent early diagnosis of extremely important diseases.

Perfectly normal individuals lose between 1 and 3 ml of blood daily in the feces,[9,10] presumably from minimal abrasions of nasopharyngeal and oral surfaces as well as from the gastrointestinal tract. Quantities of blood larger than 50 ml[7] arising high in the gastrointestinal tract darken the feces to the black appearance known as melena. To detect quantities between these two levels and to confirm that black stools really do contain blood, the peroxidase tests are essential.

Possible False Inferences. The location of bleeding cannot always be inferred from the stool color. Black stools are said to be due to conversion of hemoglobin to hematin by gastric acid, but melena can occur when blood enters the intestine below the pylorus.[7] Similarly, bright or dark blood may be seen in feces with bleeding points above the pylorus, if motility is sufficiently rapid. The general rule that black stools mean gastric bleeding and bright blood means low colonic bleeding is suggestive but hardly absolute. Similarly, superficial blood streaking on formed stool often means hemorrhoidal bleeding, but does not preclude colonic lesions, nor does it exclude simultaneous existence of a more proximal, more significant bleeding point. The existence of melena does not necessarily imply active bleeding. Up to five days after a single instillation of blood into the stomach, tarry stools can still be noted,[7] and tests for occult blood remain positive for several weeks.

Tests Employed. Of the reagents commonly used for demonstrating blood in the feces, orthotoluidine is the most sensitive. Benzidine produces somewhat fewer false positives, but is a potential carcinogen and is not in routine laboratory use. Gum guaiac solution is much less sensitive than either of these others. It is probably best for routine screening use, since there is less problem of false positives, and a meat-free diet is unnecessary. Properly made up and stored, the guaiac reagents can detect 0.5 to 1 per cent of hemoglobin in an aqueous solution, compared with 0.01 to 0.1 per cent concentrations detected with orthotoluidine.[6] These figures cannot be used to estimate fecal blood loss, since fecal findings depend not only on the amount of blood, but also on the net balance of heme degradation, competitive activity of fecal reducing substances, and the presence of interfering pigments. In addition, the test reagents must be of proper concentration. Even when stored so that deterioration is slowed, they should be made up fresh at monthly intervals.

Significance. With a test suitably standardized to avoid false positives, the finding of occult blood is nearly always diagnostically significant. Of upper gastrointestinal bleeding sites, peptic ulcers, bleeding varices, gastritis, and gastric carcinoma are the usual causes, in approximately that order,[4,7] while colitis, colon carcinoma, and diverticulitis are the commonest causes of lower intestinal bleeding. Patients can lose surprising amounts of blood without noticing, as much as 150 ml of blood per week in one study.[9] Prolonged loss of relatively small, daily quantities can produce anemia and persistently positive tests for occult fecal blood without localizing symptoms.

One precipitating factor in chronic, or sometimes acute, blood loss is aspirin ingestion. This medication, so common that patients often do not consider it a drug and fail to mention it when asked about medications, is increasingly implicated as a gastric irritant. As many as 70 per cent of patients regularly taking large doses of aspirin may have blood in their stools, averaging 5 ml per day.[8] Occasional patients, especially those with pre-existing atrophic gastritis, develop massive acute hemorrhagic gastritis after aspirin ingestion.[12]

MALABSORPTION PROBLEMS

A variety of disorders may cause excessive fecal fat excretion. Staining a fecal smear to find increased fat globules is a useful screening device, but is nonquantitative. Often the patient's history of bulky, light-colored, floating stools provides the presumptive diagnosis, although in one series of children with celiac disease, 38 out of 40 had excessive fat on a stained smear, while only 21 reported bulky or foul stools.[3]

FAT EXCRETION

To quantitate fat excretion, there must be known dietary intake and timed stool collection. The usual technique involves a diet containing 100 Gm of fat daily, with a three-day stool collection to measure total fat excretion. Excretion of more than 5 Gm per day is abnormal and values may range upwards to 50 Gm or more. In feces, most lipids are present as fatty acids, both saturated and unsaturated, since neutral fats are hydrolyzed by lipases high in the small intestine. Lipase deficiency, usually due to pancreatic disease, increases the proportion of neutral fat. In these cases, the stool usually contains excessive quantities of undigested protein, because pancreatic proteases are also deficient. Disease of liver and biliary tract severe enough to produce steatorrhea usually causes jaundice and abnormalities of blood chemistry before the steatorrhea becomes a diagnostic problem.

Fatty acids of normal fecal lipids are not precisely those of the diet. Apparently bacterial activity, epithelial desquamation, and mucosal transport mechanisms modify the excreted elements. With altered intestinal bacterial flora, increased motility, abnormal mucosal metabolism, decreased enzyme or bile salt content, or simple loss of absorbing surfaces (as from resections or fistulas), fecal fat content increases markedly and may approach more nearly the lipid composition of the diet.[11] Fecal calcium also increases, due partly to soap formation with the fatty acids, and partly to decreased transport resulting from faulty absorption of vitamin D, which is fat-soluble.

CARBOHYDRATE UTILIZATION

When celiac disease, nontropical sprue (adult celiac disease), tropical sprue, and infiltrative diseases intrinsic to the small intestine cause steatorrhea, other malabsorption problems may also be present. Carbohydrate absorption is often decreased, exacerbating the patient's nutritional problems. The complete investigation of steatorrhea usually includes one or more studies of carbohydrate metabolism. Comparing oral glucose tolerance results with intravenous glucose tolerance testing may demonstrate that intestinal malfunction is at fault rather than pancreatic deficiency. Patients with intestinal malabsorption raise their blood sugar little more than 35 mg per 100 ml after orally ingesting 100 Gm of glucose, but have a normal curve after parenteral glucose infusion. Since diabetes can sometimes cause diarrhea and malabsorption, the glucose tolerance tests may be valuable in differential diagnosis. Other metabolic abnormalities, especially excessively rapid peripheral glucose utilization, can give a potentially confusing flat GTT curve, but the intravenous GTT then has the same shape as the oral test results.

Xylose Tolerance

Glucose transport activity has large excess capacity, so GTT abnormalities develop late in malabsorption syndromes.[1] A more sensitive index of impaired carbohydrate absorption is the d-xylose tolerance test, which also assists in distinguishing pancreatic deficiency from intestinal disease as a cause of steatorrhea. After the patient ingests 25 Gm of this pentose sugar, urinary excretion is measured for five hours and the blood xylose level is determined at two hours. Normal individuals have blood levels rising to 36 ± 16 mg per 100 ml, at two hours, and in a five-hour period will excrete more than 4.5 or 5 Gm.[6] In most malabsorption syndromes, the blood level goes no higher than 15 to 18 mg per 100 ml, and urinary excretion is less than 2 Gm. Pancreatic secretions do not affect d-xylose absorption, so patients with pancreatogenous steatorrhea have normal results. Abnormally slow gastric emptying or impaired renal function can produce abnormalities resembling those with intestinal malabsorption. ^{131}I-labelled oleic acid and triolein may be useful in distinguishing pancreatic from primary intestinal malabsorption, but technical and interpretational problems have so far kept this test from achieving widespread acceptance.

PROTEIN LOSS

There is no satisfactory technique for quantitating fecal proteins and for very few patients is this a problem. The protein loss with generalized malabsorption does not require separate documentation. In occasional patients, however, severe fecal protein loss may occur, a condition to which the descriptive term *protein-losing enteropathy* has been applied.

Proteins within the intestinal lumen are reduced enzymatically to their component amino acids, which are then reabsorbed. If mucosal abnormalities prevent reabsorption, or if protein leakage exceeds reabsorptive capacity, hypoproteinemia may result. Severe ulcerative colitis, Whipple's disease, disturbances of lymphatic circulation, and intestinal lymphomas may produce this syndrome, which is suggested by hypoalbuminemia in the absence of hepatic disease or urinary protein loss. The fecal protein excretion can be documented by administering isotopically-labelled albumin or polyvinylpyrrolidone (PVP), rather than by chemical analysis of feces.

Patients with severe malabsorption may have low serum albumin levels, due partly to general malnutrition and partly to excessive fecal loss. Inadequate absorption of the fat soluble vitamins can produce low vitamin A levels, coagulation abnormalities due to vitamin K deficiency, and osteoporosis with elevated alkaline phosphatase levels due to reduced vitamin D activity.

Fecal analysis is not applied to suspected pancreatic enzyme deficiencies, except in very young children. Below age two, stool normally manifests tryptic activity; although trypsin and chymotrypsin activity is sometimes noted in adult feces, the presence or absence of enzyme activity cannot reliably be correlated with pancreatic disease. Some of the fecal enzymes may be of bacterial origin. Analysis of duodenal aspirates is more informative for pancreatic disease.

The final diagnosis of intestinal mucosal abnormality can now be made by histologic examination of biopsies obtained by peroral techniques. Biopsies, when available, are especially useful for following response to therapy, since histologic changes in most of the more common problems are reversible.

BIBLIOGRAPHY

1. FINKELSTEIN, J.D.: Malabsorption. Med. Clin. North Am. 52:1339, 1968.
2. GOSS, C.M. (ED.): Gray's Anatomy of the Human Body, ed. 27. Lea & Febiger, Philadelphia, 1959.
3. HAMILTON, J.R., LYNCH, M.J., AND REILLY, B.J.: Active celiac disease in childhood. Clinical and laboratory findings in forty-two cases. Q. J. Med. 38:135, 1969.
4. PALMER, E.D.: The vigorous diagnostic approach to upper gastrointestinal tract hemorrhage. J.A.M.A. 207:1477, 1969.
5. PETERSON, M.L.: "Constipation and diarrhea," In MacBryde, C.M. (ed): Signs and Symptoms: Applied Pathologic Physiology and Clinical Interpretation, ed. 5. J.B. Lippincott Co., Philadelphia, 1970.
6. RENCHER, J.L., AND BEELER, M.D.: "The examination of feces," In Davidsohn, I., and Henry, J.B. (eds.): Todd-Sanford Clinical Diagnosis by Laboratory Methods, ed. 14. W.B. Saunders Co., Philadelphia, 1969.
7. SCHIFF, L.: "Hematemesis and melena," In MacBryde, C.M., and Blacklow, R.S. (eds.): Signs and Symptoms, ed. 5. J.B. Lippincott Co., Philadelphia, 1970.
8. SCOTT, J.T., PORTER, I.H., LEWIS, S.M., AND DIXON, A. ST. J.: Studies of gastrointestinal bleeding caused by corticosteroids, salicylates, and other analgesics. Q. J. Med. 30:167, 1961.
9. STACK, B.H.R., SMITH, T., HYWEL JONES, J., AND FLETCHER, J.: Measurement of blood and iron loss in colitis with a whole-body counter. Gut 10:769, 1969.
10. STEPHENS, F.O., MILVERTON, E.J., HAMBLY, C.K., AND VAN DER VEN, E.K.: The effects of food on aspirin-induced gastrointestinal blood loss. DIGESTION 1:267, 1968.
11. WIGGINS, H.S., HOWELL, K.E., KELLOCK, T.D., AND STALDER, J.: The origin of fecal fat. Gut 10:400, 1969.
12. WINAWER, S.J., BEJAR, J., MCCRAY, R.S., AND ZAMCHEK, N.: Hemorrhagic gastritis. Importance of associated chronic gastritis. Arch. Intern. Med. 127:129, 1971.

CHAPTER 10

Sputum

Sputum is the material secreted in the tracheobronchial tree and brought up by coughing. Although the submucosal glands and secretory cells in the lining mucosa normally elaborate up to 100 ml of viscoelastic fluid daily, the healthy individual does not produce sputum.

NORMAL PHYSIOLOGY

Mucus secretion is part of normal bronchopulmonary cleansing. The secretions form a layer perhaps 5 microns thick,[11] immediately overlying the ciliated epithelium. By ciliary action, this semi-sticky mantle of fluid moves upward toward the oropharynx, carrying with it inhaled particles which have found their way down to the respiratory bronchioles. From the oropharynx, the secretions are swallowed so the normal person is not aware of their presence. Coughing or expectorating tracheobronchial secretions is abnormal, the quantity of material roughly paralleling the severity of the abnormality.

Besides its mechanical cleansing action, mucus attacks inhaled bacteria directly. The antibacterial effect of normal tracheobronchial mucus results largely from antibody activity, although lysozymes and slightly acid pH conditions also help maintain sterility. The antibodies are predominantly IgA, entering the mucus by direct glandular secretion rather than by transudation from plasma.[10] Despite daily exposure to innumerable organisms, the contents of the lower respiratory tract are sterile in normal individuals.

RESPONSE TO INJURY

Respiratory tract disease alters the tracheobronchial secretions and these altered secretions in turn influence the pathophysiologic process. In bacterial infections, the volume of sputum increases, the pH becomes more acid, and the chemical composition changes. Acidic pH, below 6.5, inhibits ciliary action, thereby reducing one important defense mechanism. Sputum viscosity increases, further reducing normal flow, and the number of leukocytes also rises. As in all inflammatory conditions, membrane permeability increases, so that antibiotics and other normally intravascular elements may enter the sputum. Bacterial infections result in increased DNA content, to some extent replacing normal mucopolysaccharides.[4] Besides increasing sputum viscosity, DNA also inhibits proteolytic activity. This reduces the effectiveness of drugs intended to liquefy sputum.

Sputum in quantities sufficient to be coughed up is abnormal. Some patients expectorate a mixture of nasopharyngeal secretions and saliva, but this is not sputum. Patients with chronic postnasal drip may complain of cough and expectoration, but the quality of the cough and watery nature of the material distinguish this condition from true productive coughing. In addition, microscopic examination reveals squamous epithelial cells and such characteristically oral flora as Fusobacterium fusiforme, oral spirochetes, and nonpathogenic acid-fast organisms.

SPUTUM EXAMINATION

COLLECTING THE SPECIMEN

True sputum originates from below the larynx. Some patients need instruction in deep breathing and coughing before they produce an adequate specimen. An aerosol of mucolytic agents may be helpful, or the simple mechanical maneuver of reclining the patient with his head lower than his lungs for a few minutes. Good oral hygiene improves the quality of the sputum specimen, and the patient should at least rinse his mouth thoroughly before coughing. Brushing the teeth is desirable when feasible.

Sputum is usually collected for microbiologic culture or for cytologic examination or both. In certain conditions, gross examination of the sputum and microscopic examination of stained smears are helpful. If the patient reports a change in the quantity or appearance of his sputum, this may be significant. In chronic bronchitis, which has been defined as the presence of a productive cough for at least three consecutive months a year for two consecutive years[5] patients tend to observe the sputum closely. Changing cough may signal carcinoma in these high risk patients[7] so their complaints should be accorded appropriate diagnostic attention.

Quantity and Collection

Quantitating sputum is rarely necessary. A good sputum specimen can, and in most cases should, be collected from a single episode of deep coughing. This usually results in 0.5 to 5 ml of material.[6] An early morning specimen is best, since it represents overnight accumulation, and is unlikely to contain food particles. Persons who handle the specimen should avoid contaminating themselves and avoid introducing organisms into material destined for microbiologic examination. The collecting vessels should be clean, wide-mouthed, and capable of secure closure. If day-long or 24-hour collections are made, usually when Mycobacterium tuberculosis is sought, the container should be kept closed when not immediately in use, and the patient should be especially careful not to soil the exterior. Sputum examination is indicated for suspected lower respiratory tract infections or tumors, although infarcts and noninfectious infiltrates can sometimes be spotted from sputum findings.

GROSS APPEARANCE

Descriptive terms applied to sputum include mucoid, mucopurulent, frankly purulent, blood-tinged, frankly bloody, or dust-flecked, and these characteristics correlate moderately well with the cause of cough. Purulent sputum usually accompanies acute bacterial pneumonias. In a patient with chronic bronchitis, change from mucoid to purulent or mucopurulent indicates bacterial infection overlying the chronic inflammatory process. Gradual progression from scant, sticky sputum to more abundant, loose, purulent material may signal the development of bronchiectasis. Rupture of a pulmonic abscess causes sudden expectoration of abundant purulent, often foul-smelling, pus.

MICROBIOLOGIC FINDINGS

The classical stages of pneumococcal pneumonia may be followed as the sputum changes from pink to mucoid, through reddish brown to purulent, often with gross streaks of blood. Treated pneumococcal pneumonia does not always follow this pattern, but despite changing clinical features and nonspecific sputum appearance, pneumococcus (now formally called Streptococcus pneumoniae[2]) remains one of the commonest pathogens in lower respiratory tract infections.[1,6] Other common bacterial pathogens, both in adults and children, are H. influenzae;[1,9] the gram-negative bacilli, especially in debilitated patients with other primary diseases; staphylococci;[3] and sometimes nonpneumococcal streptococci, although these more often derive from the pharynx than from the lung as a primary source.

Mycoplasma pneumoniae and the respiratory viruses are very frequent pathogens, especially when lower respiratory tract disease occurs acutely in previously healthy individuals.[1] These are difficult to isolate in the routine laboratory. The sputum in nonbacterial pneumonias tends to be less abundant, and nearly always contains fewer polymorphonuclear leukocytes than in bacterial pneumonia. Acute and convalescent serum samples may facilitate viral and mycoplasmal diagnosis, albeit in retrospect. Skin testing, as well as serologic evaluation, can be helpful in diagnosing fungal infections, especially if cultures are unrevealing. If cultures are negative, the presence of eosinophils in the sputum sometimes distinguishes an asthmatic etiology from viral or mycoplasma involvement.

PROBLEMS WITH CULTURES

Interpreting sputum cultures requires judgment, since some organisms, saprophytic and nonpathogenic in the oropharynx, acquire distinct significance when found in the lung. Candida, Actinomyces and Klebsiella pneumoniae are particular offenders, since the pulmonary infections tend to be severe and often difficult to treat. Despite obvious pulmonary infection, sputum cultures may be negative, owing to irregular distribution of organisms in the sputum. Selecting purulent or particulate material for inoculation helps circumvent this sampling error, especially when similar particles are examined on Gram-stained and acid-fast stained smears.

Homogenizing and liquefying the specimen improves sampling, especially with very viscid material. Sometimes the laboratory can treat the specimen, but intratracheal aerosol of N-acetylcysteine can result in a more voluminous, less viscid sample at the time the patient coughs. When the patient, especially a child, cannot produce an adequate specimen at all, a cough swab may be helpful. The swab is held above the larynx, while the tongue and epiglottis are depressed, and the patient coughs directly onto the swab. Bacteriologically active material can be obtained in this way, even if sputum production is minimal.

HEMOPTYSIS

Massive hemoptysis indicates blood vessel erosion by a neoplastic or inflammatory process, usually a granuloma. Streaks of blood in an otherwise purulent or mucoid sputum usually accompany more diffuse pneumonic processes, bacterial, mycoplasmal, viral, or sometimes fungal. Occasional patients with inactive tuberculosis cough up blood-streaked sputum,[8] but in general this suggests active disease. Distinct from blood-streaking or massive hemoptysis is uniform discoloration of the sputum. "Rusty" sputum accompanies chronic passive congestion, while abundant pink, frothy sputum is an immediate danger sign of acute pulmonary edema. Following nonfatal infarcts, the sputum may progress from blood streaked, through bloody, to a uniform brown tinge reflecting hemoglobin breakdown. Sputum findings are not, however, consistently helpful when infarction is part of the differential diagnosis.

MICROSCOPIC EXAMINATION

Formed elements in sputum are best studied by cytologic techniques, using the Papanicolaou technique or an appropriate modification. If detailed cellular examination is not needed, routine staining techniques are valuable. Leukocytes can be tentatively classified on Gram-stained smears and morphology alone often permits distinction between polymorphs, found in infection, and eosinophils, characteristic of asthmatic attacks. Wright's stain or other Romanowsky-type stains provide conclusive distinction. PAS and silver stains are sometimes applied to sputum in suspected pulmonary alveolar proteinosis. The characteristic compacted protein may be inside mononuclear cells or free in round or laminated clumps or in aggregates with cleft-like spaces. When round and laminated, these resemble the cysts of Pneumocystis carinii. Although both are PAS positive, only Pneumocystis takes a silver stain.

Curschmann's spirals can readily be identified on Gram-stained smears. These coiled, mucus filaments, once considered pathognomonic of asthma, are casts of small bronchi, and may occur whenever increased mucus production accompanies bronchial obstruction. Since bronchospasm and excessive secretions characterize asthmatic attacks, Curschmann's spirals are particularly to be expected, but they can also occur in other types of acute bronchitis or in bronchopneumonia, and may be found in sputum arising from small bronchi adjacent to lung carcinomas.

The cytologic evaluation of sputum specimens is beyond the scope of this chapter.

BIBLIOGRAPHY

1. HERS, J.F.P., MASUREL, N., AND GANS, J.C.: Acute respiratory disease associated with pulmonary involvement in military servicemen in The Netherlands. Am. Rev. Resp. Dis. 100:499, 1969.
2. INTERNATIONAL COMMITTEE ON NOMENCLATURE OF BACTERIA: Subcommittee on Streptococci and Pneumococci. Minutes of the meeting held in Moscow, July 21, 1966. Int. J. System. Bacteriol. 17:281, 1967.

3. KUPERMAN, A.S., AND FERNANDEZ, R.B.: Subacute staphylococcal pneumonia. Am. Rev. Resp. Dis. 101:95, 1970.
4. LIEBERMAN, J.: The appropriate use of mucolytic agents. Am. J. Med. 49:1, 1970.
5. MITCHELL, R.S., AND PIERCE, J.A.: "Cough," *In* MacBryde, C.M., and Blacklow, R.S. (eds.): Signs and Symptoms, ed. 5. J.B. Lippincott Co. Philadelphia, 1970.
6. PIRTLE, J.K., MONROE, P.W., SMALLEY, T.K. ET AL.: Diagnostic and therapeutic advantages of serial quantitative cultures of fresh sputum in acute bacterial pneumonia. Am. Rev. Resp. Dis. 100:831, 1969.
7. RIMINGTON, J.: Smoking, sputum, and lung cancer. Br. Med. J. 1:732, 1968.
8. STINGHE, R.V., AND MANGIULEA, V.G.: Hemoptysis of bronchial origin occurring in patients with arrested tuberculosis. Am. Rev. Resp. Dis. 101:84, 1970.
9. TILLOTSON, J.R., AND LERNER, A.M.: Hemophilus influenzae bronchopneumonia in adults. Arch. Intern. Med. 121:428, 1968.
10. TOMASI, T.B.: "The gamma A globulins: First line of defense," *In* Good, R.A., and Fisher, D.W. (eds.): Immunobiology. Sinauer Associates, Stamford, Conn., 1971.
11. TEAGER, H., JR.: Tracheobronchial secretions. Am. J. Med. 50:493, 1971.

CHAPTER 11

Gastric and Duodenal Contents

The stomach's purely mechanical functions of storing, mixing, and gradually emitting ingested food and fluid are usually evaluated roentgenographically and are not subject to direct laboratory investigation. The gastric mucosa has several secretory products which can be subjected to study but rarely are, namely rennin, lipase, mucus, and small amounts of nondigestive enzymes. The proteolytic enzymes, principally pepsin, undoubtedly have considerable physiologic significance, but no well-defined or generally accepted pathophysiologic tests are currently in use. Hydrochloric acid, which the gastric mucosa is capable of elaborating at concentrations as high as 160 mEq per liter,[3] is the one element of gastric origin regularly evaluated in the laboratory.

MEASURING GASTRIC ACIDITY

The complete role of gastric HCl in normal and pathologic physiology is a topic too complex for this chapter. Hydrochloric acid, along with gastric proteolytic enzymes, is important in initiating protein digestion. In the clinical syndrome called peptic ulcer disease, gastric or duodenal mucosa or both are attacked by these proteolytic activities, and gastric acidity measurements can often be correlated with clinical findings and prognosis. Measurement of gastric acid secretion is essential in diagnosing the special subgroup of peptic ulcer disease known as Zollinger-Ellison syndrome; and is often contributory in those hematologic and sometimes neurologic maladies characterized by impaired absorption of vitamin B_{12}, folic acid, or iron. Gastric hydrochloric acid is not, itself, implicated in these transport mechanisms, but deficiencies in absorptive cofactors are often mirrored in deficiencies of gastric acid secretion, a function more directly measurable.

270

Gastric secretions are collected by aspiration through a tube passed through the mouth or the nasopharynx. Fluoroscopic monitoring helps insure good intragastric placement. The tip should be at the most dependent portion of the stomach, without curling or twisting. Most gastric aspiration is performed in the morning, after an overnight fast. At this time the stomach should contain no more than 50 ml of clear or opalescent fluid, free of food particles, blood, or bile. The usual bacterial flora have little clinical significance, but tuberculous patients whose sputum contains no organisms sometimes have M. tuberculosis in cultures of overnight gastric contents. Cytologic examination of native gastric juice is usually unsatisfactory, since desquamated cells are poorly preserved. After the gastric contents have been aspirated, gastric washings can be extremely useful in documenting the presence, and sometimes the nature, of gastric neoplasms.

NORMAL PHYSIOLOGY

Under resting, unstimulated conditions, the stomach secretes a small amount of acid. Increased acidity results, physiologically, from neural and humoral stimulation; actual food intake is not required. Psychic phenomena, including emotional stimuli and the sight and smell of food, induce gastric secretion by stimulating the vagus nerve. Vagal impulses affect parietal cells directly, and also induce cells in the antrum to produce gastrin, an intense hormonal stimulus to parietal cell activity. Antral gastrin secretion is further enhanced by distention of the stomach wall, or by contact with protein breakdown products. A third, but weaker, stimulus to gastric acidity occurs when the duodenal mucosa, in contact with intraluminal digestive products, releases humoral activators. Feedback inhibition also exists, since pH levels of 1.5 or below inhibit gastrin production.[3]

Units of Measurement

In the older literature, gastric acidity was expressed as "degrees," one degree standing for each milliliter of 0.1 N NaOH needed to titrate 100 ml of gastric juice to the desired end-point. Two end-points were in common use: pH 3.5, the end-point of Topfer's reagent, and the pH 7.0 to 9.4 range obtained with phenolphthalein and neutral red. At pH levels below 3.5, all the HCl was thought to exist as dissociated or "free" acid, while above that point the hydrogen ion was thought to be buffered by organic acids and peptides.

Titratable Acidity. The concept of free and combined acid has been shown[1, 20] to have neither physiologic nor physicochemical validity, and gastric acidity is now increasingly reported simply as titratable acidity. The single end-point of titration is neutrality (pH 7.0) or physiologic neutrality (pH 7.4), and the result is expressed as milliequivalents of acid. Since one ml of 0.1 N NaOH (the usual titrant) neutralizes 0.1 mEq of HCl, calculations are very simple. The volume of 0.1 N NaOH needed to neutralize an aliquot of gastric juice, divided by 10, gives the milliequivalents of acid in the aliquot. The milliequivalents in the total specimen are easily calculated from the milliequivalents in the measured sample. The acid concentration, as milliequivalents per liter, can also be calculated from the measured number of milliequivalents in the aspirated material.

Test Meals. In older investigations, the volume and acidity of the fasting overnight collection were compared against volume and acidity of gastric juice aspirated after ingestion or intragastric instillation of a *test meal.* Besides the variability of the overnight collection period and the wide range of individual response to test meal stimulation, the crackers, meat, alcohol, or whatever was used to stimulate acid secretion introduced uncontrollable error through unpredictable buffering effect. More reproducible and intrinsically more accurate is basal collection of gastric juice during a timed period when no secretory stimuli are active. This is followed by administration of some pharmacologic stimulus known to evoke maximal or near-maximal secretion in virtually all patients.

Basal and Stimulated Sampling

Basal collection begins after removal of the fasting contents. The volume, color, and gross composition of the overnight collection should be observed, but the acid content is not measured. Once the tube is positioned and the patient is comfortable, timed collection begins. Better volume recovery occurs when suction is applied continuously, either with a pump or manually with a syringe, rather than relying on interval removal of accumulated secretions. Ordinarily, the one hour of basal observation is divided into four separate 15-minute collections, with the acid content of each combined for the report of milliequivalents per hour.

Pharmacologic Stimuli. Two stimulants are widely used to evoke maximal acid production. Histamine, usually given as histamine acid phosphate, 0.04 mg/kg body weight, is the usual stimulant in the United States, while synthetic gastrin (Pentagastrin) is widely used in Great Britain and Europe. Gastrin evokes a somewhat greater acid response than histamine,[24] and tends to produce fewer side effects.[19] Antihistamine given 30 minutes before histamine injection reduces the uncomfortable side-effects of that drug. After stimulation, 15-minute collections continue, usually for 60 minutes total. The acidity of each specimen is measured separately, and two different values may be reported. The maximal acid output (MAO) is the total amount of acid produced in the hour after pharmacologic stimulation. This is reported as mEq/hr, or as per cent increase over basal output. The peak acid output (PAO) is the sum of the two highest consecutive 15-minute values, and is reported as mEq/30 min.

Diagnostic Findings. This test of acid output after maximal stimulation provides certain types of information but not others. The principal diagnostic usefulness is demonstration of anacidity. Anacidity is best defined as failure of gastric pH to fall below 6.0 at any time, even after maximal stimulation. A modest number of individuals lose their basal acidity with advancing age, but failure to secrete acid after maximal stimulation indicates loss of parietal cell mass and strongly suggests atrophic gastritis.[16] Anacidity nearly always accompanies pernicious anemia, but it can occur without the hematologic disease. Gastric anacidity never accompanies active peptic ulcer,[14] so epigastric pain associated with anacidity must have an etiology other than peptic ulcer disease, often, but not always, gastric carcinoma.

ZOLLINGER-ELLISON SYNDROME. The histamine test is also useful in evaluating suspected Zollinger-Ellison syndrome. In this condition, gastrin-secreting pancreatic tumors bombard the parietal cells with continuous, high-level stimulation. The expected findings, then, are large volume and high acid concentration in the basal collection, with relatively little rise following exogenous histamine or gastrin. While basal acid output above 15 mEq per hour is suggestive of Zollinger-Ellison syndrome, as many as 10 per cent of patients with simple peptic ulcer disease may have outputs this high.[15] In normally responsive individuals maximal stimulation leads to appreciably increased acidity even when basal output is high. If basal acidity is 60 per cent or more of the level attained after maximal stimulation, it suggests that abnormal endogenous gastrin production is eliciting a continuous state of near-maximal secretion.

PEPTIC ULCER DISEASE. The histamine test cannot, by itself, distinguish gastric from duodenal peptic ulcer, nor can it reliably separate benign from malignant gastric ulceration. While patients with gastric carcinoma tend, as a group, to have lower basal and maximal acid production than patients with benign ulcers, test results cannot have absolute significance in any individual patient. Compared with normal individuals, patients with peptic ulcer disease have moderately high basal secretion and excessively active maximal histamine response. The normal mean basal acid output is approximately 4 or 5 mEq/hr, while several series of patients with duodenal ulcer give means of 7.1[17] and between 6 and 7 mEq/hr.[15] The range and standard deviation in all series are extremely large, however, so comparison of basal figures offers only minimally suggestive information. The extent of maximal secretory rise tends to be higher in patients with duodenal ulcer

(35 to 40 mEq/hr) than in controls (22 to 26 mEq/hr) but again the ranges overlap markedly. Patients with hiatus hernia do not differ significantly from controls,[23] nor does the postoperative prognosis of peptic ulcer patients correlate reliably with the preoperative histamine test results.

THE INSULIN TEST

Postvagotomy gastric analysis has an intent and technique different from histamine testing to diagnose ulcer. The vagus nerve is highly important in acid secretion, mediating both direct parietal cell stimulation and gastrin production. Most operations for peptic ulcer disease include sectioning the vagus nerves, in the expectation that neural stimulation to acid production will be diminished. Because of anatomic variations and the peculiarities of operative conditions, complete vagotomy is often difficult to accomplish or evaluate. The Hollander insulin test[12] attempts to document vagus inactivation by demonstrating failure to evoke gastric acid response under conditons which normally produce vagal stimulation.

PHYSIOLOGIC EFFECTS

One known, powerful stimulus to vagal activation is hypoglycemia. In the intact individual, a significant drop in the blood sugar produces increased gastric acidity by vagus-mediated stimulation. If the vagi have been completely sectioned, hypoglycemia produces little change in acid secretion. The vagotomy does not produce basal anacidity; it simply abolishes the neural stimulus to increased acid production.

Before measuring the acid response to hypoglycemia, one should determine that the patient is capable of acid production. Failure to increase posthypoglycemic acidity over a low basal level could be due to parietal cell loss or nonreactivity, rather than to absent vagal stimulation. Many workers believe that if the basal acid output is zero, histamine stimulation should be performed to document parietal cell reactivity. Once this capacity has been documented, insulin provocation can be meaningfully interpreted.

PROCEDURE

The insulin test is performed after an overnight fast, and the fasting blood glucose level is determined as well as the basal acidity. In this test, comparisons are usually made on the basis of acid concentration, expressed in mEq/L in each of eight 15-minute collections, rather than on volume or total output. Blood sugar must be tested at intervals, since blood glucose levels remaining above 45 mg per 100 ml (some workers say 50 mg per 100 ml) prove that hypoglycemia has not been adequate. Patients with low fasting blood glucose levels should manifest a drop to one half the fasting value. The usual insulin dose is either 0.2 units per kilogram body weight or 20 units, administered intravenously.

Hollander originally proposed that if any of the 15-minute aliquots had an increment of 20 or more mEq/L over basal acid concentration, then vagus function persisted. If the initial sample was anacid, then a rise to 10 mEq/L in any postinsulin sample was considered a positive result. Most later workers have used these criteria, although the time at which the test is performed and the size and sex of the patient may affect the results. It has become common to separate positive responses according to whether they occur in one of the first four collection periods (i.e., during the first hour) or in the latter four collections. Since hypoglycemia-induced secretion depends on vagal innervation, provocation of significant acidity in either period indicates integrity of at least some vagal fibers.

INTERPRETATION

The timing of postoperative testing is important, for it appears that false negative results are fairly common in tests done one week to three months after vagotomy.[13,19] Whether this is due to regeneration of marginally traumatized nerve fibers or to temporary aberrations of motility and secretion is difficult to say.

Another problem is evaluating the patient with high postoperative acid secretion. The results of insulin testing are given in concentration of acidity per liter. The total amount of acid is not recorded. Mason and Giles[18] have found that if total acid output is high (above 20 mEq per hour), the comparison of concentration before and after hypoglycemia has much less predictive value. As a rule, vagotomy and pyloroplasty reduce, but do not abolish, basal and stimulated acidity.[7] Persistence of high total acid output carries a poor prognosis for recurrence.

Among ulcer patients with normal or reduced basal acidity after vagotomy, the value of the insulin test in predicting recurrence is somewhat questionable. A negative test done at a suitably late time after the operation carries a good but not absolute prognosis for no recurrence.[7,13] but positive results are more difficult to interpret.[5,19,25] As complex as are the etiologic factors in peptic ulcer disease, it is hardly surprising that a single test of a single variable provides no absolute answer.

DUODENAL FLUID

Collecting duodenal secretions is more difficult and time-consuming than gastric aspiration, since the tube must pass the pylorus and locate itself close to the ampulla of Vater. Fluoroscopic monitoring is virtually essential. A double lumen tube is customary, with one portion remaining in the stomach to aspirate acidic gastric juice which, if it passed the pylorus, would contaminate the alkaline duodenal secretions.

Physiology

The duodenum normally secretes 1200 to 1500 ml per day of enzyme-rich clear fluid, with pH 8 to 8.5 and containing up to 145 mEq/L of bicarbonate ion.[9] Pancreatic enzymes split fats, carbohydrates, and proteins, the major constituents being lipase, amylase, trypsin, and chymotrypsin. Secretions of bicarbonate ion and of enzymes have different physiologic provocation, although both are mediated hormonally.

When acidic gastric contents enter the duodenum, the fall in pH stimulates mucosal cells to produce secretin. Secretin calls forth watery pancreatic secretion with high bicarbonate content. Enzyme production is provoked by pancreozymin, also elaborated by small intestinal mucosa, but the stimulus to pancreozymin secretion is the presence of digestive products in the lumen. Distention by volume alone inspires a small amount of pancreozymin secretion, but sustained pancreozymin production is best evoked by polypeptides or micellar fatty acids or both in the small intestinal contents.[8]

SECRETIN TESTING

Both secretin and pancreozymin are available in pharmacologic forms, although the latter has not been approved for unregulated clinical use.[2] Prior to intravenous injection, intradermal tests should be done to ensure that there is no sensitivity to these foreign proteins. The usual dose of secretin is one clinical unit per kilogram body weight, but the dose of pancreozymin, when this is used, is more subject to individual preference.

The secretin test is performed after a 20-minute basal collection of duodenal secretions, the initial fasting contents having been aspirated and examined. The presence of bile, blood, undigested food particles, and cholesterol crystals in the duodenal fluid is abnormal. The postinjection samples are collected in 20-minute aliquots, with the volume and bicarbonate concentration measured separately for each sample. Dreiling and Janowitz[6] originally collected for 80 minutes, but many workers now use a 60-

minute collection. The volume and, to some extent, the bicarbonate output vary with the size of the patient, so results are usually expressed per kilogram body weight.

Volume

Dreiling and Janowitz[6] consider a cumulative volume of 2 ml output per kilogram body weight over the total collecting period to be the lower limit of normal. Another group,[11] using a larger secretin dose by constant infusion, reached approximately the same lower limit. Patients with chronic pancreatitis tend to secrete reduced volumes, but the range of variation is wide.[22] Thus, secretion of less than 2 ml/kg points to fairly severe pancreatic destruction, either inflammatory or neoplastic, but values above that do not invalidate these diagnoses.

Bicarbonate

The concentration of bicarbonate in secretin-stimulated pancreatic secretion usually reaches a peak value of 90 to 100 mEq/L during at least one of the collection periods.[6,11,22] This value is significantly and reliably lower in patients with chronic pancreatitis, often in the range of 40 mEq/L. The reserve capacity of the pancreas is considerable, so again, a lower figure has affirmative value, while a normal or low-normal result must be interpreted along with clinical findings. The total output of bicarbonate can, of course, be calculated from the concentration and the volume. Diagnostically this offers no advantage over determining the peak concentration,[11] but may provide more reproducible results if serial testing is done on the same individual.[22]

Enzyme Content

Secretin does not stimulate enzyme release. If enzyme activity is to be measured, pancreozymin must be administered, usually after the secretin-stimulated secretions have been collected. The results ordinarily parallel the findings in secretin testing, i.e., reduced enzyme activity in patients with pancreatic damage due to inflammation or widespread neoplastic destruction. The combination of pancreozymin with secretin may afford slightly increased diagnostic sensitivity.[10] Amylase is the easiest of the pancreatic enzymes to assay accurately, although trypsin and lipase can also be measured.

In evaluating pancreatic insufficiency, fecal enzyme determinations tend to be difficult and variably reliable, so when the clinical condition suggests enzyme abnormalities, pancreozymin provocation may be valuable. A simpler and reasonably effective way to estimate enzyme production is to look for abnormal quantities of fat and inadequately digested meat in feces.[2] The usefulness of this procedure depends upon how experienced the examiner is in evaluating normal and abnormal observations, but in skilled hands, simple microscopic examination gives good correlation with more detailed tests of pancreatic function.[4,21]

BIBLIOGRAPHY

1. BOCK, O.A.A.: The concepts of "free acid" and "total acid" of the gastric juice. Lancet 2:978, 1962.
2. BROOKS, F.P.: Testing pancreatic function. New Engl. J. Med. 285:300, 1972.
3. CANNON, D.C.: "Examination of gastric and duodenal contents," In Davidsohn, I., and Henry, J.B. (eds.): Clinical Diagnosis by Laboratory Methods, ed. 14. W.B. Saunders Co., Philadelphia, 1969.
4. CERDA, J.J., AND BROOKS, F.P.: Relationships between steatorrhea and an insufficiency of pancreatic secretion in the duodenum in patients with chronic pancreatis. Am. J. Med. Sci. 253:38, 1967.
5. DIGNAN, A.P.: A laboratory appraisal of the effects of truncal and selective vagotomy. Br. J. Surg. 57:249, 1970.
6. DREILING, D.A., AND JANOWITZ, H.D.: The laboratory diagnosis of pancreatic disease: Secretin test. Am. J. Gastroenterol. 28:268, 1957.
7. GILLESPIE, G., ELDER, J.B., GILLESPIE, I.E. ET AL.: The long term stability of the insulin test. Gastroenterology, 58:625, 1970.
8. GO, V.L.W., HOFMANN, A.F., AND SUMMERSKILL, W.H.J.: Stimulation of pancreozymin secretion by digestive products in man. J. Clin. Invest. 49:1558, 1970.
9. GUYTON, A.C.: Textbook of Medical Physiology, ed. 3. W.B. Saunders Co., Philadelphia, 1966.
10. HANSCOM, D.H.: Diagnostic tests in pancreatic disease. Med. Clin. North Am. 52:1483, 1968.
11. HARTLEY, R.C., GAMBILL, E.E., ENGSTROM, G.W., AND SUMMERSKILL, W.H.J.: Pancreatic exocrine function. Am. J. Dig. Dis. 11:27, 1966.
12. HOLLANDER, F.: Laboratory procedures in the study of vagotomy (with particular reference to the insulin test). Gastroenterology 11:419, 1948.
13. JOHNSTON, D., THOMAS, D.G., CHECKETTS, R.G., AND DUTHIE, H.L.: An assessment of postoperative testing for completeness of vagotomy. Br. J. Surg. 54:831, 1967.
14. JORDAN, P.H., JR.: Clinical aspects of gastric secretion and gastric analysis. Med. Clin. North Am. 52:1305, 1968.
15. KAYE, M.D., RHODES, J., AND BECK, P.: Gastric secretion in duodenal ulcer, with particular reference to the diagnosis of Zollinger-Ellison syndrome. Gastroenterology 58:476, 1970.
16. KIRKPATRICK, J.R., DAVIS, G.T., JACOBS, A., AND WILLIAMS, S.W.: The recognition of atrophic gastritis. Br. J. Surg. 56:742, 1969.
17. MARKS, I.N., BANK, S., MOSHAL, M.G., AND LOUW, J.H.: The augmented histamine test—a review of 615 cases of gastroduodenal disease. S. Afr. Med. J. 1:53, 1963.
18. MASON, M.C., AND GILES, G.R.: The postoperative insulin test: failure to detect incomplete vagotomy in patients with high acid levels. Br. J. Surg. 55:865 (abstr.), 1968.
19. MASON, M.C., AND GILES, G.R.: Evaluation and simple modification of the gastrin test. Gut 10:375, 1969.
20. MOORE, E.W., AND SCARLATA, R.W.: The determination of gastric acidity by the glass electrode. Gastroenterology 49:178, 1965.

21. MOORE, J.G., ENGLERT, E., JR., BIGLER, A.H. ET AL.: Simple fecal tests of absorption: a prospective study and technique. Am. J. Dig. Dis. 16:97, 1971.
22. PETERSEN, H.: The duodenal aspirate following secretin stimulation. A variance study in man. Scand. J. Gastroenterol. 4:407, 1969.
23. SILBER, W.: Augmented histamine test in the treatment of symptomatic hiatal hernia. Gut 10:614, 1969.
24. THOMPSON, J.C.: Gastrin and gastric secretion. Annu. Rev. Med. 20:291, 1969.
25. WEINSTEIN, V.A., HOLLANDER, F., LAUBER, F.U., AND COLP, R.: Correlation of insulin test studies and clinical results in a series of peptic ulcer cases treated by vagotomy. Gastroenterology 14:214, 1950.

CHAPTER 12

The Cerebrospinal Fluid

Lumbar puncture and examination of the aspirated fluid are ordinarily diagnostic tools, though at times the entire procedure itself may have therapeutic implications. Lumbar puncture, a procedure which inspires more respect in physicians and trepidation in patients than many other manipulations, constitutes a vitally important technique in many conditions.

ANATOMY AND PHYSIOLOGY

ORIGIN OF THE FLUID AND ITS CONTENTS

The cerebrospinal fluid (CSF), originating from the choroid plexus of the ventricles, occupies the ventricles and the subarachnoid space over the surfaces of the brain and around the spinal cord. Whether the CSF is a dialysate of plasma or a secretion of the choroid plexus is a debate which need not concern us unduly.

The concentration of many but not all of the CSF electrolytes varies with changes in plasma levels, but some appear to be independent. Most constituents of the CSF are present in equal or lower concentrations than in plasma, but the chloride concentration is normally higher. Under pathologic conditions, elements ordinarily restrained by the so-called blood-brain barrier may enter the spinal fluid.

Red cells and white cells can enter the CSF either from rupture of vessels or from meningeal reaction to irritation. Bilirubin, normally absent from CSF, may be found in the spinal fluid of nonjaundiced patients after intracranial hemorrhage. The bilirubin is in the unconjugated prehepatic form, suggesting that hemoglobin can be locally catabolized within the central nervous system.

PRESSURE RELATIONS

The brain, spinal cord, and cerebrospinal fluid are enclosed in a rigid container composed of skull and vertebral column. Normal pressure is maintained by absorption of CSF in amounts equal to production, the absorption occurring primarily through the arachnoid villi and pacchionian corpuscles. Many factors regulate the level of CSF pressure, but the venous pressure is the most important, for ultimately the resorbed fluid drains into the venous system.

ANATOMIC RELATIONS

Despite continuous production and resorption of the fluid and exchange of substances between CSF and blood, considerable stagnation occurs in the lumbar sac. For this reason, the protein concentration and cell count of lumbar fluid exceed the values found in ventricular or cisternal fluid. The lumbar sac is, however, the usual site for routine puncture, since in this caudal area only the filum terminale occupies the spinal canal, and damage to the nervous system is unlikely to occur. In children, the spinal cord persists more caudally than in the adult, so a low lumbar puncture should be made.

INDICATIONS FOR LUMBAR PUNCTURE

Before undertaking lumbar puncture, the physician should define his diagnostic objectives. This will avoid unnecessary manipulation and permit rational selection of laboratory tests. In many conditions, the primary goal is examination of the spinal fluid itself. This goal is paramount in cases of suspected meningitis, in subarachnoid or other intracranial hemorrhage, in certain cases of suspected tumor or brain abscesses, and in cases of undiagnosed neurologic disease when these conditions must be ruled out.

In other patients, the level of CSF pressure is sought, and the goal may be to document impairment of CSF flow or to lower pressure by removing a volume of fluid. Still another reason for entering the subarachnoid space is to introduce anesthetics or other medication or radiographic contrast media.

DANGER FROM INCREASED PRESSURE

Lumbar puncture should be done with extreme caution, if at all, when intracranial pressure is elevated, especially when papilledema is present. The reason for caution is that rapid removal of fluid from the lumbar sac alters the pressure relationships within the subarachnoid space, and the brain stem can be dislocated from a region of high pressure (within the skull) to a region of lower pressure (through the foramen magnum into the spinal canal), a potentially fatal phenomenon known as herniation or "coning." In some cases of increased intracranial pressure, the need to establish a diagnosis outweighs the danger of the procedure, so that each case must be decided individually. An example of this dilemma is the comatose patient in whom intracranial bleeding or meningitis is suspected.

OTHER PROBLEMS

Serious spinal deformities or extreme age may make lumbar puncture difficult, and infection or severe dermatologic disease in the lumbar area should also contraindicate the procedure. Cisternal puncture can be used in such cases or in cases of spinal block, but this procedure requires a sure and experienced hand. A relative, though certainly not absolute, contraindication to lumbar puncture is the existence of severe personality problems in the patient. Many patients point to a previous lumbar puncture as the origin of "the miseries" for years afterward.

EXAMINATION OF CEREBROSPINAL FLUID

Certain observations should be made every time lumbar puncture is performed. The pressure should be measured, and in a few cases it may be desirable to document the dynamic relationships with the Queckenstedt procedure (see p. 284). The CSF should be examined for general appearance, consistency, and tendency to clot. A cell count should be performed, with an attempt to distinguish the types of cells present. In many cases, protein and sugar concentrations are desirable. Other tests done when the patient's condition dictates are: examination of Gram-stained or acid-fast stained smears of the CSF sediment; culture for pyogenic bacteria, tubercle bacilli, or fungi; differential tests employing colloidal suspensions or protein partition; serologic tests for syphilis; and miscellaneous chemical determinations such as bilirubin, urea, chlorides, bromides, or various enzymes.

Table 15.   Normal CSF Values for Children and Adults

	Adults	Infants and Young Children
Quantity (Total)	100-150 ml	Varies with size
Appearance	Clear	Clear
Pressure	75-200 mm H$_2$O	50-100 mm H$_2$O
Cells	0-5	0-20
	All lymphocytes	All lymphocytes

Table 15 shows some of the normal values for CSF examination in which a difference may exist between adults and children.

GENERAL APPEARANCE

Normal spinal fluid has the clarity and consistency of water. Slight color change may be difficult to note, and it is helpful to compare a sample of the CSF with a tube of water. The consistency need not ordinarily be specially examined, because conditions which increase the viscosity nearly always cause fairly conspicuous color change. Turbidity signifies the presence of leukocytes, usually neutrophils, in considerable numbers; lymphocytes alone rarely produce a grossly visible change. Yellowish discoloration, called xanthochromia, usually signifies previous bleeding.

Blood in CSF

It may be difficult to evaluate the significance of fresh blood in the specimen, since damage to an intraspinal vessel may cause a "bloody tap," even though the spinal fluid is intrinsically perfectly clear. If the blood is due to local trauma, the admixture diminishes as CSF is removed, and the fluid in the third tube tends to be appreciably lighter than in the first. If the proportion of blood remains constant, it is probable that the bleeding preceded the puncture.

Subsequent examination of the specimen may clarify the problem of bloody tap versus genuinely bloody fluid. After centrifugation, the supernatant fluid is colorless if the blood came from traumatic lumbar puncture, and is pale-to-deep yellow if the blood was in the fluid initially. Xanthochromia begins within four or five hours after subarachnoid hemorrhage, and usually clears approximately three weeks after the event.[7]

Clotting

In conditions of spinal subarachnoid block, the fluid may be dark yellow with a tendency toward rapid and spontaneous clotting, but spontaneous clotting can occur whenever the protein content is high. It is conversion of fibrinogen to fibrin that produces the clot. Fibrinogen is absent from the normal CSF, but when protein increases significantly, fibrinogen as well as globulins and increased quantities of albumin cross the blood-brain barrier.

CSF PRESSURE

In recumbent adults, the CSF pressure in the lumbar sac varies from 75 to 200 mm of water, with a mean normal value of 120 mm of water. If lumbar puncture is done with the patient seated, the fluid in the manometer normally approaches the level of the foramen magnum. Slight elevation of spinal fluid pressure may occur if an anxious patient involuntarily holds his breath or tenses his muscles. If the knees are flexed too firmly against the abdomen, venous compression may cause spurious elevation, especially in obese patients.

Pathologic decrease of CSF pressure is rare, but may occur in conditions of dehydration or following previous aspiration of CSF.

More significant is elevation of CSF pressure, which may be a conspicuous finding in patients with intracranial tumors or with purulent or tuberculous meningitis. Less marked elevation to approximately 250 to 500 mm of water may accompany low-grade inflammatory processes, encephalitis, or neurosyphilis.

The Queckenstedt Procedure

Since the ventricular spaces, intracranial subarachnoid space, and vertebral subarachnoid space are part of the same closed system, pressure change in one area should be reflected in other areas as well. If local change is not transmitted, existence of a block can be inferred. In the Queckenstedt test, the jugular veins are compressed while lumbar CSF pressure is monitored. Temporary occlusion of both jugular veins impedes the absorption of intracranial fluid and produces an acute rise in intracranial CSF pressure. If CSF flow is unobstructed, the pressure elevation is transmitted to the lumbar fluid, which rises in the manometer and then returns to previous levels when venous occlusion is released. Total or partial spinal block is diagnosed if the lumbar pressure fails to rise when both jugular veins are compressed, or if the pressure requires more than 20 seconds to fall after compression is released. This procedure is risky in patients with increased intracranial pressure or with highly reactive carotid body receptors. Radiologic examination with contrast material (myelogram) is safer and gives far more information.

Opening and Closing Pressures

Removal of cerebrospinal fluid produces a fall in CSF pressure. Although no absolute figure can apply, an expected range is 5 to 10 mm drop for every milliliter of fluid removed from the lumbar sac. If, for example, 10 ml are removed for examination, the closing pressure would be 50 to 100 mm of water less than the opening pressure. A conspicuously small drop in pressure suggests that the total quantity of spinal fluid is increased, as in hydrocephalus; a disproportionately large pressure drop indicates a small CSF pool, as might occur with tumors or spinal block.

CELL COUNT

The normal spinal fluid is virtually free of cells, although up to five small lymphocytes per mm^3 are considered normal. In children, the upper limit of normal may be as high as 20 lymphocytes per mm^3. The presence of granulocytes or large mononuclear cells is never normal, nor should red cells be present. If red cells are present in the CSF, they may be due to a hemorrhagic process or to trauma during the puncture. In distinguishing these events, the red cells should be examined closely. Crenation of the cells indicates they have been in the CSF for some little time. A decrease in the RBC count between the first and last fluid to be aspirated indicates a traumatic puncture.

Sometimes it is necessary to evaluate the leukocyte or protein content of spinal fluid known to be contaminated by traumatic bleeding. A rough rule for discounting adventitious blood is that simple contamination adds one or two white cells for every 1000 red cells, so that a bloody spinal fluid that contained, for example, 20,000 red cells per mm^3 should be expected to contain no more than 30 to 40 white cells. Unless the blood has an unusually high white cell count, demonstration of more than 45 cells in such a fluid would indicate preexisting pleocytosis.

Differential White Count

When cells are counted, they should also be identified as to type. Spinal fluid for cell counts is usually diluted with some compound that accentuates the nucleus and permits rapid differentiation between mononuclear cells and granulocytes. For more detailed morphologic study, the centrifuged sediment can be smeared and examined, and techniques are available for concentrating cells on a fine-gauge filter or in an induced fibrin clot.

Significance of Elevation

White cell counts below 300 to 500 per mm³ usually consist largely of mononuclear cells and may indicate viral infection (including poliomyelitis and "aseptic meningitis"), syphilitic involvement of the central nervous system, tuberculous meningitis, multiple sclerosis, or some localized irritative process such as a tumor or abscess. Above 500 per mm³, the white cells tend to be predominantly granulocytes arising from a purulent infection.

Neutrophils Plus Monocytes. A puzzling finding may be a mildly or moderately elevated count with significant numbers of both lymphocytes and neutrophils. This may reflect developing tuberculous meningitis or can be found in the CSF when there is a brain abscess. Localized tumors contribute relatively few cells to the CSF, but massive leukemic infiltration of the central nervous system may cause significant pleocytosis.

Cryptococcus. In occasional cases, an erroneous diagnosis of "moderate numbers of lymphocytes" may be made if cryptococcal organisms (torula) are in the CSF. These fungi are small and round and may be numerous without provoking a significant cellular response. Cryptococci are easily demonstrated by adding India ink to the spinal fluid, for the cryptococcal capsule stands out as a transparent disk surrounded by black carbon particles.

CHEMICAL TESTS

SPINAL FLUID PROTEINS

The spinal fluid normally contains very little protein, for serum proteins are large molecules which do not cross the blood-brain barrier. The normal concentration, 15 to 45 mg per 100 ml, is well below 1 per cent of the normal serum levels of 5 to 8 Gm per 100 ml (see Table 16). The proportion of albumin to globulin is even higher in spinal fluid than in plasma, for the albumin molecule is significantly smaller and can more easily pass through endothelial barriers. This situation is comparable to the passage of serum proteins across the glomerular filter, and urinary protein tends to be largely albumin in all but the most florid renal disorders.

Table 16.   Normal Values for Some Commonly Measured
            Substances in Cerebrospinal Fluid

	CSF Level	Compared with Plasma Level
pH	7.32-7.35	Very slightly lower
Glucose	45-85 mg/100 ml	50-80 per cent
Protein	15-45 mg/100 ml	0.2-0.5 per cent
A/G Ratio	8:1	3-4 times higher
Chloride	110-125 mEq/liter	115-125 per cent
Urea nitrogen	10-15 mg/100 ml	Same

Source of Abnormal Proteins

Protein concentration may rise for a number of reasons. One source is increased permeability of the blood-brain barrier due to inflammation. In severe meningitis, all types of serum protein may enter the CSF, including fibrinogen which is a very large molecule indeed. In purulent meningitis, the CSF protein is further increased because bacteria and cells, both intact and disintegrated, contribute protein to the medium. In most diseases, cell count and protein concentration tend to change in parallel.

Effect of Added Blood. When there is blood in the spinal fluid, the CSF protein level is necessarily elevated, but preexisting protein levels must sometimes be evaluated in a spinal fluid contaminated by a bloody tap. The rough calculation of 1 mg protein for each 1000 red cells can be subtracted from the measured protein concentration. A chronic subdural hematoma may contribute a small amount of protein to the CSF without introducing red cells.

Protein Without Cells

When protein concentration rises and relatively few cells are present, degenerative disease of the central nervous system should be suspected. The Guillain-Barré syndrome, or ascending polyneuritis, characteristically affects the spinal fluid proteins, and multiple sclerosis and neurosyphilis may increase the globulin content, adding only a few mononuclear cells. Conditions of subarachnoid block, especially when caused by a spinal tumor, permit protein accumulation in the fluid distal to the block, and the fluid may clot upon aspiration. Superficially located tumors, notably acoustic neuroma and meningioma, may cause a moderate increase in CSF protein.

Techniques

Since the protein concentration in CSF is so much lower than in blood, different means must be used for measurement. The most popular, quick qualitative test for increased protein is the Pandy test, in which dilute phenol solution added to the specimen produces turbidity proportional to the protein concentration. Greater accuracy can be achieved by using sulfosalicylic acid and quantitating the turbidity with a colorimeter.

Electrophoresis. More detailed information about proteins can be achieved by electrophoresis. The CSF proteins derive largely from serum proteins, and, as might be expected from molecular sizes, albumin is the predominant protein in normal CSF. The gamma globulin fraction is normally very low, but when serum globulin levels are high, the CSF gamma peak may increase. Occasionally, elevated CSF immunoglubulin without parallel serum levels suggests a central nervous system plasmacytoma.[9] Increased CSF levels of all plasma proteins characterize the *capillary permeability pattern,* a finding associated with, but hardly specific for, inflammation, neoplasms, diabetes, Guillian-Barré syndrome, and some cerebrovascular disease. A so-called degenerative pattern has been described in which the β_2-globulins are disproportionately increased. This has been reported[1] in some cases of cerebral atrophy, syringomyelia, and amyotrophic lateral sclerosis, but cannot be considered a reliable diagnostic finding.

GLUCOSE

Cerebrospinal fluid glucose concentration is normally 50 to 80 per cent of the blood glucose level, and changes in the blood sugar are reflected in the CSF after a 30 to 60 minute lag.[7] The normal CSF glucose level is between 40 and 80 mg per 100 ml, but critical evaluation of CSF glucose determination requires comparison against a blood sample drawn, if possible, 30 to 60 minutes before lumbar puncture is done.

The most dramatic drop in CSF sugar occurs with purulent meningitis, when the combination of bacterial and leukocytic activity may reduce the CSF glucose to zero. Glucose metabolism is an active process which continues after the sample has been aspirated, so that sugar should be determined promptly in samples that are suspected to contain granulocytes or microorganisms. Because all types of organisms consume glucose, a decreased sugar content may indicate the presence of fungi, protozoa, or tubercle bacilli, as well as pyogenic bacteria. Less change in CSF sugar accompanies lymphocytic meningitis, brain abscesses, degenerative diseases, and most tumors. Occasional superficial tumors may lower the sugar content, and the glucose level in neurosyphilis may vary slightly from normal in either direction.[8]

CHLORIDES

Unlike most other CSF constituents, chlorides are present in higher concentration than in plasma. The ratio is approximately 1.2 to 1, so that normal CSF chloride values are 110 to 125 mEq per liter. The plasma chloride level is quite labile, and changing plasma values are reflected promptly in the CSF; thus, any condition that alters the plasma chloride will also affect the CSF level. Spinal fluid chloride determination receives less attention now than it used to. Its chief diagnostic value is in tuberculous meningitis, in which there may be nonspecific neurologic findings and mild elevation of proteins and mononuclear cells in the CSF. The CSF levels of sugar and chlorides are, in these cases, significantly depressed. Other types of meningitis may cause a decrease in the CSF chloride, while syphilis, tumors, encephalitis, and brain abscesses do not affect this ion. If the patient is receiving an intravenous infusion of electrolyte solutions, the chloride values in the CSF are invalidated.

UREA

The urea levels in blood and spinal fluid are approximately equal, and CSF urea increases in uremia. Urea is sometimes injected intravenously in patients with acutely elevated intracranial pressure. In such cases, the induced uremia results in markedly increased CSF osmolality, which may relieve cerebral edema by shifting fluid from brain to hyperosmolal spinal fluid. Following infusion of 0.5 to 1.0 gram of urea per kilogram of body weight, the urea levels of blood and spinal fluid require 24 to 48 hours to return to physiologic levels.

CALCIUM

The spinal fluid contains only half as much calcium as the blood contains. This is entirely predictable, since approximately one-half of the serum calcium is bound to protein, and protein does not diffuse freely into the spinal fluid. When CSF protein is increased, the calcium level increases also.

ENZYMES

Such serum enzymes as lactic dehydrogenase (LDH), glutamic oxalacetic transaminase (GOT), and glutamic pyruvic transaminase (GPT) have been measured in the spinal fluid and are present in slightly lower concentrations in the CSF than in serum. Although many workers have found that mild-to-moderate enzyme changes accompany various neurologic disorders, CSF enzyme levels are not, at present, measured under routine conditions. The enzyme most often affected is glutamic oxalacetic transaminase, which rises in inflammatory, hemorrhagic, or degenerative diseases of the central nervous system.[8]

MICROORGANISMS

Significant numbers of bacteria, fungi, or protozoa in the CSF can be identified by examining the stained sediment after centrifugation. Whenever there is a question of meningitis or central nervous system infection, smears of the CSF sediment should be stained with a Gram stain and with an acid-fast stain. The pyogenic bacteria and many fungi can be demonstrated by examination of a good smear, but failure to isolate organisms on smear should not be interpreted to mean that organisms are absent. Unless the cause of the central nervous system disorder is self-evident, steps should always be taken to rule out the presence of tubercle bacilli, because tuberculous meningitis can develop insidiously and presents few clear-cut diagnostic signs.

CULTURING THE CSF

The spinal fluid should be cultured on several media since it is always advisable to rule out bacterial, fungal, and tuberculous infections, and more than one organism may be present. The meningococcus (Neisseria meningitidis) prefers a high carbon dioxide atmosphere and special media, so that separate plates should be inoculated to isolate this organism. Sometimes an aliquot of the original sample can be incubated at 37°C for 24 hours permitting the organisms to multiply in the spinal fluid before incubation of a second set of cultures.

Immunologic Tests

Immunologic techniques are now being applied to CSF microbiology in some laboratories. The cryptococcal antigen test[5] uses a strong, specific anticryptococcus antibody to identify antigenic elements which may be in CSF even when organisms are undetectible. Several bacterial antigens have been demonstrated by counter-immunoelectrophoresis,[2] a technique which can, in little more than an hour, give extremely specific documentation of bacterial invasion. This technique is still experimental, but has tremendous potential application.

Serologic Tests for Syphilis

Blood tests used in diagnosing syphilis are of two types: the nonspecific types which demonstrate syphilitic reagin, and the specific types which demonstrate antitreponemal antibodies. The nonspecific tests, which are cheaper, more readily available, and do not require a specialized laboratory, are most widely used for spinal fluid testing. Biologic false positives are fairly rare on CSF specimens. The pronounced alterations in protein proportions that accompany encephalitis, hemorrhage, acute meningitis, or even a bloody tap, may sometimes give reactive results in flocculation tests, such as the Venereal Disease Research Laboratory (VDRL) test.[6] The older techniques of colloidal gold or gum mastic testing relied upon these syphilis-induced protein alterations to produce diagnostic changes in suspension stability. These tests have largely been abandoned, since syphilis can more accurately be diagnosed immunologically, and other protein aberrations are better documented by electrophoresis.

Although nonspecific tests (see Chap. 2) are usually applied to CSF, they are considerably less sensitive than the fluorescent treponemal antibody (FTA) test for detecting neurosyphilis.[4] Because of the low antibody levels involved, absorption with nonsyphilitic treponemal antigen (FTA-ABS) may remove CSF reactivity. If neurosyphilis is a serious diagnostic consideration, the FTA constitutes a more reliable screening test than the VDRL.

BIBLIOGRAPHY

1. CAWLEY, L.P.: Electrophoresis and Immunoelectrophoresis. Little, Brown & Co., Boston, 1969.
2. COONROD, J.D., AND RYTEL, M.W.: Determination of aetiology of bacterial meningitis by counterimmunoelectrophoresis. Lancet 1:1154, 1972.
3. DUBLIN, W.B., AND DUBLIN, A.B.: Cerebrospinal fluid pH, carbon dioxide tension, standard bicarbonate. Bull. Los Angeles Neurol. Soc. 28:157, 1963.
4. ESCOBAR, M.R., DALTON, H.P., AND ALLISON, M.J.: Fluorescent antibody tests for syphilis using cerebrospinal fluid: Clinical correlations in 150 cases. Am. J. Clin. Pathol. 53:886, 1970.
5. GOODMAN, J.S., KAUFMAN, L., AND KOENIG, M.G.: Diagnosis of cryptococcal antigen. New Engl. J. Med. 285:434, 1971.
6. HEYMAN, A.: "Syphilis," *In* Wintrobe, M.M., Thorn, G.W., Adams, R.D. et al. (eds.): Harrison's Principles of Internal Medicine, ed. 6. McGraw-Hill Book Co., New York, 1970.
7. JENKINS, R.G.: The cerebrospinal fluid. GP 27:130, 1963.
8. SPIEGEL-ADOLF, M.: Cerebrospinal fluid. Progr. Neurol. Psychiatry 20:455, 1965.
9. WEINER, L.P., ANDERSON, P.N., AND ALLEN, J.C.: Cerebral plasmacytoma with myeloma protein in the cerebrospinal fluid. Neurology 16:615, 1966.

Part 2

CLINICAL FINDINGS

CHAPTER 13

Diseases Affecting
Red Blood Cells

Most of this chapter is devoted to consideration of the many disorders that result in anemia, or deficiency of the total hemoglobin-red cell mass. A brief section is devoted to several conditions in which the hemoglobin-red cell mass is increased. In terms of clinical significance, deficiency of oxygen-carrying power far outweighs the few disorders in which oxygen-carrying capacity is increased.

Table 17 is a summary attempt to classify anemias by their etiology and physiologic impact. Anemias can never be fully grouped into mutually exclusive, comprehensive categories, since the etiology, morphology, or

Table 17.   Physiologic Classification of Anemias*

ANEMIAS CAUSED BY INCREASED LOSS OR DESTRUCTION OF HEMOGLOBIN-RED CELL MASS

I. Anemia resulting from blood loss, internal or external
   A. Acute
   B. Chronic

II. Anemia resulting from excessive destruction of red cells
    A. Owing to intracorpuscular defects
       1. Hereditary defects of red blood cells
          a. Hemoglobinopathies
          b. Thalassemia
          c. Primaquine-sensitive hemolytic disease (G-6-PD deficiency)
          d. Hereditary spherocytosis
          e. Hereditary nonspherocytic disease
          f. Hereditary elliptocytosis

* Adapted, with permission, from Tables 5.2 and 5.3 in Harris, J.W., and Kellermeyer, R.W.: The Red Cell, rev. ed. The Commonwealth Fund, Harvard University Press, Cambridge, Mass., 1970.

Table 17   (Continued)

2. Acquired defects of red blood cells
   a. Thermal injury
   b. Paroxysmal nocturnal hemoglobinuria
   c. Deficiency diseases
      (1) Vitamin B_{12}
      (2) Folic acid
      (3) Iron

B. Owing to extracorpuscular abnormalities
   1. Immune mechanisms with demonstrable antibodies
      a. Blood group antibodies
      b. Cold agglutinins
      c. Cold hemolysins

   2. "Autoimmunity" with or without demonstrable antibodies
      a. Idiopathic acquired hemolytic anemia
      b. Secondary acquired hemolytic anemia
         (1) Lupus erythematosus
         (2) Lymphomas
         (3) Others

   3. Nonimmune mechanisms
      a. Chemicals toxic to normal cells
      b. Thermal injury
      c. Infectious agents

   4. Unknown mechanisms
      a. Splenomegaly
      b. Acute and chronic infections
      c. Acute and chronic renal disease
      d. Malignant neoplasms

ANEMIAS CAUSED BY DECREASED PRODUCTION OF HEMOGLOBIN-RED CELL MASS

  I. Anemia of primary bone marrow failure

 II. Anemia resulting from bone marrow failure secondary to other diseases

III. Anemia resulting from endocrine abnormalities

IV. Anemia resulting from specific deficiencies

   A. Vitamin B_{12}

   B. Folic acid

   C. Vitamin C

   D. Iron

physiologic change in many conditions may overlap or shade into any one of several other disease states. The organization of the table represents only one of several possible approaches to classifying the anemias.

ANEMIAS CAUSED BY INCREASED LOSS OR DESTRUCTION OF HEMOGLOBIN—RED CELL MASS

BLOOD LOSS

Acute Blood Loss

When more than 15 per cent of the blood volume is lost rapidly, the initial clinical symptoms result from hypovolemia, which the body combats with prompt vascular constriction and tachycardia. If these changes do not adequately compensate for the lost volume, blood pressure falls. Up to 48 hours are required before sufficient fluid transfer occurs to replace the lost volume, and during this period hemoglobin concentration and hematocrit may not reflect the acute changes.

A few hours after acute blood loss, the number of circulating platelets rises, and the white count may go as high as 20,000 per mm^3 within 24 hours. Once volume is replaced, a normochromic, normocytic anemia occurs. Reticulocytosis occurs within one or two days, reaching a peak at four to seven days. If reticulocytosis is marked, as it may be following massive blood loss, corpuscular indices may indicate a macrocytic condition, because reticulocytes are significantly larger than mature red cells. Similarly, reticulocytes may adsorb antiglobulin (Coombs) serum, and the direct Coombs test may be weakly positive in conditions of rapid erythropoiesis. If bleeding does not recur, reticulocytosis ceases within 30 days, so that an elevated reticulocyte count beyond that period suggests continuing blood loss. If blood is shed within the body—into the gastrointestinal tract, peritoneal cavity, soft tissues, and the like—degradation of the stagnant hemoglobin may raise serum levels of bilirubin and urea. With external loss, naturally, these signs of hemoglobin and protein breakdown are absent.

Chronic Blood Loss

Since the anemia of chronic blood loss is due to iron deficiency, a brief consideration of iron metabolism is necessary before discussing the clinical manifestations of iron lack.

Iron Metabolism. Iron, the central molecule in the body's oxygen-carrying compounds, performs a critical role in metabolism. The body contains between 2 and 6 Gm of iron, depending on size. Free ionized iron is toxic, so some means of binding and transport are vital. One half to two thirds of the body's iron is in hemoglobin; most of the remaining iron exists in ferritin and hemosiderin, storage forms of iron bound to protein. A small amount circulates in the iron-binding globulin of plasma, and still smaller amounts exist in myoglobin, the cytochromes, and other compounds concerned with intracellular oxygen metabolism.

INTAKE. Iron is derived solely from dietary ingestion, except for the 350 to 500 mg that the infant receives in fetal life. Iron is present in meats, eggs, leafy vegetables, and fortified cereal products; an average adult who eats a normal diet ingests, but does not absorb, 10 to 30 mg of iron per day. In the adult male, iron loss through feces, bile, sweat, and epidermal desquamation averages 0.5 to 1.5 mg daily and approximately this quantity is absorbed from the diet. Menstruating females lose approximately 16 to 32 mg of iron monthly, imposing an average additional daily loss of 0.5 to 1.0 mg. Growing children have greater iron requirements than adults, and a pregnancy exacts 350 to 500 mg from the mother. Lactation drains an additional 0.5 mg per day, although the nursing infant obtains relatively little iron from milk.

ABSORPTION. Iron is absorbed across the mucosa of the duodenum and proximal jejunum, in a manner not fully understood. In the blood stream, iron is carried by a β_1-globulin known as transferrin, or iron-binding globulin. Sufficient transferrin is normally available to carry approximately 300 mcg of iron per 100 ml of blood, but the normal level of circulating iron is approximately 100 mcg/100 ml, or one third of the potential iron-binding capacity. Transferrin levels may vary with changes in tissue oxygenation and also with changes in generalized protein synthesis. The serum iron level and per cent saturation of iron-binding globulin are guides to the state of iron metabolism.

Iron enters the developing erythrocyte either directly from the transferrin molecule or indirectly through the action of reticuloendothelial cells. Rare individuals with congenital absence of transferrin have a severe, refractory iron-deficiency anemia.

STORAGE. Potentially usable iron is stored as hemosiderin and ferritin. Although the bulk of stored iron is in the liver, enough iron is normally present in bone marrow so that marrow sections stained for iron granules can indicate the condition of iron stores. Quantitative experiments have established that normal adult males have total available stores of 1000 to 1500 mg.[19] Excessive iron intake, as from repeated blood transfusion, causes increased deposition primarily in reticuloendothelial cells, whereas in idiopathic hemochromatosis, iron is deposited in parenchymal cells of such organs as the liver, heart, and pancreas.

IRON EXCESS. Patients who receive repeated whole blood transfusions gradually acquire large iron stores. Each 500 ml unit of blood contains approximately 200 to 250 mg of iron and since the cause for transfusion is usually refractory anemia, the iron is not reused for hemoglobin synthesis. The excess iron is deposited primarily in the reticuloendothelial cells but may accumulate in parenchymal cells as well, and death may be caused by iron-induced myocardial damage. Because venesection would aggravate the underlying anemia, therapy with chelating agents has been suggested, but experience has not shown this to be fully effective.[49]

Iron-Deficiency Anemia. Insufficient iron supply results in hypochromic microcytic anemia of varying degree, accompanied by varying degrees of clinical debility. Several factors, alone or in combination, may produce iron deficiency: poor dietary intake, inadequate absorption, increased requirement, or loss of blood.

The most common victims of inadequate dietary intake are small children reared on little but milk during the critical first two years, when their body's red cell mass should be increasing rapidly. In the United States, fortified food products and generally varied diet make poor intake alone a rare cause of iron deficiency. A borderline intake may, however, become inadequate under conditions of increased requirement, such as rapid growth spurts, onset of menstruation, or repeated pregnancies. For adult males and postmenopausal women, dietary deficiency alone very seldom produces significant iron lack. In less developed countries, the combination of poor diet, frequent parasitic infestations, and repeated pregnancies makes iron-deficiency anemia a widespread and pressing health problem.

COMMON ETIOLOGIES. Certain gastrointestinal disorders or operations, such as total gastrectomy, ileostomy, and steatorrhea and other forms of chronic diarrhea, may impair iron absorption; however, other stresses may contribute to reducing effective iron intake. Increased iron utilization, combined with borderline intake or impaired absorption or both, produces most of the iron-deficiency conditions of adolescent and mature women in the United States and elsewhere. The severe anemia formerly called "chlorosis" was iron-deficiency anemia occurring during the adolescent growth spurt and frequently aggravated by excessive or irregular blood loss during the first few years of menstruation.

Chronic blood loss is the commonest cause of iron-deficiency anemia, and almost the only cause in adult men and postmenopausal women. Except for the special cases of pregnancy and menstruation, bleeding from the genitourinary tract or gastrointestinal tract causes the overwhelming majority of iron-deficiency anemias. In countries where intestinal parasites are encountered, infestation is a frequent cause of occult bleeding, while, in the United States, malignant neoplasms are the commonest offender, followed by chronic ulcers and benign neoplastic growths.

DIAGNOSTIC FINDINGS. Iron-deficiency anemia should be considered if anemia is hypochromic and microcytic, often with bizarrely shaped red cells on blood smear. No significant abnormalities of white cells or platelets occur, but reticulocyte counts are low. Bone marrow examination frequently reveals normoblastic hyperplasia, but the cells are small, poorly filled with hemoglobin, and bizarrely shaped. No stainable iron is found in the bone marrow, and serum iron levels are decreased below 40 mcg/100 ml. Serum iron-binding capacity is increased, so the percent saturation is low, usually below 15 per cent of total capacity.[14] Iron deficiency is the only condition in which iron-binding capacity is high and the serum iron level is low. Other hypochromic microcytic anemias—such as thalassemia, pyridoxine-responsive anemia, and anemias of chronic infection and lead poisoning—are associated with normal or increased iron stores and with serum transferrin levels that are normal or decreased. Urinary and fecal urobilinogen are decreased with iron deficiency, indicating diminished hemoglobin metabolism.

When iron therapy is given, reticulocytosis begins by the third day and increases steadily for the next week or so, after which it tends to level off at a higher than normal rate until normal hemoglobin values are attained. Hemoglobin level begins to rise by the end of the second week, but subjective clinical improvement may occur before a rise is detectable. It is not enough simply to treat iron-deficiency anemia, because the anemia is a symptom, not a primary disease. The cause of the deficiency must be established and treated.

Other Conditions of Disordered Iron Metabolism. SIDEROBLASTIC ANEMIA. Several other anemias resemble that of simple iron deficiency, but have somewhat different causes. Certain hereditary and acquired conditions may cause impaired iron utilization. In the congenital type, anemia develops quite early, and hemochromatosis and splenomegaly develop gradually. The acquired type is similar, but anemia develops much later in life and may be idiopathic or secondary to a variety of chronic debilitating illnesses, drug ingestion, or other primary hematologic disorders.[18] In both forms, the marrow contains many erythrocyte precursors with virtually no cytoplasmic hemoglobin and an accumulation of coarse siderotic granules which may surround the nucleus. These cells are called sideroblasts or "ringed" sideroblasts. Both serum iron and iron-binding capacity are high, and plasma iron turnover is increased. Urinary levels of coproporphyrin, porphobilinogen, and other hemoglobin precursors are high, but fecal and urinary urobilinogen and serum bilirubin do not reach levels suggestive of increased hemoglobin breakdown. The condition termed sideroblastic or sideroachrestic anemia is diagnosed when sideroblasts are prominent in the marrow.

PYRIDOXINE-RESPONSIVE ANEMIAS. In a few patients with hypochromic red cells and hyperplastic, sideroblast-containing bone marrows, the problem is not refractory sideroblastic anemia. The red cells are variable in size and have a slightly decreased life span. Large doses of pyridoxine, up to 200 mg orally, may induce hematologic improvement, even though no dermal, neurologic, or mucosal signs of pyridoxine deficiency have been noted. A familial incidence, largely in males, has been reported in the so-called classic form,[18,20] but the majority of these rather rare cases form a heterogeneous population.

HEMOGLOBIN METABOLISM

Adequate erythropoiesis requires that functioning hemoglobin be produced and then transported in suitable containers—the red cells—to the body's oxygen-consuming tissues. Failure at any point in this process may have serious physiologic consequences. Hemoglobin is a complex molecule consisting of four identical heme units and a globin portion which consists of four polypeptide chains, two identical alpha chains, and two identical beta chains.

Heme Synthesis

The heme portion of hemoglobin consists of an iron atom covalently linked to four ring structures called pyrroles. The unit of four pyrrole rings is common to a group of substances called porphyrins. Heme is produced when iron is added to the last of this series, protoporphyrin IX. Anything that interferes with porphyrin synthesis necessarily impairs heme production. Since the iron-containing heme complex is joined to globin, defects in globin synthesis also impair normal hemoglobin production.

Porphyrin Production. The pyrroles of the heme unit derive initially from glycine and succinyl coenzyme A which in turn originates from the tricarboxylic acid cycle. Numerous thoroughly documented steps occur in heme synthesis which we will summarize only by listing. Succinyl coenzyme A and glycine combine to form alpha-amino, beta-keto adipic acid, which is decarboxylated to form delta-amino levulinic acid (ALA). This straight-line compound is the first recognizable heme precursor of diagnostic significance. Two molecules of ALA combine to form porphobilinogen, a molecule with a single-ring configuration. Four porphobilinogen rings condense to form the tetrapyrrole uroporphyrinogen. Subsequent steps in synthesis are conversion of uroporphyrinogen to coproporphyrinogen, conversion of coproporphyrinogen to protoporphyrin, and coupling of proto-porphyrin with iron for the happy ending—the production of heme.

Uroporphyrin and Coproporphyrin. Uroporphyrinogen and coproporphyrinogen, as indicated by their names, can be converted to uroporphyrin and coproporphyrin, but these end products do not engage in heme synthesis. Normally, only small quantities of coproporphyrin and uroporphyrin are found in urine and feces, but in certain metabolic disorders excess porphyrins accumulate (see Porphyrias, p. 243). Uroporphyrinogen and coproporphyrinogen and their end products uroporphyrin and coproporphyrin exist in two isomeric forms, III and I. The type III isomers participate in heme synthesis, while the type I substances are by-products and usually exist in rather small quantities in urine and feces.

Heme Catabolism

Before considering the steps involved in globin synthesis and the linkage of heme to globin, we shall complete the cycle traced by the heme molecule. Heme destruction begins with liberation of hemoglobin from the red cells. When red cells are destroyed, their hemoglobin is degraded within the reticuloendothelial system. The iron atoms are split off and transported to hematopoietic centers to be incorporated in later hemoglobin synthesis. The globin portion returns to the body's protein pool for possible reuse. The remaining porphyrin component is converted from the ring structure to a straight-line molecule of four pyrrole rings. This line of pyrrole rings is called biliverdin—one of the pigments responsible for the lurid green hue of a resolving bruise—but most biliverdin is rapidly reduced to bilirubin.

Bilirubin. Bilirubin is insoluble, and only when it is bound to serum albumin can it be transported through the blood. In this form, it is measured by the indirect or delayed van den Bergh reaction. From the reticuloendothelial system, bilirubin is carried to the liver, where enzymatic reactions conjugate it with glucuronic acid and other compounds and render it soluble. This soluble conjugated form is measured by the direct or immediate van den Bergh reaction, and is capable of passing through the glomerular filter into the urine.

Urobilinogen. Most of the conjugated bilirubin passes from the liver cells into the bile, which enters the duodenum. Within the intestine, bacteria degrade the conjugated bilirubin to a variety of colorless compounds called, collectively, urobilinogen. Much of the urobilinogen is excreted in the feces, where it is oxidized to the colored compounds stercobilin and urobilin. A modest proportion of fecal urobilinogen, however, is reabsorbed through the intestinal wall to reenter the blood stream. The urobilinogen normally present in urine probably derives from this reabsorbed

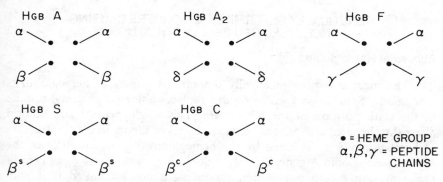

Figure 13. Schematic representation of composition of normal and more common abnormal hemoglobins.

component. Most of the reabsorbed urobilinogen reenters the liver and retraces the excretion route through the bile into the feces. The quantity of fecal and urinary urobilinogen mirrors the quantity of heme available for degradation. The quantity of bilirubin in the blood may also reflect hemoglobin breakdown, although bilirubin levels are affected by many nonhematologic problems.

Globin Synthesis

Incomparably more frequent than disorders of heme metabolism are genetically determined disorders of globin synthesis. The term *hemoglobinopathy* is used to describe conditions in which genetic defects of polypeptide synthesis result in production of abnormal hemoglobin. The two pairs of polypeptide chains in the globin moiety are produced under separate genetic control. Alpha chain production results from one locus, and beta chain production from another. In uterine life, the fetus elaborates a hemoglobin different from the normal adult form. This is called fetal hemoglobin, or hemoglobin F, which contains two alpha chains but has two gamma chains instead of the beta chains in adult hemoglobin. At about 36 weeks' gestation, the fetal marrow starts producing hemoglobin A instead of hemoglobin F. At birth, 70 per cent of the baby's hemoglobin is type F, a proportion that falls rapidly to adult levels of 5 per cent or less by one year. The normal adult has small amounts, usually 1 to 3 per cent of total levels, of still a third hemoglobin. Called hemoglobin A_2, this consists of two alpha chains and two delta chains. Each of these four chains mentioned—alpha, beta, gamma, and delta—has a highly specific sequence of peptide linkages controlled by the base sequence in the genetic locus (Fig. 13). Abnormal hemoglobins appear to result from single alterations in genetic sequence, which alter the peptide sequence of the globin chain.

GENETICALLY DETERMINED DISORDERS CAUSING
INCREASED RED CELL DESTRUCTION

Abnormal Hemoglobins

The most common genetically determined abnormal hemoglobin is hemoglobin S, in which a valine residue replaces a normal glutamyl residue in the sixth position of the beta chain. This single peptide substitution alters the chemical and physical characteristics of the molecule. Production of hemoglobin S is mediated by the hemoglobin S gene, an allele of the normal hemoglobin A gene. The hemoglobin S gene occurs in 8 per cent of the American Negro population, producing a non-sex-linked trait with incomplete dominance. If the gene is present in single dose, 20 to 40 per cent of the individual's hemoglobin is the S form, while the individual with a double dose has no hemoglobin A, only hemoglobin S, and a small, variable quantity of hemoglobin F. Possession of the hemoglobin S gene in single dose causes sickle trait, in which the abnormal hemoglobin can be demonstrated in the laboratory, but the individual suffers virtually no serious ill effects. Occasional patients with sickle cell trait manifest painless hematuria,[52] and at very low oxygen tensions, notably in unpressurized airplanes, splenic infarction has been reported.[44] Individuals with a double dose, approximately 0.2 per cent of the American Negro population, have the full syndrome of sickle cell disease.

Varieties of Hemoglobin. Hemoglobin S was the first abnormal hemoglobin to be identified, and it has a characteristic pattern of electrophoretic and chromatographic migration. Each normal and abnormal hemoglobin, of which more than twenty are now recognized, has its own pattern and can be identified in pure form and in combinations by suitable control of electrophoretic conditions. The proportion of hemoglobins F and A_2 in a mixture can be determined by chemical means.

Most hemoglobin abnormalities exist as beta chain defects, but a variety of combinations and permutations are recognized. Most are of interest primarily to geneticists and biochemists; only hemoglobin S and hemoglobin C present significant clinical problems in the United States. The remainder occur largely in Africa, Asia and the near East. Of American Negroes, 2.3 per cent are estimated to be heterozygous for hemoglobin C, and 1 in 6000 is homozygous.[53] The hemoglobin S trait is present in 8 to 11 per cent of American Negroes and the homozygous form exists in 2 to 3 American Negroes per thousand. The heterozygous form combining one hemoglobin S gene and one hemoglobin C gene also exists, and it produces a clinical condition somewhat less severe than unmodified hemoglobin S disease.

THE SICKLING PHENOMENON. Hemoglobin S differs from hemoglobin

A by a single amino acid residue. Normal hemoglobin has glutamic acid, a negatively-charged residue, at the sixth position of the beta chain; hemoglobin S has the uncharged amino acid valine. When oxygen-saturated, the molecules exist at random dispersion in a homogeneous solution. In the deoxygenated state, however, the altered charge permits individual molecules to link together in chains, which then align to form rigid, boat-shaped tactoids which are markedly insoluble. Whether free in solution or confined within red cells, hemoglobin S forms a viscous semi-solid gel upon deoxygenation, and resumes its soluble configuration when reoxygenated.

Individuals homozygous for the abnormal gene have only hemoglobin S in their red cells, and oxygen tensions no lower than those sometimes found in venous blood may induce sickling. The cells of heterozygotes contain 60 to 70 per cent hemoglobin A, along with 30 to 40 per cent hemoglobin S.[31] At this intracellular concentration of hemoglobin S, much lower oxygen tensions are needed to induce sickling. Such tensions occur only under conditions of laboratory manipulation, and in vivo sickling in heterozygotes has been reported only at extremely low oxygen tensions.[40]

Because sickling appears to result from abnormal intramolecular configurations and consequent formation of intermolecular bonds,[33] attempts have been made to prevent or reverse sickling by physical or chemical manipulations which hinder bond formation. Under intensive study are the physical, physiologic, and potential therapeutic effects of urea,[34] cyanate,[6] and carbamyl phosphate[25] on hemoglobin S, both in laboratory solutions and in the red cells of afflicted patients.

LABORATORY FINDINGS IN SICKLE CELL DISEASE. Laboratory diagnosis of sickle cell anemia and sickle cell trait relies principally on hemoglobin electrophoresis. Red cells can be made to sickle by exposure to a reducing agent such as sodium metabisulfite, but this screening device is often misleading and is rarely definitive. Other laboratory findings in sickle cell anemia include hemoglobin levels ranging from 5 to 9 Gm per 100 ml, with normal cell indices but markedly abnormal size and shape of stained red cells (Fig. 14). Marked reticulocytosis and normoblastic bone marrow hyperplasia testify to continuing red cell destruction and production, but during sickle cell crises red cell destruction continues while erythropoiesis slows disastrously. Serum iron and body iron stores are high. Moderate leukocytosis and a slight increase in platelets are often noted. Serum unconjugated bilirubin and fecal urobilinogen are elevated. The erythrocytes have a markedly shortened life span and are characterized by increased mechanical fragility and decreased osmotic fragility.

The disease follows a chronic course characterized by intermittent aplastic crises, hyperhemolytic crises, and repeated episodes of painful

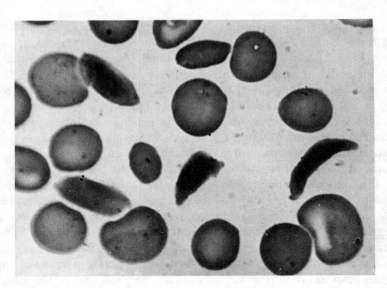

Figure 14.   Sickle forms in blood of patient with sickle cell disease. This smear of peripheral blood was made when the patient was in a sickle cell crisis.

vascular occlusion. Thrombosis probably results from the altered size, shape, and compressibility of the sickled cells. Once capillary occlusion occurs, the resultant stasis permits increased deoxygenation which aggravates the sickling and permits the occlusion to enlarge. Numerous other manifestations in bones, joints, abdominal cavity, nervous system, and skin combine to make the disease unremitting and subject to frequent exacerbations.

HEMOGLOBIN C DISEASE. Homozygous hemoglobin C disease may clinically resemble sickle cell anemia but tends to be milder. A mild to moderately severe hemolytic anemia is accompanied by splenomegaly, rather than the small spleen seen in late sickle cell anemia. The blood contains large numbers of target cells, and osmotic fragility is decreased. In combined hemoglobin S and hemoglobin C disease, sickling can be induced, and target cells are present on smears. Aplastic crises may occur, but the hemolysis is usually well compensated, producing hyperplastic bone marrow, decreased red cell survival, and increased levels of serum bilirubin and fecal urobilinogen.

Thalassemia. Thalassemia was originally considered a severe hypochromic, microcytic anemia affecting children of Mediterranean origin. Subsequent discovery of less severely affected older persons led to division into *thalassemia major* and *thalassemia minor,* representing homozygous and heterozygous states of the abnormality. The number of known variants has grown enormously. The term *thalassemia syndromes* is now used to describe a series of conditions with disordered hemoglobin synthesis resulting in decreased hemoglobin stores in circulating red cells.

THE GENETIC DEFECT. A common defect appears to underlie all the syndromes, namely diminished synthesis of the polypeptide chains comprising normal globin moieties. Individually abnormal genes transmit defective polypeptide synthesis for each chain, and affected individuals may be homozygous or heterozygous for one or another thalassemia gene and other hemoglobinopathies as well. The beta chain is most frequently affected, with alpha chain involvement being less common but far more clinically severe in the homozygous state. Defective delta chain synthesis has been described,[37] but has little clinical impact.

The three types of normal hemoglobin are A ($\alpha_2\beta_2$), A_2 ($\alpha_2\delta_2$) and F ($\alpha_2\gamma_2$). The alpha chain is common to all. The β chain appears most vulnerable to genetic vagaries, since the two most common hemoglobinopathies, hemoglobin S and hemoglobin C, also involve genetically determined abnormalties of the β chain. In the thalassemias, the chains are not abnormally constructed, as they are in hemoglobin S and hemoglobin C. Instead, production is markedly depressed, so insufficient building blocks exist for globin synthesis. If β chain output is depressed, δ or γ chain output or both may rise, resulting in increased amounts of hemoglobin A_2 or F to compensate for diminished hemoglobin A. Another result is accumulation of redundant α chains, which precipitate as insoluble inclusions in mature and developing red cells. These inclusions render the cells liable to deformity and splenic destruction, and also produce membrane abnormalities involving sodium and potassium transport.[35]

Different genes transmit different degrees of unbalanced chain production. The severity of clinical manifestations varies with the particular genes involved, as well as with the state of homozygosity or heterozygosity. The molecular basis for the defects may well reside in the quantity or function of messenger RNA but the specific aberration has not been identified.[35]

CLINICAL FINDINGS. The clinical consequences of defective globin synthesis are decreased circulating hemoglobin, ineffective erythropoiesis, and increased destruction of those cells which do circulate. Tremendous marrow hyperplasia results, producing skeletal deformities, and there may be enormous splenomegaly. Homozygous children (thalassemia major, Cooley's anemia) have severe anemia, with erythrocytes that are markedly microcytic, hypochromic, variable in shape, and unusually resistant to osmotic hemolysis. A characteristic finding is leptocytosis, the presence of target cells (literally, thin cells). Following splenectomy, erythrocytes are less variable in shape, but Heinz bodies, containing precipitated excess globin chains, become prominent.

Reticulocytosis, nucleated red cells, and leukocytosis between 10,000 and 25,000/mm³ all testify to marrow hyperactivity. Iron utilization is defective, and total serum iron and transferrin saturation are both high. Increased iron stores characterize even the untreated state. Following the blood transfusions necessary to maintain reasonable activity, there may be symptomatic hemosiderosis. In heterozygote individuals (thalassemia minor), rather marked morphologic changes and microcytosis accompany relatively mild degrees of anemia, and the other signs of hemolysis (bilirubinemia, reticulocytosis, increased fecal and urinary urobilinogen, and increased iron binding saturation) are present to variable degrees.

Glucose-6-Phosphate Dehydrogenase Deficiency

Another genetically determined hemolytic condition arises from an enzymatic defect in the red cell itself, being distinct from abnormalities of hemoglobin. The condition was discovered when hemolytic reactions occurred in individuals exposed to small or therapeutic doses of a variety of ordinarily nontoxic agents. The defect was traced to the red cells, and the pattern of drug-induced hemolysis was shown to be a sex-linked characteristic of rather high incidence. Several genetic variants exist, but the most common gene has an incidence of approximately 11 per cent among American Negroes.[4] The list of drugs implicated is long and includes antimalarial drugs such as primaquine, certain sulfonamides, nitrofurans, antipyretics, analgesics, and miscellaneous drugs including vitamin K. Viral and bacterial infections, septicemia, and diabetic acidosis may also precipitate hemolytic episodes.[4]

The Biochemical Problem. The red cell defect is a deficiency of the enzyme glucose-6-phosphate dehydrogenase (G-6-PD). Lacking this enzyme, the cells cannot oxidize glucose-6-phosphate and generate adequate quantities of reduced nicotinamide adenine dinucleotide phosphate (NADPH), which results as the obligate coenzyme in this step of the hexose monophosphate shunt.[3] The resultant deficiency of reduced NADP and reduced glutathione impairs the cell's normal balance of oxidation and reduction. The affected cell cannot prevent excessive oxidation of essential components, and the result is that the oxygen-carrying iron portion of the hemoglobin molecule is oxidized and eventually the hemoglobin is irreversibly denatured.

Laboratory Findings. The clinical results of this inborn defect vary with the state of challenge. In health, there are no readily detectable hematologic abnormalities except, perhaps, slightly shortened red cell survival.[4] Reduced levels of G-6-PD and reduced glutathione can be demonstrated by suitable techniques, and Heinz bodies—clumps of denatured hemoglobin readily noted on stained smears—can be induced by incubating the red cells with ascorbic acid or phenylhydrazine at high oxygen tension (see p. 20).

Hemolytic crises occur after two to three days of exposure to a suitable drug. Evidence of intravascular hemolysis becomes more pronounced over the next seven to ten days, and then, even though the drug is continued, recovery begins. With continued drug administration at a constant level, an equilibrium is reached between red cell destruction and production, but increasing the drug dosage provokes another hemolytic episode. This occurs because younger cells contain higher levels of the enzyme. With obliteration of the older cells and replacement by a large population of younger cells, the red cell level can become stabilized. Increasing the dose presents a greater challenge, and the older members of the young cell population are then attacked.

The results of drug exposure are much worse if the patient is already seriously ill, and renal disease, hepatic disease, or diabetic acidosis may dramatically intensify the process.

Favism. The biochemical defect in favism appears to be similar to primaquine sensitivity, although the clinical course is somewhat different. Exposure to the fava bean or its pollen seems to produce or activate a circulating blood factor which destroys the sensitive erythrocytes.[23] Deficiency of G-6-PD has been demonstrated in affected individuals, and sex-linked genetic transmission is apparent. Sensitive individuals thus have abnormal erythrocytes and, in addition, a serum abnormality which probably has an immune origin. During the initial phases of the hemolytic episode, the red cells transiently exhibit a positive direct Coombs test. Heinz bodies can be induced in cells from sensitive individuals.

Hereditary Spherocytosis

Laboratory Findings. This genetically determined form of hemolytic anemia is unusual in that both intracorpuscular and extracorpuscular factors influence the clinical findings. There is usually mild anemia; the red cells appear small and deeply stained on smears, but have a normal corpuscular volume. These spherocytes have a small diameter, but lack the biconcavity that gives normal erythrocytes their central pallor. The hemoglobin intensity thus appears uniform throughout the cells and the mean corpuscular hemoglobin concentration may be higher than the normal 32 to 36 per cent.[39] Other findings include reticulocyte counts ranging from 10 to 20 per cent with wide variation between patients; normoblastic bone marrow hyperplasia; slightly elevated serum bilirubin; moderately elevated fecal urobilinogen; and relatively high serum iron levels.

Clinical Course. The clinical severity of the disease varies; most patients are asymptomatic most of the time, although aplastic crises and severe episodes of infection may occur. A frequent concomitant is cholelithiasis, and radiolucent pigment stones have been described in children as young as 3 years. The incidence increases with age, and the occurrence of radiolucent gallstones in a patient with mild anemia and splenomegaly should provoke strong suspicion of spherocytosis.

The Cellular Defect. OSMOTIC FRAGILITY. Spherocytes are more susceptible than normal cells to osmotic and mechanical trauma. Lacking normal concavity, the spherocyte cannot expand if intracellular water increases. It already has maximum volume relative to the surface area, and additional water causes rapid hemolysis. If increased osmotic fragility is not demonstrated under standard conditions, sterile incubation of the spherocytes at 37°C for 24 hours before performing an osmotic fragility test nearly always produces an abnormal osmotic fragility curve. A control test on normal cells should accompany both the standard and the incubated osmotic fragility tests.

AUTOHEMOLYSIS. Another indication of spherocytic abnormality is marked autohemolysis when the patient's cells are incubated under sterile conditions at 37°C for 48 hours. In normal blood, only 6 per cent of the cells hemolyze during this time; but in spherocytosis, up to 20 per cent hemolysis may occur. Incubating normal cells with added glucose decreases hemolysis from 6 per cent to about 1 per cent; the protective effect of glucose on spherocytes is more marked, reducing the degree of hemolysis from 20 per cent to approximately 3 per cent.[55]

BIOCHEMICAL DEFECTS. The actual nature of the red cell defect is not fully understood. The cells are more than normally permeable to sodium, and they appear to require a faster than normal rate of glycolysis to maintain a viable level of metabolism, thus requiring large amounts of glucose.[22] Not yet understood is the basis for these abnormalities or the nature of the genetic alteration. The genetic pattern appears to be autosomal dominance, or partial dominance, and the heterozygotes manifest the abnormality. The severity varies within and between kindreds.

IN VIVO HEMOLYSIS. Two conditions must be fulfilled before in vivo hemolysis occurs in spherocytosis: The cells must be abnormal, and they must circulate through the spleen. Normal cells transfused into a patient with spherocytosis survive normally. Normal survival occurs when spherocytic cells are transfused into an otherwise normal individual whose spleen has been removed. But spherocytic cells transfused into a normal recipient with a normal spleen survive only 16 to 20 days. Splenectomy corrects the clinical anemia of patients with spherocytosis, but the red cells remain abnormal.

Nonspherocytic Hemolytic Anemias

This wastebasket category includes various hereditary conditions in which erythrocyte life span is shortened, but there is no abnormal hemoglobin, no evidence of immunologic attack, no spherocytosis, no abnormal osmotic fragility in fresh blood, and no increase in red cell survival following splenectomy. Common to many of these are genetically-transmitted enzyme deficiencies which impair metabolic equilibrium. Since mature erythrocytes possess no nucleus and no organelles, they cannot synthesize protein and their original enzyme supply must serve for their whole life span. These enzymes metabolize glucose through the anaerobic Embden-Meyerhof pathway and, to a smaller extent, through the oxidative hexose monophosphate shunt. Besides supplying energy, these enzyme-mediated processes enable the cells to resist methemoglobin formation and prevent oxidative damage resulting in hemoglobin denaturation.

Enzyme Deficiencies. It sometimes seems that wherever an enzyme has been identified, a congenital enzyme deficiency can be discovered. Of the red cell enzymes, a glucose-6-phosphate dehydrogenase (G-6-PD, see above) deficiency is overwhelmingly the most common abnormality. Additional defects, however, have been localized to other enzymes of the hexose monophosphate shunt, to enzymes of the Embden-Meyerhof pathway, and to enzymes involved in maintaining the integrity of glutathione. All of these result in a lifelong hemolytic process in homozygous persons (or male hemizygotes, in the X-linked deficiencies), although clinical severity is highly variable within single enzyme categories or even in a single family. Most of these are rare, and diagnosis depends on specific biochemical documentation.

Pyruvate kinase (PK) deficiency is the most common of these less common disorders and can be used as a paradigm. Approximately 95 cases have been reported.[26] Transmitted by an autosomal recessive gene, the deficiency is partial in heterozygous persons. All the usual findings of partially compensated hemolysis are present—reticulocytosis, elevated serum haptoglobin, moderate anemia (usually 6 to 12 Gm hemoglobin per 100 ml), and increased propensity to gallstone formation. Splenomegaly usually accompanies severely symptomatic cases, and splenectomy may lessen or abolish the need for transfusions, without affecting the basic defect or significantly increasing mean red cell life span.[48] The other deficiency states give comparable clinical pictures and are diagnosed by biochemical analysis.

Hereditary Elliptocytosis

This rare red cell defect is determined by an autosomal dominant gene and is characterized by oval or elliptical red cells easily diagnosed on stained smears. In most cases, there are no marked clinical abnormalities, although a minority of affected individuals have a relatively mild, compensated hemolytic condition.[7] A fairly severe hemolytic condition occasionally occurs in individuals who may well be homozygous for the gene.

HEMOLYSIS OF RED CELLS WITH ACQUIRED DEFECTS

Changes Accompanying Various Disorders

Red cells abnormally susceptible to hemolysis are produced in a variety of conditions. The anemias of folic acid, vitamin B_{12} or iron deficiencies are often associated with shortened erythrocyte life span, and cell survival is somewhat diminished in myeloid metaplasia.[54] Following severe burns of more than 20 per cent of the body surface, circulating red cells are altered, and hemolysis occurs during the first week after the burn. Superimposed upon red cell destruction may be bone marrow hypoplasia in the second and third weeks, resulting in severe anemia which requires replacement of red cells as well as large quantities of plasma.[16]

Paroxysmal Nocturnal Hemoglobinuria

Laboratory and Clinical Findings. This rare disorder is characterized by red cells unusually sensitive to slight decreases in pH. Since the disorder occurs in middle life and has no familial incidence or racial or sex predilection, it may be an acquired red cell abnormality, but the cause is unknown. A chronic hemolytic condition exists, with anemia, reticulocytosis, hemoglobinemia, hemoglobinuria, and serum bilirubin elevation to about 5 mg per 100 ml. Leukopenia is common, predisposing the patient to severe infection, and thrombotic episodes are frequent. Hemosiderin is present in the renal parenchyma as well as in the urine, and excretion of this iron-containing compound may lead to a superimposed iron-deficiency anemia.

The Biochemical Defect. The characteristic finding is intense sensitivity to complement-mediated hemolysis. Of interest is the fact that not all cells of the affected individual are involved. Two populations of cells exist. The complement-sensitive cells may constitute between 1 and 90 per cent of the red cell population.[42] Apparently due to a membrane defect, the nature of the abnormality is obscure. Diminished levels of erythrocyte acetylcholinesterase are thought to be a manifestation, not a cause, of the abnormality.[18,26]

The defect is readily demonstrated by the Ham acid-hemolysis test, in which hemolysis occurs when the cells are incubated with fresh serum acidified to pH 6.4 to 6.7. If the proportion of susceptible to nonsusceptible cells is low, this test may not be sufficiently sensitive, but most cases do not require the more accurate procedure involving a specific antibody in addition to complement.[42] In affected patients, younger cells are more susceptible to complement than older cells, and the hemolytic crises sometimes precipitated by iron therapy may be due to pronounced, sudden reticulocytosis.[26] Hemolytic crises may also follow transfusion of ordinary bank blood, but infusion of normal cells washed and resuspended in saline ordinarily causes no ill effects.

DESTRUCTION OF RED CELLS DUE TO EXTRACORPUSCULAR FACTORS

Immune Mechanisms with Demonstrable Antibodies

The most readily demonstrated antibodies are those associated with the red cell blood groups. Except in autoimmune states, the antibodies destroy transfused cells rather than the patient's own erythrocytes. The blood group antibodies are commonly divided into two groups: the *naturally occurring isoagglutinins* that are present in nearly everyone, without a recognizable immunizing event; and *immune antibodies* stimulated by transfusion or pregnancy. Blood group antibodies, transfusion reactions, and hemolytic disease of the newborn are discussed in Chapter 3.

"Cold" Antibodies

Antibodies with maximum activity at temperatures below 37°C are often termed *cold,* whatever their origin. Many have optimum in vitro activity at temperatures between 18° and 25°C and are associated with blood group specificity. Others have greatest activity at 4°C and seem to have immunologic significance outside the blood group systems.

Cold Agglutinins. Individuals of all blood types possess small quantities of antibody which agglutinates group O red cells at 4°C. Sometimes antiglobulin serum is necessary to demonstrate the existence of the antibody-red cell reaction, but in many normal individuals, serum diluted as much as 1:8 will agglutinate group O cells at cold temperatures. Warming the cell-serum mixture to 37°C reverses the agglutination.

Under certain conditions, this cold agglutinin may reach very high titers, and it may be potent enough to cause agglutination at body temperature. Patients with a cold agglutinin titer in the tens of thousands may suffer from intravascular agglutination after exposure to the cold, causing such problems as frostbite, focal gangrene, and Reynaud's phenomenon. In a few patients, exposure to cold may produce generalized intravascular hemolysis, accompanied by hemoglobinemia, hemoglobinuria, bilirubinemia, and falling hematocrit.

Cold agglutinin disease sometimes occurs spontaneously in older people, with high antibody titers persisting for years. Certain neoplastic diseases, especially lymphomas, produce high titers of cold agglutinins which subside with remissions. A more common cause of cold agglutinin production is viral (primary atypical) pneumonia, and a simple serologic test for the presence of cold agglutinins is often used in diagnosing the disease. Although the antibody usually causes no clinical problems, occasional patients with viral pneumonia have episodes of overt hemolysis. Within several months of recovery, the antibody disappears.

Cold Hemolysin (Donath-Landsteiner Antibody). Agglutination, not hemolysis, is the hallmark of the nonspecific cold antibody described above. A rare but interesting cold antibody routinely causes hemolysis both in the test tube and in the patient. This is the Donath-Landsteiner antibody which causes paroxysmal cold hemoglobinuria (PCH). Its mode of action is biphasic. At cold temperatures and in the presence of complement, the antibody fixes itself to the red cell. When the cell–complement–antibody complex is warmed to 37°C, rapid lysis occurs. When the patient is exposed to cold temperatures, or even if a single extremity is chilled and then warmed, intravascular hemolysis may occur. These patients do not have high titers of the nonspecific cold agglutinin, and their antibody is identified by the Donath-Landsteiner test, in which the cell–serum mixture is first chilled and then warmed.

The Donath-Landsteiner antibody and paroxysmal cold hemoglobinuria are remarkable in several respects. Patients who have the antibody nearly always have a positive serologic test for syphilis (STS), but the antibody is not the same as reagin. Although many such patients have had acquired or congenital syphilis, PCH is not exclusively associated with syphilis. Antiluetic therapy may sometimes suppress the antibody.

CHARACTERIZATION OF THE DEFECT. Another peculiarity is Levine's observation[29] that the antibody has blood group specificity. Cells that are negative for the P antigen (P + P₁) are not affected, but such cells are extremely rare, and the P antigen is always present on the patient's cells. Another unexplained observation, and one which seems unrelated to the blood group specificity, is that the patient's own cells are appreciably more susceptible to hemolysis than cells from other donors.[51] Except for this peculiarity, there are no hematologic abnormalities between attacks. During and immediately after a hemolytic episode, a direct Coombs test on the patient's red cells may have a positive result, and the acute episode is also characterized by early leukopenia, followed by leukocytosis.

"Autoimmune" Hemolytic Disease With or Without Demonstrable Antibodies

In some forms of hemolytic disease, the patient's serum proteins are active against his own red cells, significantly shortening their life span. When this condition accompanies some other disease, the hemolytic activity is termed *secondary* or *symptomatic* even though the anemia may in some cases dominate the clinical picture. In another group of patients, no illness other than the hemolytic condition can be identified, and this type of hemolytic anemia is described as *idiopathic or primary*. In both types, the term *autoimmune* is used because the protein–erythrocyte interaction resembles processes which have a clearly immune origin, and the immune activity is directed against the patient's own red cells.

The Direct Coombs Test. The unifying factor among these sometimes diverse clinical states is the presence of abnormal globulins in the serum or on the cells. Before the antiglobulin test was known, the existence of a self-directed erythrocyte-destroying agent was inferred. Refinement of the antiglobulin test now permits identification of a variety of globulins and protein fragments coating the cells. In most cases of primary and secondary autoimmune hemolytic disease, a "warm" antibody, or 7S immunoglobulin, can be identified on the cells and sometimes also in the serum. In other cases, the red cells are coated by 19S globulin or other protein elements.

The Indirect Coombs Test. The life span of coated erythrocytes is shortened. As a general rule, cells coated with 7S globulins are primarily destroyed in the spleen, while the larger immunoglobulins cause either intravascular agglutination or hepatic destruction or both.[10] Antibodies, though present on the red cells, are frequently absent from serum, possibly because erythrocytes and other tissues "mop up" enough antibody that no surplus remains in circulation. Cold-active antibodies more often remain in the serum than warm ones, and a significant serum titer of warm antibody occurs only in severe disease. By elution techniques, the antibody can sometimes be removed from the cells to be identified and used for cross-matching.

Diseases Causing Hemolytic Anemia. The diseases most likely to cause secondary hemolytic anemia are the lymphomas, lymphocytic leukemia, and disseminated lupus erythematosus. In infectious mononucleosis and viral pneumonia, there may be transient autoimmune hemolysis; and tuberculosis, sarcoidosis, generalized carcinoma, and certain ovarian tumors have sometimes been implicated. Although idiopathic primary autoimmune hemoloysis can persist without other associated disease, many apparently idiopathic hemolytic anemias prove to be the initial symptom of slowly developing systemic illness. In other cases, patient morbidity and ultimate survival is surprisingly little affected,[43] and there is no way to predict from the presenting signs what the outcome will be.

Laboratory Findings. Diagnosis of autoimmune hemolytic disease depends, first, on demonstration of hemolysis: shortened red cell survival time, increased fecal urobilinogen, elevated serum bilirubin, and the absence of inborn cellular defects such as abnormal hemoglobin or enzyme deficiency. A positive direct Coombs test is a customary finding, but the indirect Coombs test is often negative since no antibody is demonstrable in the serum. Except in aplastic crises, the bone marrow is hyperactive and there are peripheral reticulocytosis and leukocytosis. Occasional cases of thrombocytopenia are the exception; the platelet count is usually normal.

Nonimmune Types of Erythrocyte Destruction

Systemic Diseases. In certain patients who are seriously ill from widespread carcinoma, chronic infections, or renal disease, the red cells have a shortened life span. If erythropoiesis is diminished, progressive anemia results. The exact mechanism is not known, but it does not appear to be immune in nature. A severe type of hemolytic disease sometimes occurs in uremia, especially in children. Marked reticulocytosis, anisocytosis, and marrow hyperplasia characterize this uncommon complication.

Splenomegaly. Splenomegaly of any origin may be associated with shortened red cell survival, and sometimes also with leukopenia or thrombocytopenia or both. The cause of red cell destruction in these cases is unclear, and may in fact differ with various causes for the splenomegaly.

Drugs. Certain drugs provoke hemolysis of all red cells, not just defective ones. These drugs are often oxidant compounds, and a few, notably benzene and trinitrotoluene, cause bone marrow depression as well as hemolysis. Ingested lead, in addition to its hemolytic effects, inhibits heme synthesis, so that the rather mild hemolysis is not adequately compensated by increased erythropoiesis.

Infections. Certain specific infectious agents cause overt hemolysis. Malarial infections cause episodic intravascular hemolysis when the parasitized erythrocytes are lysed by maturing plasmodia. Blackwater fever is the especially severe hemolytic type caused by P. falciparum infection, but the recurrent attacks caused by other species have a hemolytic component. Clostridial infections, even relatively localized, may cause widespread intravascular hemolysis due to circulation of bacterial hemolysins. Bartonella bacilliformis, etiologic agent of Oroyo fever, adheres to the red cell surface, causing splenic trapping and destruction in a manner reminiscent of antibody adherence.[18]

ANEMIAS DUE TO INADEQUATE PRODUCTION OF HEMOGLOBIN—RED CELL MASS

BONE MARROW FAILURE

A condition of relative bone marrow failure exists whenever body requirements outstrip the production of functioning erythrocytes. Following internal or external blood loss, the normal bone marrow can increase its production by a factor of six to eight.[9] Red cell production is stimulated by erythropoietin, the name used for a circulating activity whose exact nature is still under study. The kidney and possibly other sites are involved in its production which occurs in response to altered tissue oxygenation.[18] Inadequate erythropoiesis may result if the stimulatory mechanism is defective or if the bone marrow responds poorly to normally produced erythropoietin.

Types of Failure

Although bone marrow failure is often called *aplastic anemia,* the aspirated marrow may contain normal or even increased numbers of cells. Early descriptions of bone marrow failure emphasized the increased proportion of adipose tissue and reduced numbers of hematopoietic elements, but functional aplasia can accompany a normally cellular marrow. Aplastic anemia, refractory anemia, aregenerative anemia, and anemia of bone marrow failure are synonymous terms for the same condition. All these terms refer to a hematologic problem in an individual without other disease. If the hematologic problem is part of another disease, it should be classified and treated as the primary condition.

The clinical condition described as aplastic anemia may develop suddenly or slowly. It may be clearly associated with some chemical, pharmacologic, or physiologic agent, or it may appear without a recognizable cause. The last-named type is described as *idiopathic aplastic anemia,* while the former conditions are described as *secondary aplastic anemias.* Frequently, bone marrow failure affects all elements simultaneously and results in pancytopenia, but sometimes the red cells only, or the red cells in combination with either white cells or platelets, are selectively depressed.

Laboratory Findings. Diagnostic laboratory procedures are relatively simple, despite the complexity of physiologic events. There is usually severe anemia, which tends to be normocytic or occasionally slightly macrocytic.

The reticulocyte count is low or zero, and there frequently is an absolute neutropenia with little change in the absolute number of lymphocytes. Platelet counts are depressed, but those platelets present are morphologically normal. The laboratory signs of hemolysis, hemoglobinopathy, and specific deficiencies are absent. The bone marrow usually contains decreased numbers of precursor cells and increased numbers of mature lymphocytes, but some marrows appear normocellular. No morphologic changes can be identified in the aspirated cells. Plasma iron content is normal or high, and iron binding capacity is normal or slightly decreased, so that per cent saturation may be high.

Aplastic Anemia of Childhood

Idiopathic or secondary bone marrow failure is described as acquired if it develops in late childhood or adult life, but certain erythrocyte defects and pancytopenias occur in early childhood and appear to be congenital.[13] Unlike the anemias of later onset, these may be markedly improved by adrenal steroids or testosterone. Some patients with acquired aplastic anemias in childhood may also respond to steroid therapy; there is no present explanation for either the defect or the therapeutic response.

Secondary Aplastic Anemia

In adults, aplastic anemia often follows exposure to chemical and physical agents. Some agents—such as ionizing radiation, mustard compounds, antimetabolites, and benzene—consistently depress the marrow of any individual with sufficient exposure. Other agents—such as chloramphenicol, mesantoin, and certain gold preparations—have been implicated in enough cases that some causal connection is probable, but the mechanism is unclear. Many other agents—including antibiotics, antihistamines, anticonvulsants, and antithyroid drugs—have accompanied scattered cases of bone marrow depression, but a causal relationship has not been demonstrated.

Idiopathic Aplastic Anemia

In approximately 50 per cent of patients with acquired bone marrow failure there has been no known exposure to injurious agents and these patients are said to have idiopathic, or primary, aplastic anemia. The diagnosis of idiopathic aplastic anemia must often be discarded later, because anemia may be the first sign of a slowly developing systemic disease. The two conditions that most often appear as aplastic anemia are early leukemia and miliary tuberculosis. After weeks, months, or occasionally years of seemingly "idiopathic" bone marrow failure, some patients develop all the signs and symptoms of acute leukemia. Until the transformation occurs, careful diagnostic studies reveal no clues to the coming catastrophe. Miliary tuberculosis, on the other hand, can usually be demonstrated by bone marrow culture or observation of granulomata in tissue sections of bone marrow. In every case of aplastic anemia, the marrow should be cultured, and sections of fixed material should be carefully examined. Occasional patients with acquired red cell depression have a thymoma, and the anemia improves following thymectomy, but these cases are rare.

Anemia Accompanying Other Diseases

Infections. Aplastic anemia occasionally accompanies or follows tuberculosis or hepatitis. Patients with chronic compensated hemolytic conditions are especially liable to various infections, which tend either to exacerbate the hemolytic process or produce marrow aplasia with consequent rapid clinical deterioration.

Long-standing infections of any kind consistently produce an anemia which stabilizes at a modest level rather than continuing inexorably as the infection persists. The anemia is normochromic and normocytic, with hemoglobin levels between 5 and 10 Gm per 100 ml and low or zero reticulocyte counts. Both serum iron and total iron binding capacity are low, but neither injected iron nor infused transferrin correct the marrow hypoplasia.[2]

Renal Disease. The uremia of chronic renal disease is always accompanied by anemia, which tends to worsen parallel with the uremia until the BUN exceeds 100 mg per 100 ml at which point the anemia stabilizes.[12] Both shortened red cell survival and decreased marrow activity contribute. Diminished erythropoietin production may be at least in part at fault, but circulating, dialyzable elements are probably also involved.

Liver Disease. In chronic liver disease and in cases of moderately or far advanced neoplastic disease, red cell survival is somewhat shortened, and the bone marrow compensates poorly for increased destruction. Since there is some response, the marrow failure is relative, not absolute. Encroachment on marrow tissue by bone growth or neoplastic invasion may cause immature or bizarre cells to enter the circulation. When extramedullary hematopoiesis occurs, there may be striking immaturity of the circulating cells.

Anemias Associated with Endocrine Abnormalities

In hypothyroidism, anemia is frequent, usually normocytic and normochromic, but occasionally either macrocytic or microcytic. Numerous defects contribute to this result. Marked hypothyroidism may depress production of intrinsic factor and acidic gastric juice, and may depress iron absorption as well. In addition to these rather variable changes, there may, in females, be blood loss from menometrorrhagia, so that any combination of megaloblastic and iron-deficiency anemia may result.

Hypometabolism in Hypothyroidism. Hypothyroid patients most frequently have a normochromic, normocytic anemia of moderate degree. This probably represents an equilibrium between red cell production and tissue oxygen requirements, for the hypometabolism of marked hypothyroidism affects the entire organism. This metabolic depression seems to fix the hemoglobin level; if superimposed iron deficiency or vitamin B_{12} deficiency is corrected, the hemoglobin increases only to the preexisting hypothyroid level.[27] If tissue oxygen demands are increased by dinitrophenol, red cell production increases with no change in thyroid function[32]; and following acute blood loss, brisk reticulocytosis occurs even though the patient remains hypothyroid.

Adrenal and Pituitary Deficiencies. Both pituitary and adrenal hypofunction are associated with mild to moderate normochromic, normocytic anemia. This may result from decreased oxygen needs or from inadequate bone marrow stimulation or both. The anemia of Addison's disease is accompanied by relative lymphocytosis, increased numbers of eosinophils, and decreased numbers of neutrophils, but platelets are not significantly affected.

MACROCYTIC ANEMIAS

Effective erythropoiesis requires orderly nuclear development as well as adequate hemoglobin production. In a group of anemic conditions, mature red cells are abnormal because nuclear development is deranged in the precursor marrow cells. Normal production of nucleic acids, both ribonucleic acid (RNA) and desoxyribonucleic acid (DNA), requires vitamin B_{12} (cyanocobalamin) and folic acid (pteroylglutamic acid). The interrelationship of these two substances is somewhat unclear, as is the exact role each one plays. Both participate in the transfer of small molecular groups and are important in the synthesis of purines and pyrimidines.[46] Each substance has been isolated in a chemically stable form, but these stable compounds are probably not the biologically active forms. There is some evidence that vitamin B_{12} may be necessary to convert folic acid into its biologically active form.[8] Their interdependence can be inferred from the fact that massive doses of either vitamin B_{12} or folic acid can partially compensate for deficiencies of the other; but, as small doses of either substance cannot correct the changes caused by deficiency of the other, they appear to be individually unique.

Vitamin B_{12} and Intrinsic Factor

Castle's early work demonstrated conclusively that the normal diet contained a substance (extrinsic factor) necessary for hematopoiesis, and that adequate absorption required some substance (intrinsic factor) present in normal gastric juice but deficient in juice from patients with pernicious anemia. The hematopoietic activity of parenterally administered liver extract was ascribed to an anti-pernicious anemia principle richly present in liver. Subsequently, extrinsic factor and anti-pernicious anemia principle were identified as the same substance, namely, vitamin B_{12}.

Synthesis. Vitamin B_{12} is synthesized by microorganisms. Although bacteria in the human intestine can manufacture the vitamin, the body cannot utilize its own product, which is produced too far distally in the gut. The body must rely on dietary sources of preformed vitamin; liver is especially rich in it, but most meats, fish, eggs, and milk contain more than enough to meet the normal daily requirement of one microgram.

Absorption. Since binding is necessary for vitamin B_{12} absorption and since binding requires an acid medium, the critical steps in vitamin B_{12} absorption occur in the stomach. Here, intrinsic factor is produced which, in the acid medium of gastric juice, splits the vitamin from ingested food and binds it firmly. The intrinsic factor–vitamin B_{12} complex progresses through the digestive tract to the distal ileum where a calcium-dependent reaction transfers vitamin B_{12} across the mucosa. The vitamin synthesized by intestinal flora, not being bound to intrinsic factor, cannot be absorbed. In pernicious anemia, the gastric mucosa supplies no intrinsic factor, and ingested vitamin B_{12} is excreted unchanged in the feces. If the concentration of vitamin B_{12} is high enough, some can enter the blood stream by passive transfer without intrinsic factor. Early regimens for treating pernicious anemia by feeding the patient huge quantities of liver were effective for this reason. Parenteral injection of vitamin B_{12} bypasses the faulty transport mechanism and delivers the required principle to the blood-producing organs.

Folic Acid

Requirement of another hematopoietic agent was demonstrated when Wills used yeast preparations to alleviate certain megaloblastic anemias which liver extract had not cured. This substance has now been identified as folic acid, which occurs in yeasts, leafy vegetables, eggs, meats, and other elements of a well-balanced diet. Dietary supplies of folic acid enter the circulation by passive diffusion, probably in the jejunum.

Interrelationship of Vitamin B_{12} and Folic Acid

The erythropoietic abnormalities of vitamin B_{12} and folic acid deficiency are identical, although the total clinical situations are quite different. Chromatin development is abnormal, causing abnormal nuclear division and increased nuclear size. Because of these abnormalities, large red cells are produced, with shortened life span and impaired oxygen-carrying capacity. Thus, much erythropoietic effort is expended, with relatively few functioning red cells to show for it.

Absolute Requirement of Vitamin B_{12}. Although both substances are necessary for normal nuclear development, vitamin B_{12} deficiency causes physiologic abnormalities that do not occur in pure folic acid deficiency. These lesions in the nervous system and alimentary tract are not corrected and may even be aggravated by large doses of folic acid which correct the hematologic defect. Quite possibly, in such cases, the folic acid overcomes the erythropoietic block, so the body's limited B_{12} supply is consumed by hematopoiesis, and other tissues are further deprived of their B_{12} requirements. Deficiency of folic acid or vitamin B_{12} also causes white cell abnormalities probably related to altered DNA and RNA synthesis. Folic acid antagonists used in treating leukemia may produce megaloblastic bone marrow changes, as may anticonvulsant drugs of the hydantoin group.[15]

Genetic Considerations

The basic physiologic defect in pernicious anemia is failure to secrete intrinsic factor, resulting in a body-wide deficiency of vitamin B_{12}. This defect appears to be genetically determined, and is associated with gastric abnormalities including gastric mucosal atrophy and achylia gastrica. A familial incidence is reported to be as high as 22 per cent, [18] and patients' asymptomatic relatives have greater than normal incidence of gastric parietal cell antibodies, intrinsic factor antibodies, depressed vitamin B_{12} absorption, and achlorhydria. The genetic pattern appears to be consistent with transmission as an autosomal dominant, with incomplete penetrance.[18]

Autoantibodies. Patients with pernicious anemia and significant gastric mucosal changes very frequently manifest antibodies against gastric parietal cells. The significance of this finding is somewhat tempered by the demonstration of parietal cell antibodies in patients with conditions not involving vitamin B_{12} absorption. Antibody activity against intrinsic factor, on the other hand, nearly always signals pernicious anemia, but many patients with well-documented impairment of intrinsic factor activity have no demonstrable antibodies.[43] A further complicating feature is the association of thyroglobulin antibodies or other endocrine autoantibodies or both with pernicious anemia and in the relatives of affected patients.[11]

Diagnosis of Macrocytic Anemias

The diagnosis of pernicious anemia depends on demonstration of inadequate intrinsic factor, inadequate vitamin B_{12} absorption, and the characteristic gastric changes. *Achylia gastrica* is a more descriptive term than achlorhydria in reference to the gastric abnormality, because total gastric secretion, not just hydrochloric acid, is decreased. Since acid production normally declines with age, achlorhydria alone does not establish the diagnosis of pernicious anemia in older patients.

Gastric Findings. Achylia gastrica is diagnosed when subcutaneous administration of histamine *does not* cause an increase in either the volume or acidity of the gastric juice. Within an hour of histamine stimulation, normal individuals produce more than 100 ml of gastric juice which contains more than 50 clinical units of free acid. Patients with pernicious anemia produce small volumes of thick, cloudy fluid with an essentially neutral pH and no titratable acidity.

Vitamin B_{12} Absorption—The Schilling Test. Principle. The cobalt portion of vitamin B_{12} can be radioactively tagged with ^{57}Co, providing a marker for studying B_{12} metabolism. Normal individuals absorb a large portion of an oral dose of vitamin B_{12} and, within 24 hours, excrete a large proportion of the absorbed material in the urine. Excretion is increased if unlabelled vitamin B_{12} is also injected, as a "flushing dose" that apparently saturates the body's current requirements. Patients with pernicious anemia absorb little of the oral dose, and thus have little radioactive material to excrete in the urine. Fecal radioactivity levels demonstrate that patients with pernicious anemia excrete, by the fecal route, far more of the administered dose than do normal controls. Either urinary or fecal determinations can be used in the Schilling test, but collection and measurement of urine is far easier and is generally employed.

PERFORMANCE OF THE TEST. Following oral administration of 0.5 or 1.0 mcg of ^{57}Co-labelled vitamin B_{12} and parenteral injection of 1000 mcg of unlabelled material, urine output is monitored for 24 hours. Complete collection and accurate measurement are important, for the test depends upon total quantity of radioactivity excreted. At the end of 24 hours, the radioactivity of an aliquot of urine is determined. Total excreted radioactivity is then calculated and expressed as per cent of the total administered dose of radioactive ^{57}Co. Normal individuals excrete from 15 to 40 per cent of the smaller (0.5 mcg) dose, and 5 to 40 per cent of the larger (1.0 mcg) dose within 24 hours. Patients with pernicious anemia excrete up to 7 per cent of the smaller dose and 0 to 3 per cent of the larger dose.

PROBLEMS IN INTERPRETATION. This procedure, like other tests depending upon urinary excretion, is difficult to interpret in patients with severe renal disease. If urinary excretion is impaired, urine volume is smaller and less radioactive material is excreted in the allotted time. If renal disease is known to be a problem, the test can be prolonged to a 48 or 72 hour collection, because eventually nearly all the absorbed material will be excreted. Another problem is the patient who fails to collect all urine in the 24 hour period, resulting in the total sample and total radioactivity being smaller than they should be.

ADDITION OF INTRINSIC FACTOR. When vitamin B_{12} absorption is shown to be impaired, the next step must be to document the cause. The Schilling test can be repeated in the presence of 60 mcg of intrinsic factor given orally with the vitamin B_{12}. If urinary ^{57}Co excretion rises to normal when intrinsic factor is added, the diagnosis of intrinsic factor deficiency is established. A second low excretion indicates some other cause of malabsorption, either intestinal disease or abnormal competition for vitamin B_{12} in the bowel lumen.

Before a Schilling test is done, other diagnostic procedures should already have been completed. The priming dose of 1000 mcg of vitamin B_{12} produces therapeutic effects and can induce marked bone marrow changes. Bone marrow aspiration should precede the Schilling test, and the subsequent reticulocytosis that may occur additionally supports the diagnosis.

Other Clinical and Laboratory Findings. Patients with untreated pernicious anemia sometimes may have the full-blown syndrome of extreme pallor, weakness, glossitis, neurologic deficits, angina, and mental aberrations. More often the disease is less florid, and laboratory procedures are more important.

PERIPHERAL BLOOD. Frequently the red cell count is lower than the patient's reasonably good clinical condition might indicate. The red cells are larger than normal (mean corpuscular volume 100 to 160 cubic micra compared with normal volume of 80 to 94 cubic micra); examination of the stained smear often reveals marked irregularity of red cell size and shape,

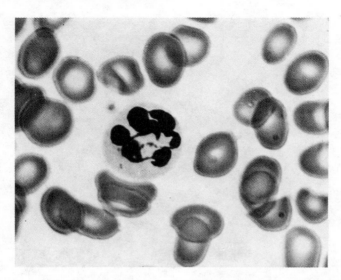

Figure 15.   Large hypersegmented neutrophil in blood of patient with pernicious anemia.

and basophilic stippling or retained nuclear fragments may be present. Large and somewhat oval cells, deeply colored and lacking a zone of central pallor are the macrocytes, or megalocytes, which give the condition macrocytosis its name. Neutrophils are decreased, and often the remaining granulocytes are abnormally large and have tangled and "hypersegmented" nuclei (Fig. 15). These changes probably reflect the same nucleic acid abnormalities that affect erythrocyte physiology. A slight decrease in platelets may occur, but bleeding disorders are relatively rare in this condition. The total white count is low, with a relative lymphocytosis.

BONE MARROW. The bone marrow is hypercellular, containing a large number of abnormal red cell precursors. These have the characteristic megaloblastic pattern which certify the diagnosis (Fig. 16). Neutrophilic precursors are also abnormally large, and giant metamyelocytes are especially conspicuous. Patients who take "tonics" or multivitamin preparations may have obtained just enough vitamin B_{12} or folic acid to alter the morphology so that few or minimal morphologic changes can be seen, but the biochemical and absorption defects remain as diagnostic aids.

OTHER ABNORMALITIES. Other findings include shortened red cell survival, slightly increased serum bilirubin levels, markedly increased urinary and fecal urobilinogen, and very high serum levels of lactic dehydrogenase. These findings testify to the shortened life span of the adult red cells and of the precursors that never fully mature. Serum iron is high, and

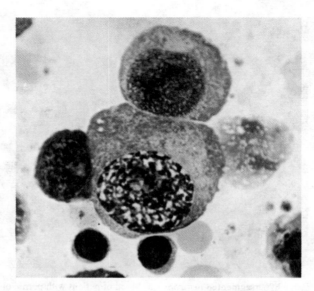

Figure 16.   Megaloblasts in bone marrow of patient with untreated pernicious anemia.

large stores of iron can be found in the reticuloendothelial system. Contributing to the hemolytic condition are abnormalities of both the red cells and serum. Red cells from patients with pernicious anemia have a shortened life span when given to normal recipients, and normal red cells have a shorter than normal survival when given to patients with pernicious anemia.[17]

Differential Diagnosis. In the differential diagnosis of macrocytic anemias, the etiologic factors in Table 18 should be considered. Extensive laboratory tests may not be necessary after considering the presence or absence of these factors. Bioassays, using bacterial indicators, are available for both vitamin B_{12} and folic acid.[30] In folic acid deficiency, the metabolic precursor *formiminoglutamic acid* (FIGLU) accumulates in the urine and this, too, can be bioassayed. Therapeutic trial is an acceptable tool to differentiate folic acid deficiency from vitamin B_{12} deficiency, because physiologic doses of each fail to correct the morphologic changes of the other deficiency. Since massive doses of either will correct the megaloblastic abnormality, only small doses should be given for diagnostic purposes—i.e., 25 to 400 mcg of folic acid or 5 mcg of vitamin B_{12}—compared with pharmacologic doses of 5 to 15 mg of folic acid and 1000 mcg of vitamin B_{12}.

CONDITIONS WITH INCREASED HEMOGLOBIN—RED CELL MASS

Polycythemia is any condition in which the number of circulating erythrocytes rises above normal. When red cell mass increases in response to an identifiable physiologic or pathologic stimulus, the condition is called secondary polycythemia. If no etiology can be documented, the change is considered primary, and is described as polycythemia vera (true polycythemia) or polycythemia rubra vera.

SECONDARY POLYCYTHEMIA

The primary function of the red cells is to carry oxygen. If the body lacks sufficient oxygen, it invokes homeostatic mechanisms to produce more red cells so that more oxygen can be carried. Presumably erythropoietin mediates this process. In any condition associated with hypoxia, there may be reactive polycythemia. The most common cause is disease of the cardiopulmonary system such as chronic interference with effective pulmonary exchange, congenital or acquired heart lesions which chronically depress arterial oxygen saturation, and chronic cardiac insufficiency. Increased red cell mass develops in individuals living at high altitudes or exposed for long periods to low atmospheric oxygen. Chronic exposure to chemicals which produce significant proportions of sulfhemoglobin or methemoglobin may also cause polycythemia.

Laboratory Findings

The characteristic laboratory finding in secondary conditions is an increase in circulating red cell mass with a less striking increase of total blood volume. The elevated hematocrit reflects both absolute increase in red cells and relative decrease in plasma volume, although plasma volume does increase to some extent. White cells and platelets tend to be normal. Arterial oxygen determinations reveal low saturation, and other laboratory findings are compatible with the primary disease. Because of high red cell volume and decreased plasma content, clot retraction is poor, but other tests of clotting function are normal.

POLYCYTHEMIA VERA

This primary hematologic disease of unknown cause is characterized by markedly increased red cell mass and increased total blood volume. The disease occurs most commonly in middle life, and men are somewhat more susceptible than women. The onset is gradual, and symptoms usually derive from vascular congestion and thrombotic phenomena. An unex-

Table 18.   Classification of Vitamin B_{12} and Folic Acid Abnormalities*

VITAMIN B_{12} ABNORMALITY (DEFICIENCY)

I. Inadequate intake (extrinsic factor defect)
   A. Vegans
   B. Chronic alcoholism (usually folate deficiency)
   C. Poverty, newborns or nursing infants of deficient mothers

II. Defective absorption
   A. Defective production of intrinsic factor
      1. Genetic failure to synthesize intrinsic factor (no gastric atrophy)
      2. Genetic failure to secrete adequate amount of intrinsic factor (gastric atrophy)
      3. Gastric atrophy as end stage of multiple causes (inadequate amount of intrinsic factor)
      4. Endocrine disorders (polyendocrinopathies)
      5. Surgical: total or subtotal gastrectomy
      6. Gastric mucosal destruction: malignancy, chemical, radiation, freezing
   B. Malabsorption syndromes
      1. Primary: sprue, gluten-induced enteropathy, lack of IF-B_{12} receptors, lack of "releasing factor"
      2. Secondary: ileitis, surgical removal, strictures or anastomoses, pyloric stenosis, malignancies or granulomatous lesions of small intestine, pancreatic insufficiency, calcium chelating agents, PAS, colchicine, B_{12} deficiency, folate deficiency
   C. Lack of availability of ingested vitamin B_{12}
      1. Fish tapeworm competition (*Diphyllobothrium latum*)
      2. Bacterial competition: blind loop, diverticula, etc.

III. Increased requirement
   A. Increased hematopoiesis: hemolysis, myeloproliferative disorders
   B. Hyperthyroidism
   C. Growth: infancy, pregnancy, lactation, malignancy
   D. Abnormal binding capacity
      1. Tissue (liver), plasma protein deficiency, altered binding capacity (chronic myelogenous leukemia, myeloproliferative)

FOLIC ACID ABNORMALITY (DEFICIENCY OR ALTERED UTILIZATION)

I. Inadequate intake
   A. Megaloblastic anemia of infancy: abnormal diet, avitaminosis C, goat's milk anemia
   B. Megaloblastic anemia of pregnancy and puerperium
   C. Nutritional megaloblastic anemia: avitaminosis C
   D. Chronic alcoholism (with or without liver disease)

II. Defective absorption
   A. Malabsorption syndromes
      1. Primary: sprue, gluten-induced enteropathy, Crohn's disease
      2. Secondary: surgical resection (extensive), drugs (anticonvulsants), malignancy, Paget's disease
   B. Lack of availability of ingested folates
      1. Bacterial competition: blind loop, etc.

Table 18 (Continued)

III. Inadequate utilization
   A. Folic acid antagonists
   B. Vitamin C deficiency
   C. Enzyme deficiency
      1. Acquired: liver disease
      2. Inborn error
   D. Alcohol, vitamin B_{12}, chloramphenicol

IV. Increased utilization
   A. Increased hematopoiesis: hemolysis, polycythemia, myeloproliferative disorders, chronic dermatitis
   B. Hyperthyroidism
   C. Growth: infancy, pregnancy, malignancy
   D. Febrile states
   E. Chronic dialysis, renal failure

---

* Reprinted, with permission, from Table 7.4 *in* Harris, J. W., and Kellermeyer, R. W.: The Red Cell, rev. ed. Commonwealth Fund, Harvard University Press, Cambridge, Mass., 1970.

plained symptom is generalized pruritus. Splenomegaly nearly always occurs in long established cases.

Laboratory Findings

The characteristic laboratory findings are elevation of hematocrit and red blood cell count, above 55 per cent and 6 million per cu mm respectively. Unlike secondary polycythemia, polycythemia vera is often associated with leukocytosis and increased numbers of platelets. Immature leukocytes, including myelocytes, may be found in the circulating blood, and the leukocyte alkaline phosphatase content is high. The bone marrow is usually hyperplastic, with both erythroid and myeloid hyperplasia. The arterial oxygen saturation is normal, whereas in secondary polycythemia it is low.

Other laboratory findings are altered, but these tests are seldom necessary to make the diagnosis. There may be slight hyperbilirubinemia and increased fecal and urinary urobilinogen excretion, reflecting excessive erythropoiesis, and plasma iron turnover is increased. The erythrocytes sediment more slowly than normal, and clot retraction is poor. The basal metabolic rate is moderately elevated. Uric acid metabolism is abnormal; although serum uric acid may or may not be increased, urinary uric acid levels tend to be high, and polycythemia occurs in association with gout at a frequency above chance occurrence.[53]

Association with Leukemia

The relationship of polycythemia to leukemia is unclear. The clinical course of polycythemia vera is long and, in most patients, the hematocrit can be adequately controlled by venesection or marrow suppression by irradiation or a combination of both. In some patients, the disease terminates in severe anemia, associated with thrombocytopenia and the appearance of increasingly immature leukocytes in the blood. Estimates of the tendency for polycythemia to develop into acute or chronic myelogenous leukemia vary and depend to some extent on the diagnostic criteria for leukemia.

In differentiating myelogenous leukemia from polycythemia vera, it is useful to recall that the leukocyte alkaline phosphatase value is markedly decreased in the former and is high in the latter. Erythrocyte response to erythropoietin in bone marrow cultures is decreased in cells from patients with polycythemia and unaltered in cells from the leukemics tested in an interesting recent study.[56] Chromosome changes have not been reported in polycythemia. Some authorities consider polycythemia to be a precursor stage of myelogenous leukemia, while others state that bone marrow irradiation for polycythemia predisposes to the development of leukemia. Many patients with polycythemia vera survive for years and die of some unrelated ailment or of thromboembolic or hemorrhagic manifestations.[44]

BIBLIOGRAPHY

1. BAGLIONI, C.: "Correlations between genetics and chemistry of human hemoglobins in molecular genetics," *In* Taylor, J. H. (ed.): Molecular Genetics: Advanced Treatise, Part I. Academic Press, New York, 1963.
2. BARRETT-CONNOR, E.: Anemia and infection. Am. J. Med. 52:242, 1972.
3. BEUTLER, E.: Abnormalities of the hexose monophosphate shunt. Semin. Hematol. 8:311, 1971.
4. BEUTLER, E.: "Glucose-6-phosphate dehydrogenase deficiency," *In* Stanbury, J.B., Wyngaarden, J.B., and Frederickson, D.S. (eds.): The Metabolic Basis of Inherited Disease, ed. 3. McGraw-Hill Book Co., New York, 1972.
5. BIECHL, A., STAPLETON, J.E., WOODBURY, J.F.L., AND READ, H.C.: Anemia in rheumatoid arthritis: I. Red cell survival studies. Can. Med. Assoc. J. 86:401, 1962.
6. CERAMI, A., AND MANNING, J.M.: Potassium cyanate as an inhibitor of the sickling of erythrocytes in vitro. Proc. Natl. Acad. Sci. USA 68:1180, 1971.
7. COOPER, R.A., AND SHATTIL, S.J.: The red cell membrane in hemolytic anemia. Mod. Treat. 8:329, 1971.
8. COX, E.V., MEYNELL, M.J., COOKE, W.T., AND GADDIE, R.: Folic acid and cyanocobalamin in pernicious anemia. Clin. Sci. 17:693, 1958.
9. CROSBY, W.H.: The metabolism of hemoglobin and bile pigment in hemolytic disease. Am. J. Med. 18:112, 1955.
10. DACIE, J.V.: Haemolytic Anaemias-Congenital and Acquired, Part II. The Auto-Immune Haemolytic Anaemias, ed. 2. Grune & Stratton, New York, 1962.
11. DONIACH, D., ROITT, I.M., AND TAYLOR, K.B.: Autoimmunity in pernicious anemia and thyroiditis: A family study. Ann. N.Y. Acad. Sci. 124:605, 1965.
12. ERSLEV, A.J., AND SHAPIRO, S.S.: "Hematologic aspects of renal failure," *In* Strauss, M.B., and Welt, L.G. (eds.): Diseases of the Kidney, ed. 2. Little, Brown & Company, Boston, 1971.

13. ESTREN, S., AND DAMESHEK, W.: Familial hypoplastic anemia of childhood. Am. J. Dis. Child. 73:671, 1947.
14. FAIRBANKS, V.F.: Diagnostic tests for iron deficiency. Ann. Intern. Med. 75:640, 1971.
15. FLEXNER, J.M., AND HARTMANN, R.C.: Megaloblastic anemia associated with anticonvulsant drugs. Am. J. Med. 28:386, 1960.
16. HAM, T.H., SHEN, S.C., FLEMING, E.M., AND CASTLE, W.B.: Studies on the destruction of red blood cells in thermal injury. Blood 3:373, 1948.
17. HAMILTON, H.E., SHEETS, R.F., AND DEGOWIN, E.L.: Studies with inagglutinable erythrocyte counts: VII. Further investigation of the hemolytic mechanism in untreated pernicious anemia and the demonstration of a hemolytic property in the plasma. J. Lab. Clin. Med. 51:942, 1958.
18. HARRIS, J.W., AND KELLERMEYER, R.W.: The Red Cell, rev. ed. Commonwealth Fund, Harvard University Press, Cambridge, Mass., 1970.
19. HASKINS, D., STEVENS, A., JR., FINCH, S., AND FINCH, C.A.: Iron metabolism: iron stores in man as measured by phlebotomy. J. Clin. Invest. 31:543, 1952.
20. HORRIGAN, D.L., AND HARRIS, J.W.: Pyridoxine-responsive anemia: Analysis of 62 cases. Adv. Intern. Med. 12:103, 1964.
21. HYNES, M.: The iron reserve of a normal man. J. Clin. Pathol. 2:99, 1949.
22. JANDL, J.H., AND COOPER, R.A.: "Hereditary spherocytosis," *In* Stanbury, J.B., Wyngaarden, J.B., and Frederickson, D.S. (eds.): The Metabolic Basis of Inherited Disease, ed. 3. McGraw-Hill Book Co., New York, 1972.
23. KANTOR, S.F., AND ARGESMAN, C.E.: Serologic studies on favism. J. Allergy 30:114, 1959.
24. KIRKMAN, H.N.: Enzyme defects. Progr. Med. Genet. 8:125, 1972.
25. KRAUS, L.M., AND KRAUS, A.P.: Carbamyl phosphate inhibition of the sickling of erythrocytes in vitro. Biochem. Biophys. Res. Commun. 44:1381, 1971.
26. LEAVELL, B.S., AND THORUP, O.A.: Fundamentals of Clinical Hematology, ed. 3. W.B. Saunders Co., Philadelphia, 1971.
27. LEAVELL, B.S., THORUP, O.A., AND MCCLELLAN, J.E.: Observations on the anemia in myxedema. Trans. Am. Clin. Climatol. Assoc. 68:137, 1956.
28. LESSIN, L.S., AND ROSSE, W.F.: Diagnostic approach to hemolytic anemias. Mod. Treat. 8:321, 1971.
29. LEVINE, P., CELANO, M.J., AND FALKOWSKI, F.: The specificity of the antibody in paroxysmal cold hemoglobinuria (P.C.H.). Transfusion 3:278, 1963.
30. LUHBY, A.L., AND COOPERMAN, J.M.: Folic acid deficiency in man and its interrelationship with vitamin B_{12} metabolism. Ad. Metab. Disord. 1:264, 1964.
31. MATIOLI, G.T., AND NIEWISEH, H.B.: Electrophoresis of hemoglobin in single erythrocytes. Science 150:1825, 1965.
32. MULDOWNEY, F.P., CROOKS, J., AND WAYNE, E.J.: Total red cell mass in thyrotoxicosis and myxedema. Clin. Sci. 16:309, 1957.
33. MURAYAMA, M.: Structure of sickle cell hemoglobin and molecular mechanism of the sickling phenomenon. Clin. Chem. 14:578, 1967.
34. NALBANDIAN, R.M., SHULTZ, G., LUSHER, J.M. ET AL.: Sickle cell crisis terminated by intravenous urea in sugar solutions—a preliminary report. Am. J. Med. Sci. 261:309, 1971.
35. NATHAN, D.G.: Thalassemia. New Engl. J. Med. 286:586, 1972.
36. NATHAN, D.G., STOSSEL, T.B., GUNN, R.B. ET AL.: Influence of hemoglobin precipitation on erythrocyte metabolism in alpha and beta thalassemia. J. Clin. Invest. 48:33, 1969.
37. NECHELES, T.F., ALLEN, D.M., AND GERALD, P.S.: The many forms of thalassemia: Definition and classification of the thalassemia syndromes. Ann. N.Y. Acad. Sci. 165:5, 1969.
38. OSGOOD, E.E.: Contrasting incidence of acute monocytic and granulocytic leukemias in P^{32} treated patients with polycythemia vera and chronic lymphocytic leukemia. J. Lab. Clin. Med. 64:560, 1964.
39. PRICHARD, R.W.: A reason for a high MCHC, Letter to the editor. Am. J. Clin. Path. 45:751, 1966.
40. RANNEY, H.M.: Sickle cell disease. Blood 39:433, 1972.

41. ROITT, I.M., DONIACH, D., AND SHAPLAND, C.: Autoimmunity in pernicious anemia and atrophic gastritis. Ann. N.Y. Acad. Sci. 124:644, 1965.
42. ROSSE, W.F., AND LOGUE, G.L.: Immune hemolytic anemias. Mod. Treat. 8:379, 1971.
43. SILVERSTEIN, M.N., GORNES, M.R., ELVEBACK, L.R. ET AL.: Idiopathic acquired hemolytic anemia. Arch. Intern. Med. 129:85, 1972.
44. SILVERSTEIN, M.N., AND LANIER, A.P.: Polycythemia vera, 1935-1969. An epidemiologic study in Rochester, Minnesota. Mayo Clin. Proc. 46:751, 1971.
45. SMITH, E.W., AND CONLEY, C.L.: Sicklemia and infarction of spleen during aerial flight: electrophoresis of the hemoglobin in 15 cases. Johns Hopkins Med. J. 96:35, 1955.
46. STOKSTAD, E.L.R., AND KOCH, J.: Folic acid metabolism. Physiol. Rev. 47:83, 1967.
47. SUTHERLAND, D.A., EISENTRAUT, A.M., AND MCCALL, M.S.: The direct Coombs test and reticulocytes. Br. J. Haematol. 9:68, 1963.
48. VALENTINE, W.N.: The hereditary hemolytic anemias associated with erythrocyte enzyme deficiencies. Adv. Intern. Med. 16:303, 1970.
49. VAN DER WEYDEN, M., AND FIRKIN, B.G.: The management of aplastic anemia in adults. Br. J. Haematol. 22:1, 1972.
50. WEATHERALL, D.J.: "The thalassemias," In Stanbury, J.B., Wyngaarden, J.B., and Frederickson, D.S. (eds.): The Metabolic Basis of Inherited Disease, ed. 3. McGraw-Hill Book Co., New York, 1972.
51. WEINTRAUB, A.M., PIERCE, L.E., DONOVAN, W.T., AND RATH, C.E.: Paroxysmal cold hemoglobinuria. Arch. Intern. Med. 109:589, 1962.
52. WELT, L.G., AND LYLE, C.B., JR.: "The kidney in sickle cell anemia," In Strauss, M.B., and Welt, L.G. (eds.): Diseases of the Kidney, ed. 2. Little, Brown & Co., Boston, 1971.
53. WINTROBE, M.M.: Clinical Hematology, ed. 6. Lea & Febiger, Philadelphia, 1966.
54. WINTROBE, M.M., AND BOGGS, D.R.: "Diseases of the spleen and reticuloendothelial system," In Wintrobe, M.M., Thorn, G.W., Adams, R.D. et al. (eds.): Harrison's Principles of Internal Medicine, ed. 6. McGraw-Hill Book Co., New York, 1970.
55. YOUNG, L.E., IZZO, M.J., ALTMAN, K.I., AND SWISHER, S.N.: Studies on spontaneous in vitro autohemolysis in hemolytic disorders. Blood 11:977, 1956.
56. ZUCKER, S., HOWE, D.M., AND WEINTRAUB, L.R.: Bone marrow response to erythropoietin in polycythemia vera and chronic granulocytic leukemia. Blood 39:341, 1972.

CHAPTER 14

Disorders of White Cells

White cell disorders run the gamut from too few to too many, and they involve qualitative as well as quantitative changes. Although primary hematologic diseases cause the most dramatic of the leukocyte disorders, common alterations of white cell behavior result from other systemic diseases. The numbers and morphology of the circulating leukocytes provide valuable diagnostic and prognostic tools in a wide variety of diseases.

WHITE CELL CHANGES SECONDARY TO NONHEMATOLOGIC CONDITIONS

PHYSIOLOGIC LEUKOCYTOSIS

Elevated white cell counts, due largely to increased numbers of neutrophils, regularly follow certain physiologic stresses. If the elevation is sudden, some immature cells may appear in the circulation. This physiologic neutrophilia should be considered when routine white cell counts prove unexpectedly high. Counts as high as 15,000 to 25,000 per cu mm have been noted following strenuous exercise, paroxysmal tachycardia, convulsions, emotional stress, and parturition.[15] Within an hour after stress subsides, the white count should return to normal.

PATHOLOGIC CHANGES

Certain characteristic hematologic responses to various diseases, listed earlier in Chapter 1 (see Tables 4 and 5), are presented here. Lymphocytes ordinarily respond to physiologic stimuli rather differently from granulo-

333

Table 4.   Conditions That Affect Neutrophils*

A. Increased neutrophil counts accompany:
   1. Infections: Especially with pyogenic bacteria; either localized as appendiceal abscess, or generalized as septicemia.
   2. Other disorders associated with acute inflammation or cellular necrosis: Infarction, collagen disease, acute hemolysis.
   3. Neoplasms: Leukemia, carcinoma, lymphomas, especially with areas of tissue necrosis and widespread metastases.
   4. Intoxications: Drugs; chemicals, especially in poisonings with liver damage.
   5. Acute hemorrhage.
B. Decreased neutrophil counts accompany:
   1. Infections: Acute viral (rubeola, infectious hepatitis); bacterial (brucellosis, typhoid fever); protozoal (malaria, kala-azar); and overwhelming infections (septicemia).
   2. Bone marrow damage: Aplastic anemia or neutropenia due to unknown cause; irradiation; toxic drugs and chemicals (benzol, mustard drugs, antimetabolic agents); drug idiosyncrasy (amidopyrine, sulfonamides, and others).
   3. Disorders associated with splenomegaly: Congestive splenomegaly; diseases of the reticuloendothelial system (parasitic diseases, chronic infections, neoplasms); Felty's syndrome.
   4. Other disorders: Disseminated lupus erythematosus; anaphylaxis; "aleukemic" leukemia.
   5. Nutritional deficiency: Vitamin B_{12}; folic acid.

* Adapted, with permission, from Leavell, B.S., and Thorup, O.: Fundamentals of Clinical Hematology, ed. 3. W.B. Saunders Co., Philadelphia, 1971.

cytes; this is not surprising, since the lymphocytes are produced at a different site and by a different cellular system. If the number of circulating lymphocytes remains constant while the number of granulocytes diminishes, the differential leukocyte count will indicate lymphocytosis. This constitutes a relative, rather than an absolute, lymphocytosis and should be considered as a primary change in granulocytes.

Absolute lymphopenia, in which the number of circulating lymphocytes diminishes, is rather infrequent, characteristically occurring in lupus erythematosus, adrenal cortical hyperactivity, and sometimes in Hodgkin's disease.[31]

LEUKEMOID REACTIONS

Occasionally such massive leukocytosis accompanies a systemic disease as to simulate leukemia. Tuberculosis is a noteworthy offender, causing hypercellularity of the granulocytic, monocytic, or lymphocytic series. Marked variation of cellular maturity combined with anemia can cause a vexing diagnostic problem.[27] A predominantly granulocytic picture may accompany a variety of conditions: pneumococcal or meningococcal sep-

Table 5.   Conditions That Affect Other Leukocytes*

A. Lymphocytosis may accompany:
    1. Infections
        a. Acute: Infectious mononucleosis, pertussis, infectious lymphocytosis, other viral and bacillary infections.
        b. Convalescence: Especially from viral infections.
        c. Chronic: Tuberculosis, brucellosis, syphilis.
    2. Neoplasms: Lymphocytic leukemia, lymphosarcoma.
    3. Metabolic disease: Hyperthyroidism.
B. Monocytosis may accompany:
    1. Infections
        a. Bacterial: Tuberculosis, subacute bacterial endocarditis, brucellosis, typhoid fever.
        b. Protozoal: Malaria, kala-azar.
        c. Rickettsial: Rocky Mountain spotted fever.
    2. Neoplasms: Monocytic leukemia, Hodgkin's disease, reticuloendotheliosis.
    3. Recovery from infections and agranulocytosis; polycythemia vera.
C. Eosinophilia may accompany:
    1. Allergic reactions: Bronchial asthma, drug reactions, allergic dermatitis, hay fever, angioneurotic edema.
    2. Parasitic infestation: Intestinal (hookworm, tapeworm, ascaris, *Taenia echinococcus*); especially with muscle invasion by trichina.
    3. Skin diseases: Exfoliative dermatitis, pemphigus, dermatitis herpetiformis.
    4. Neoplasms: Metastatic carcinoma, myelocytic leukemia, Hodgkin's disease.
    5. Other diseases: Periarteritis nodosa, eosinophilic granuloma.

* Adapted, with permission, from Leavell, B.S., and Thorup, O.: Fundamentals of Clinical Hematology, ed. 3. W.B. Saunders Co., Philadelphia, 1971.

sis; such toxic states as eclampsia, mercury poisoning, or severe burns; and dissemination of malignant neoplasms, particularly if there is widespread tissue necrosis or bone marrow replacement. Following massive hemorrhage or a severe hemolytic episode, immature white cells may enter the blood along with early erythrocytic forms. A lymphocytic leukemoid picture is far less common, but may complicate whooping cough, chickenpox, and typhoid fever. The lymphocytic changes in infectious mononucleosis sometimes resemble very closely those of lymphocytic leukemia.

Distinction from Leukemia

In distinguishing leukemoid reactions from leukemia, a helpful observation is that orderly cellular maturation exists in the benign condition even though the number of immature cells is greatly increased. Usually the red cells and platelets are less abnormal than in acute leukemia. When immature forms outnumber mature leukocytes and the primary process has also affected red cells and platelets, differentiation becomes difficult indeed. In such cases it may be helpful to determine leukocyte alkaline phosphatase levels, since this enzyme increases in leukemoid reactions and diminishes or disappears in acute leukemia.[18] Cytogenetic studies to demonstrate chromosomal abnormality may also aid in diagnosing leukemia (see Philadelphia chromosome, p. 346). If the underlying condition is not apparent or if the blood picture is particularly suggestive, the diagnosis may have to be withheld pending some change in clinical condition.

INFECTIOUS MONONUCLEOSIS

This disease, long suspected of having a viral etiology, has recently been very closely linked to the Epstein-Barr virus (EBV), a herpes-like virus also associated with Burkitt's lymphoma. The evidence is largely serologic, resting on the time sequence of antibody production, rather than on isolation and transmission studies of the type classically used to fulfill Koch's postulates.

The word *infectious* in the name is probably accurate, but the time-honored designation *mononucleosis* is misleading. The proliferating cells, which can be found in tonsils, lymph nodes, spleen, and other organs as well as blood, are of lymphocytic origin. The synonymous term *glandular fever* acknowledges that fever and lymph node enlargement are the most common findings, but it does not convey the protean forms the disease may take. Pharyngitis, splenomegaly, malaise, headache, hepatomegaly, abdominal pain, bleeding disorders, and neurologic disorders tend to occur, in order of descending frequency.

Viral Etiology

EBV has been incriminated through two sets of findings. One is that, in college student populations known to be prime risks for the disease, infectious mononucleosis (IM) occurs largely[25] or exclusively[7,20] in individuals without pre-existing EBV antibodies. These susceptibles, negative for EBV antibodies before the illness, almost uniformly develop high and persisting EBV antibody titers afterwards. A second pertinent observation is that EBV has been cultured from peripheral leukocytes taken from patients with IM.[6] Neither of these data proves that EBV is the etiologic agent for infectious mononucleosis, but the virus definitely seems involved. Instead of the primary etiologic agent, it could be a latent infection, activated by the febrile disease, or a cross-reactor with whatever the causative agent is, or simply a fellow traveller that accompanies some still-undiscovered infection.

Hematologic Changes

Hematologic changes are numerous and somewhat variable. Early, there may be mild leukopenia, but by the second week the white cell count reaches 15,000 to 30,000 per cu mm, with an absolute lymphocytosis. Characteristic atypical lymphocytes comprise 15 to 60 per cent of the white cells in the second through fourth weeks of the illness. These cells may take any one of several forms, with coarse chromatin pattern, irregularly shaped nucleus, and basophilic, sometimes vacuolated, cytoplasm. When these cells are present in large numbers, the hematologic picture may resemble acute lymphocytic leukemia. Although occasional cases of hemolytic anemia and of thrombocytopenia have been reported, red cells and platelets are usually normal. The most useful information to be gained from examining the bone marrow is demonstration that leukemic changes are absent.

The Heterophil Test

The most useful tool for diagnosing infectious mononucleosis makes use of a peculiar serologic entity called the heterophil antibody. There is, in normal human serum, an antibody that agglutinates sheep and other mammalian red cells. This antibody is present at low titers (below 1:112) and can be removed from the serum by absorption with the Forssman antigen (guinea pig or horse kidney). In patients with infectious mononucleosis, the titer of sheep-cell agglutinating antibody rises to levels of 1:224 and usually higher. The antibody in infectious mononucleosis is not quite the same as the normally present antibody, for it cannot be removed from serum by absorption with the Forssman antigen; it can, however, be removed by absorption with bovine red cells. Rising titers of sheep-cell agglutinating antibody also occur in serum sickness and occasionally after viral infections. In these cases, the antibody is susceptible to absorption with the Forssman antigen, and it may or may not be removed by contact with bovine red cells. The heterophil titer does not rise in leukemia.

Differential Test. The presumptive test for the heterophil antibody measures activity against raw sheep cells. When elevated levels of sheep-cell agglutinating antibody have been demonstrated, the problem of determining the cause remains. The Davidsohn differential test distinguishes between the antibody in serum sickness and the antibody in infectious mononucleosis by testing their susceptibility to absorption. After the titer of anti-sheep-cell activity has been documented, two aliquots of serum are incubated, one with bovine red cells and the other with Forssman antigen. The incubated sera are then retested against sheep cells to determine if the activity has diminished. The serum from patients with infectious mononucleosis characteristically retains a titer greater than 1:56 after absorption with the Forssman antigen, and loses virtually all its activity following exposure to bovine cells. In serum sickness, on the other hand, the titer declines sharply after exposure to the Forssman antigen, while absorption with bovine cells causes variable and unpredictable results.

Approximately 70 per cent of patients with infectious mononucleosis have a positive heterophil test in the first three weeks of illness. The height of the titer does not parallel the severity of the disease, and elevation may persist despite clinical improvement. Serologic tests for syphilis often become positive in the active stages of the disease.

Spot Test. A more rapid procedure is used in many laboratories for diagnosing most uncomplicated cases. The effect of IM serum on horse red blood cells seems to be as diagnostic as that for sheep cells, producing agglutination on a slide or tile within one minute.[17] Differential absorption is combined with this rapid test by mixing one aliquot of the serum or plasma under test with a guinea pig kidney reagent and another aliquot with a beef red cell antigen. Horse erythrocytes are added to each after the brief mixing procedure; in IM serums, the aliquot absorbed with the Forssman antigen retains its activity, while the one treated with bovine erythrocytes gives a much weaker reaction.[16]

Other Changes

Patients with infectious mononucleosis often have abnormal liver function tests even without clinical evidence of hepatitis. Serum lactic dehydrogenase (LDH) rises the most dramatically, out of proportion to changes in transaminases. Rather than reflecting occult liver damage, the excess LDH may well derive from the same cellular influences that induce lymphocytic abnormalities. Positive cephalin flocculation tests, increased Bromsulphalein (BSP) retention, and elevated alkaline phosphatase levels occur in a significant number of cases. Other nonspecific laboratory abnormalities may occur, including mild hematuria and albuminuria. The spinal fluid may be under slightly elevated pressure and may contain a few lymphocytes.

ACUTE INFECTIOUS LYMPHOCYTOSIS

This condition, occurring chiefly in children, is characterized by rather marked elevation (up to 40,000/cu mm) of circulating lymphocytes. The lymphocytes do not have the morphologic changes of infectious mononucleosis; the heterophil test is negative; and the constitutional symptoms are rather slight. This lymphocytosis lasts several weeks and then disappears, leaving no residual changes and no characteristic laboratory findings.

CONDITIONS PRIMARILY AFFECTING WHITE CELLS

AGRANULOCYTOSIS

Since the normal white count is 5,000 to 10,000/cu mm, values below 5,000/cu mm must be considered abnormal. The term leukopenia, however, is reserved for counts below 3,000/cu mm, and it is nearly always the granulocytes that are reduced. Of the remaining white cells, 98 or 99 per cent may be lymphocytes, and when counts are extremely low, the number of circulating lymphocytes is also reduced.

Onset and Etiology

Acute agranulocytosis is usually discovered after the sudden onset of severe, intractable infections, frequently in the mouth but sometimes at other sites. Careful history often discloses exposure to one of a variety of drugs or chemicals. In patients being treated with marrow-suppressing drugs, agranulocytosis is an expected result though no less dangerous for being predictable. A more challenging diagnostic problem is the patient who develops acute granulocytopenia after exposure to small or unremarkable doses of some ordinarily innocuous compound. These idiosyncratic responses probably have an allergic basis. Many of the same drugs have been implicated in thrombocytopenia, anemia, and in such common allergic manifestations as pruritus, edema, and urticaria.

Several different mechanisms are implicated with different drugs. Reduced granulocyte production may result from interference with purine or pyrimidine metabolism, with DNA synthesis, or with other, unknown sites. X-ray and radiomimetic drugs reliably produce neutropenia, and the effect is dose-dependent. A long list of drugs, including phenothiazines, sulfonamides, anticonvulsants, and numerous others, are thought to interfere with DNA synthesis and to result both from dose-related and host-related factors.[8] Idiosyncratic reactions occur unpredictably, often, but not always, in individuals who have had some previous exposure to the drug or related compounds. Chloramphenicol-induced marrow aplasia is of this type, and shorter-lived but similar reactions may accompany the use of quinine derivatives, thiazides, and others. The role of drug-induced or drug-associated leukocyte antibodies is fairly well documented in aminopyrine sensitivity,[19] but remains unproven, though tantalizing, in other contexts.

Laboratory Findings

Laboratory diagnosis of agranulocytosis is self-evident from the total and differential white cell count. In patients with fulminating infection, the disparity between the expected and actual white count may be dramatic. The bone marrow usually contains normal or increased numbers of very immature white cell precursors, with few myelocytes or later forms. In most cases, erythropoiesis and thrombopoiesis are normal, but some patients have complete bone marrow depression. The infecting pathogen should be identified by appropriate cultures. The infected sites are characteristically ulcerated, necrotic, and reddened but, because granulocytes are absent, there is virtually no pus and little tendency to wall off or to localize the infection. Rarely, unsuspected lymphoma, tuberculosis, or subacute bacterial endocarditis may cause moderate granulocytopenia, but hematologic, bacteriologic, and radiologic tests usually reveal these underlying causes.

LEUKOCYTE ANTIBODIES

White blood cells do not share most erythrocyte antigens, but possess a complicated set of antigens also present in other tissues. The major white cell antigens have been subsumed into a system known as HL-A, standing for Human Leukocyte locus-A.[34] Following multiple pregnancies or blood transfusions, patients may develop antileukocyte antibodies, which can be demonstrated by cytotoxicity or agglutination techniques. These antibodies may be responsible for a proportion of febrile reactions noted after blood transfusions,[4] and immunocompetent patients who receive platelet transfusions often develop HL-A antibodies which seriously impair subsequent transfusion therapy.[12,32] The principal clinical application of HL-A typing and antibody identification is in organ transplantation, for the HL-A locus appears to be the strongest determinant of histocompatibility presently available for study.[26]

LEUKEMIA

The leukemias are a group of uniformly fatal diseases of unknown cause, exhibiting a great variety of clinical pictures, but usually characterized by excessive production of leukocytes and their precursors. Every type of leukocyte has been incriminated in both acute and chronic forms of the disease, and clinical findings are so diverse that multiple causes may well be involved. Ionizing radiation is known to be leukemogenic; many drugs and infectious agents have been proposed as etiologic agents; genetic predisposition and acquired chromosomal abnormalities are associated with the disease, although not necessarily causally; and viral infection or interaction may play a role in certain cases.[11,24,33] Despite the variety of cell types and possible causes, the leukemias can profitably be classified under two clinical headings: acute and chronic.

Acute Leukemias

Immature leukocytes, with a high percentage of blast forms, dominate the blood and bone marrow in acute leukemias. The blast forms may be myelocytic, lymphocytic, or monocytic, and in some cases the distinction is difficult. Although commonly a disease of childhood, acute leukemia can occur at any age, and chronic leukemic processes often terminate in an acute episode. In early childhood, acute leukemia is usually lymphoblastic; myelogenous and monocytic forms are more likely to affect adults.[31]

The prognosis of acute leukemia is changing as increasingly vigorous therapeutic regimens achieve widespread use. Before effective chemotherapy, mean survival after diagnosis was four months,[14] and nearly all died within a year. In most current series, successful induction of at least one remission has become the rule, rather than the exception. Unfortunately, predicting repeated remission and long-term prognosis remains difficult and correlation with morphologic or chromosomal patterns is variable.[10,28] Alterations in immune mechanisms have shown fair correlation with clinical course,[13] but the clinical application remains unsettled.

The symptoms of acute leukemia are severe, and progress rapidly. Initially there may be only malaise, fever, or anorexia, but rapid deterioration is usually accompanied by anemia, thrombocytopenia and a concomitant bleeding diathesis, intractable infections, and complaints relating to the central nervous system. On physical examination, pallor and hemorrhagic manifestations are almost universally found, and splenomegaly, hepatomegaly, and lymphadenopathy are common.

Hematologic Changes. The most consistent laboratory finding in acute leukemia is anemia, with hemoglobin values sometimes as low as 2 or 3 Gm per 100 ml. The anemia tends to be normochromic and normocytic, but there may be reticulocytes and nucleated red cells in the circulating blood. The platelet count is reduced, sometimes markedly so, and bizarre forms may be present. The low platelet count affects coagulation tests based on platelet function (e.g., bleeding time, tourniquet test, and clot retraction), but the tests of plasma coagulative functions remain normal.

The white count is highly unpredictable and may vary in the same patient over a relatively short period of time. White counts in acute leukemia range from extremely low levels (aleukemic leukemia) to counts above 100,000/cu mm. Wintrobe[31] reports that 8.4 per cent of his series of 163

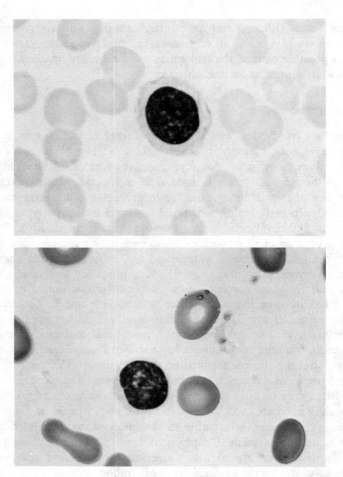

Figure 17.   *Upper,* Blast cell in the blood of a patient with acute leukemia. Note the similarity in size and appearance to the normal lymphocyte in the lower photograph.

cases had counts below 2,500/cu mm, and 38.3 per cent had counts above 25,000. Of the remaining 53.3 per cent, 13.8 per cent had white counts in the normal range. Regardless of cell count, the morphology is abnormal and many immature forms and blasts are present. When the white count is low, examination of smears may be misleading, for the abnormal cells with small, dark nuclei may unwittingly be called lymphocytes. As lymphocytes predominate in cases of agranulocytosis, the mistake is easy to make unless thin, carefully stained smears are examined with a critical eye (Fig. 17). In agranulocytosis and aplastic anemia, unlike leukemia, the remaining cells of the myelocytic series tend to be mature neutrophils and blasts are rare.

To determine in which series of cells the blast forms belong, thorough knowledge of white cell morphology is essential. Certain clues may be helpful, such as demonstration of Auer bodies and peroxidase-positive granules in young cells of the monocytic and myelocytic series. In a residual group of cases, no distinction can be made and these are termed *stem cell leukemia.*

Bone Marrow. The bone marrow in well-developed cases contains increased numbers of blast and immature forms, while mature members of the affected series may be totally absent. In early cases, only the presence of an increased proportion of blasts (over 2C per cent of the developing white cells[5]) may be suggestive of the diagnosis. Aspiration is sometimes difficult when the abnormal cells are tightly packed, and a "dry tap" or aplastic marrow is suspected after marrow puncture. Tissue fragments obtained in these cases consist of closely adherent masses of blasts.

Other Changes. Other laboratory findings are seldom necessary to diagnose acute leukemia, but many abnormalities exist. The basal metabolic rate is elevated though thyroid function is usually normal. The erythrocyte sedimentation rate is elevated out of proportion to the degree of anemia. Uric acid levels tend to be high in patients with high white counts, while successful therapy may cause serum and urine uric acid concentrations to reach levels potentially dangerous to the kidneys. Serum lactic dehydrogenase may be elevated, but the serum alkaline phosphatase and other enzymes are not consistently altered. If a bleeding tendency occurs, there may be hematuria, but urinary findings are usually not striking. With central nervous system involvement, spinal fluid pressure may rise, and leukocytes and protein enter the fluid.

Chronic Leukemias

While acute leukemias characteristically have a short clinical course and involve highly immature cells, the chronic leukemias run a variable course and involve all stages of maturing cells. The predominant cell type is rarely in doubt. The onset is insidious, so that it may be difficult to state exactly when the disease began. In some patients, unexplained anemia and leukocytosis are noted during examination for some other cause; other patients present themselves with only an ill-defined history of prolonged weakness or irritability. Wide variation exists from patient to patient, and the clinical manifestations may reflect leukemic infiltration of any organ system. The gastrointestinal tract and the genitourinary tract of both sexes are common sites of involvement, and lymphadenopathy and splenomegaly usually occur quite early in the disease. Generalized lymphadenopathy is an especially striking sign in chronic lymphocytic leukemia, and splenomegaly is almost always found in the course of the disease. In clinical practice, the most noteworthy cases of splenomegaly are those accompanying chronic myelocytic leukemia.

Chronic leukemia may derive either from lymphocytic or from myelocytic elements. In general terms, chronic myelogenous leukemia occurs more often in early and middle adult years, while chronic lymphocytic leukemia becomes increasingly common in older people. Chronic myelogenous leukemia does occur, though rarely, in children, and a very few cases of chronic lymphocytic leukemia in childhood have been reported. Ordinarily, chronic lymphocytic leukemia runs a longer and less dramatic course than chronic myelogenous leukemia.

Hematologic Changes. The diagnosis of chronic leukemia is usually made without great difficulty from the total and the differential white count. Aleukemic chronic leukemia does not occur, so that leukocytosis is the initial finding. This may range from mild (15,000-20,000/cu mm) to astronomic (as many as one million white cells per cu mm)[3] and may occasionally persist for some time before other signs and symptoms develop.

The differential count in chronic lymphocytic leukemia presents very little challenge; the classic description is of a "monotonous picture of adult lymphocytes." Indeed, chronic lymphocytic leukemia is the only leukemia in which immature leukocytes may be totally absent from the circulating blood. Characteristically, many disintegrating cells—"smudge" or "basket" cells—are seen in the smear.

In chronic myelogenous leukemia, the blood smear has more to offer the interested examiner. The field is crowded with large numbers of myelogenous cells in all stages of development, and blood smears may in some cases be virtually indistinguishable from smears of bone marrow (Fig. 18). The predominant cell tends to be the myelocyte, but all forms, both earlier and later, may be numerous. Circulating myeloblasts, if present, are relatively rare. Since eosinophilic and basophilic forms are also increased, the smear becomes a crowded sampler of cells in all sizes, shapes, and colors.

Anemia, an almost universal accompaniment of chronic leukemia, tends to be less severe than in the acute form of leukemia. In both myelogenous and lymphocytic chronic leukemia, the hematocrit may prove a better index of clinical condition and therapeutic requirements than the white count. The anemia is ordinarily normochromic and normocytic, but immature and nucleated red cells may circulate in chronic myelogenous leukemia. Late in lymphocytic leukemia, abnormal serum proteins may develop, and the course may be complicated by hemolytic anemia, with or without a positive direct Coombs test and isoagglutinins or autoagglutinins.

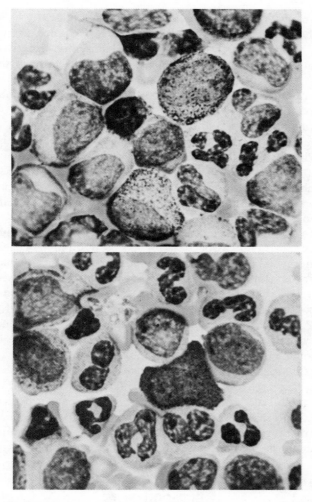

Figure 18.   Blood smear (upper photograph) and bone marrow smear (lower photograph) from patient with chronic myelogenous leukemia.

The platelet count varies greatly. Early in the chronic myelogenous form, the count may rise to 800,000 or 1,000,000 per cu mm, or there may be little alteration throughout most of the disease. Mild platelet depression may occur early in chronic lymphocytic leukemia. In the later phases of either type, thrombocytopenia and bleeding complications are frequent.

Bone Marrow. Bone marrow cellularity resembles the blood. Adult lymphocytes, normally rather rare in the bone marrow, may overrun the marrow in cases of chronic lymphocytic leukemia, but early in the disease they may be present only in small and localized clumps. As the disease progresses, the lymphocytes in both blood and bone marrow become larger, younger, and more atypical, resembling adult lymphocytes less and less closely. In chronic myelogenous leukemia, the percentage of immature forms rises progressively, and the proportion of basophilic and eosinophilic forms is elevated.

Philadelphia Chromosome. A remarkably uniform feature of chronic myelogenous leukemia is the presence of the so-called Philadelphia chromosome (Ph[1]) in blood and bone marrow cells.[22] Approximately 90 to 95 per cent of patients with chronic myelogenous leukemia have this small, abnormal chromosome, thought to be a chromosome 21 which has lost half its longer arm.[21] The abnormality is not constitutional, but appears with the disease and affects only the neoplastic hematopoietic cells. Although chronic myelogenous leukemia and its blastic crises are the neoplasms with which Ph[1] is consistently associated, Ph[1] has been found in occasional cases of neoplasm involving each of the other marrow elements, including acute lymphocytic leukemia.[23] Such observations inevitably raise speculations about the relationship of marrow elements to some pluripotent stem cell, and the etiology of all hematopoietic neoplasms. For practical diagnostic purposes, Ph[1] should be considered a sign of chronic myelogenous leukemia. During remissions, cells from the blood cease to show the Ph[1] abnormality although marrow elements retain this trait.[30]

Other Changes. Other laboratory determinations contribute relatively little to the diagnosis. The basal metabolic rate is elevated, and weight loss may be pronounced. Urinary findings are insignificant except with renal infiltration. With massive skeletal infiltration, the serum alkaline phosphatase may rise. Serum and urinary uric acid levels are high and, as with acute leukemia, dangerous acute uric acidemia may follow cytolytic therapy.

BIBLIOGRAPHY

1. BRITTINGHAM, T.E., AND CHAPLIN, H., JR.: Febrile transfusion reactions caused by sensitivity to donor leukocytes and platelets. J.A.M.A. 165:819, 1957. .
2. CAWLEY, J.C., AND HAYHOE, F.G.J.: The inclusions of the May-Hegglin anomaly and Döhle bodies of infection: an ultrastructural comparison. Brt. J. Haematol. 22:491, 1972.
3. DAMESHEK, W., AND GUNZ, F.: Leukemia, ed. 2. Grune & Stratton, New York, 1964.
4. DAUSSET, J.: Leuco-agglutinins. IV. Leuco-agglutinins and blood transfusion. Vox Sang. 4:190, 1954.
5. DIAMOND, L.K.: Clinical pathological conference, Children's Medical Center, Boston. J. Pediatr. 48:647, 1956.
6. DIEHL, V., HENLE, G., HENLE, W., AND KOHN, G.: Demonstration of herpes group virus in cultures of peripheral leukocytes from patients with infectious mononucleosis. J. Virol. 2:663, 1968.

7. EVANS, A.S., NIEDERMAN, J.C., AND MCCOLLUM, R.W.: Seroepidemiologic studies of infectious mononucleosis with EB virus. N.Engl.J.Med. 279:1121, 1968.

8. FINCH, S.C.: "Granulocyte disorders-benign, quantitative abnormalities of granulocytes," *In* Williams, W.J., Beutler, E., Erslev, A.J., and Rundles, R.W. (eds.): Hematology. McGraw-Hill Book Co., New York, 1972.

9. GALBRAITH, P.R., AND ABU-ZAHRA, H.T.: Granulopoiesis in chronic granulocytic leukemia. Br. J. Haematol. 22:135, 1972.

10. GOH, KONG-OO: Classifying acute leukemias. Ann. Intern. Med. 76:325, 1972.

11. GOODHEART, C.R.: Herpes virus and cancer. J.A.M.A. 211:91, 1970.

12. GRUMET, F.C., AND YANKEE, R.A.: Long-term platelet support of patients with aplastic anemia. Ann. Intern. Med. 73:1, 1970.

13. HERSH, E.M., WHITECAR, J.P., JR., MCCREDIE, K.B. ET AL.: Acute leukemia: Therapy, immunocompetence, immunosuppression and prognosis. N. Engl. J. Med. 285:1211, 1971.

14. KLAASSEN, D.J., CHOI, O.S., AND BARRETT, K.E.: Acute leukemia long-term survival. Cancer 29:622, 1972.

15. LEAVELL, B.S., AND THORUP, O.A.: Fundamentals of Clinical Hematology, ed. 3. W.B. Saunders Co., Philadelphia, 1971.

16. LEE, C.L., DAVIDSOHN, I., AND PANCZYSZYN, O.: Horse agglutinins in infectious mononucleosis. II. The spot test. Am.J.Clin.Pathol. 49:12, 1968.

17. LEE, C.L., DAVIDSOHN, I., AND SLABY, R.: Horse agglutinins in infectious mononucleosis. Am.J.Clin.Pathol. 49:3, 1968.

18. MEISLIN, A.G., LEE, S.L., AND WASSERMAN, L.R.: Leukocyte alkaline phosphatase activity in hematopoietic disorders. Cancer 12:760, 1959.

19. MOESCHLIN, S., AND WAGNER, K.: Agranulocytosis due to the occurrence of leukocyte agglutinins. Acta Haematol. 8:229, 1952.

20. NIEDERMAN, J.C., EVANS, A.S., SUBRAHMANYAN, L., AND MCCOLLUM: Prevalence, incidence and persistence of EB virus antibody in young adults. N.Engl.J.Med. 282:361, 1970.

21. NOWELL, P.C.: "Chromosome abnormalities in human leukemia and lymphoma," *In* Zarafonetis, C.J.D. (ed.): Proceedings of the International Conference on Leukemia-Lymphoma. Lea & Febiger, Philadelphia, 1968.

22. NOWELL, P.C., AND HUNGERFORD, D.A.: A minute chromosome in human chronic granulocytic leukemia. Science 132:1497, 1960.

23. PROPP, S., AND LIZZI, F.A.: Philadelphia chromosome in acute lymphocytic leukemia. Blood 36:353, 1970.

24. RUNDLES, R.W.: "Myeloproliferative disorders—general considerations," *In* Williams, W.J., Beutler, E., Erslev, A.J., and Rundles, R.W. (eds.): Hematology. McGraw-Hill Book Co., New York, 1972.

25. STEVENS, D.A., PRY, T.W., AND MANAKER, R.A.: Infectious mononucleosis—always primary infection with herpes-type virus? J. Natl. Cancer Inst. 44:533, 1970.

26. TERASAKI, P.I.: "Human leukocyte antigens," *In* Williams, W.J., Beutler, E., Erslev, A.J., and Rundles, R.W. (eds.): Hematology. McGraw-Hill Book Co., New York, 1972.

27. TWOMEY, J.J., AND LEAVELL, B.S.: Leukemoid reactions to tuberculosis. Arch. Intern. Med. 116:21, 1965.

28. WAGNER, H.P., COTTIER, H., AND CRONKITE, E.P.: Variability of proliferative patterns in acute lymphoid leukemia of children. Blood 39:176, 1972.

29. WOLFF, S.M.: The Chediak-Higashi syndrome: studies of host defenses. Ann. Intern. Med. 67:293, 1972.

30. WHANG, J., FREI, E., TJIO, J.H. ET AL.: The distribution of the Philadelphia chromosome in patients with chronic myelogenous leukemia. Blood 22:664, 1963.

31. WINTROBE, M.M.: Clinical Hematology, ed. 6. Lea & Febiger, Philadelphia, 1966.

32. YANKEE, R.A., GRUMET, F.C., AND ROGENTINE, G.N.: Platelet transfusion therapy. The selection of compatible platelet donors for refractory patients by lymphocyte HL-A typing. N. Engl. J. Med. 281:1208, 1969.

33. ZARAFONETIS, C.J.D. (ED.): Proceedings of the International Conference on Leukemia-Lymphoma. Lea & Febiger, Philadelphia, 1968.

34. ZMIJEWSKI, C.M., AND FLETCHER, J.L.: Immunohematology, ed. 2. Appleton-Century-Crofts, New York, 1972.

CHAPTER **15**

Hemostasis and Its Disorders

In conditions of health, fluid blood circulates in a closed vascular system. If the system is disrupted, the body attempts to restore integrity with a variety of defenses. In broadest outline, there are four major mechanisms: (1) The injured blood vessels constrict, as best they can, to seal the break; (2) the normally fluid blood coagulates in a fibrin clot to prevent further blood loss and seal the open vessels; (3) platelets aggregate into a plug which occludes the interrupted vessel; and (4) the reparative functions of tissue regrowth are set into motion. Dysfunction of any one or several of these mechanisms may produce a bleeding tendency. In discussing the mechanisms of hemostasis we shall confine the discussion to coagulative functions and platelet activity. Although vascular disorders must be mentioned in passing, complete discussion of blood vessels is not appropriate at this point, nor is consideration of tissue regeneration.

TERMINOLOGY AND OUTLINE

The complicated theories presented here are the product of innumerable experiments and inferences, and thus constitute a series of plausible hypotheses, rather than divinely revealed or immutable fact. With so many workers active in the field, it is not surprising that many terms are current for similar or identical entities. To clarify the situation, an international committee was formed in 1954 to standardize the nomenclature, and as a result of their efforts, numbers have been assigned to various clotting factors.[38] In some cases common terms have remained through long usage, but the international terminology can be consulted if confusion arises. In this discussion both the international numbers and certain common terms

348

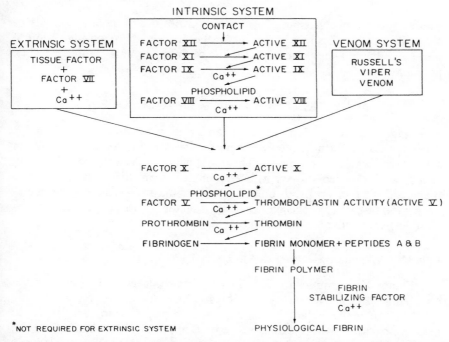

Figure 19.   Schematic representation of coagulation mechanisms. (Redrawn, with permission, from Leavell, B. S., and Thorup, O. A.: Fundamentals of Clinical Hematology, ed. 3. W. B. Saunders Company, 1971.)

will be used when each clotting factor is first mentioned. Figure 19 shows the interrelations of the various clotting factors, leading to the end-point of a firm fibrin clot.

COAGULATION OF FLUID BLOOD

When blood is shed by venepuncture or injury, some little time elapses before the fluid becomes a gelatinous clot. Although no change is visible, the "latent period" is a time of furious biochemical activity involving a bewildering number of substances and reactions. For simplicity, the clotting process is frequently divided into three stages, counting backward from the moment clotting is apparent.

CONVERSION OF FIBRINOGEN TO FIBRIN

Stage 3 is the conversion of fibrinogen to fibrin. Fibrinogen (factor I) is a large protein molecule synthesized by the liver and normally present in soluble form in the plasma. The gelatinous fibrin clot at first consists of small fibrin molecules joined together rather loosely. Through the action of fibrin stabilizing factor (factor XIII), the fibrin monomers assume a stable, permanent configuration.

ACTIVATION OF PROTHROMBIN TO THROMBIN

Stage 2 is the development of thrombin from prothrombin (factor II). Thrombin, a powerful proteolytic agent, is responsible for the cleavage in stage 3 of fibrinogen into fibrin. Thrombin is not present in the circulation as a powerful proteolytic agent, but circulates as prothrombin, an inactive precursor. To convert prothrombin to thrombin, three elements are necessary: ionized calcium, plasma accelerator factor (factor V, also called Ac-globulin), and activated Stuart factor (factor X).

Activation of Factor X—the Key Step

Factor X is produced in the liver as a fairly large and inactive molecule, subject to activation by proteolysis. Any one of several proteolytic systems can activate factor X. Simplest is direct in vitro activation by certain powerful proteolytic agents, among them trypsin, papain, and the venom of Russell's viper. Although useful for certain laboratory tests, such activation is hardly physiologic. The body appears to have two alternate systems for activating factor X: *intrinsic* and *extrinsic*. While either or both may occur in the in vivo process, the two can be separated in the laboratory. The complicated, time-consuming processes that activate Stuart factor are collectively termed stage 1.

ALTERNATE PATHWAYS FOR STAGE 1

The Extrinsic System

The extrinsic clotting system utilizes the clot-promoting properties of tissue juices, so-called tissue thromboplastin (this has been termed factor III, but the numerical designation is never used). Although most vertebrate tissues have some thromboplastic activity, there is considerable species specificity; mammalian brain, lung, and placenta are among the most potent thromboplastic agents for human plasma. To activate factor X, tissue thromboplastin requires the presence of ionized calcium and another plasma component—factor VII or pro-SPCA (serum prothrombin conversion accelerator). In the absence of factor VII the extrinsic clotting system functions poorly. Contact with tissue juices or damaged tissue activates the extrinsic clotting system.

The Intrinsic System

If blood is drawn by careful venepuncture to avoid tissue contamination, a different series of events occurs. The so-called intrinsic clotting system employs only the elements present in plasma; platelets are helpful but not essential. A series of activating events culminates in the effect on Stuart factor.

The first inactive substance is factor XII, or Hageman factor, which seems to be transformed by contact with glass or other "wettable" surfaces into an active form. Activated factor XII in turn alters factor XI (PTA, plasma thromboplastin antecedent) which, in the presence of calcium ions, converts factor IX (Christmas factor, plasma thromboplastin component, PTC) to an active form. Activated factor IX, in the presence of ionized calcium and some source of phospholipids, renders the inactive form of factor VIII (antihemophilic factor or globulin, AHF, AHG) capable of activating Stuart factor.

NATURE OF THE CLOTTING FACTORS

Phospholipids for the intrinsic system may derive either from platelets or from the circulating phospholipids of plasma. Factors II, VII, IX, and X (prothrombin, pro-SPCA, Christmas factor and Stuart factor, respectively), are all synthesized by the liver and require vitamin K for their production. All are present to some extent in serum after clotting has occurred. They can be removed from plasma by adsorption with barium sulfate or aluminum hydroxide. Factors VIII and V (antihemophilic factor and Ac-globulin) are quite labile; they disappear from plasma upon storage and are not present in serum. Factor VII is required for the extrinsic clotting system but not for the intrinsic system. Activation of factor X and the presence of calcium, factor V, fibrinogen, and fibrin stabilizing factor are necessary to form a stable clot, regardless of the initiating event.

PLATELETS

ORIGIN AND FUNCTIONS

Platelets or thrombocytes are anucleate, disk-shaped fragments 1.5 to 4.0 microns in diameter, and readily visible on stained blood smears. They originate from megakaryocytes and contain a variety of metabolically active substances, both within their cytoplasm and adsorbed on their surface in the so-called "plasmatic atmosphere." Their interaction with vascular endothelium or exposed collagen fibrils at injured sites initiates one phase of clotting, wherein the platelets adhere first to the vessel wall, and then to each other, producing a reversible mass of aggregated platelets called the temporary hemostatic plug. ADP release from platelets is critical in this aggregation, which then participates in the complex interactions of thrombin generation, starting with activation of Factor XII. Irreversible viscous metamorphosis accompanies fibrin formation, and the contractile protein of platelets mediates consolidation of the fibrin mass and clot retraction.[14]

SURVIVAL AND DISAPPEARANCE

Platelets survive a relatively short time in the circulation, estimates ranging from seven to fourteen days, depending upon the method of study.[12] Platelets may disappear rapidly if hypothermia, incompatible transfusion, extracorporeal circulation, or any other event produces intravascular clotting. Platelet activity disappears from stored blood within 48 hours, so that patients who receive large quantities of bank blood in a short time may be temporarily platelet-deficient. Decreased platelet production accompanies many leukemias, severe systemic infection, uremia, and other conditions of generalized bone marrow hypofunction. Irradiation and marrow-suppressant drugs also cause thrombocytopenia. Under physiologic conditions, the site of platelet destruction, following senescence, is probably the reticuloendothelial system.

FIBRINOLYSIS

The intricacies of clotting do not end with formation of a stable fibrin clot. A countersystem of fibrinolysis exists, the functions of which are not fully understood. Possibly it prevents intravascular fibrin deposition; possibly it protects wounds from too exuberant fibrinogenesis and eschar formation. Briefly, the fibrinolytic system exists in plasma as plasminogen (profibrinolysin), an inactive substance capable of slow activation by organic solvents, plasma fractions and tissue elements, and capable of rapid activation by enzymes found in streptococci (streptokinase) and normal human urine (urokinase). Activation results in the formation of plasmin (fibrinolysin), a potent protease which destroys fibrin. It also digests fibrinogen, other plasma clotting factors (such as VII, IX, V, and prothrombin), plasma globulins, and many hormonal proteins. Fibrinolysis is a potentially dangerous event, and abnormally active fibrinolysis has serious consequences in certain pathologic conditions.

INHIBITORS OF COAGULATION

Under certain conditions the activity of many plasma factors can be inhibited. An antiplasmin (antifibrinolysin) also exists, presumably to protect against the ill effects of unbridled fibrinolytic activity. One clinically significant inhibitor of coagulation is heparin. This mucopolysaccharide is produced by the liver and directly antagonizes thrombin as well as inhibiting thromboplastin generation. In pharmacologic doses heparin has countless other effects, and when occasional patients produce a heparin-like anticoagulant, there may be a variety of physiologic alterations. Heparin or a heparin-like substance appears to reside in platelets and in a variety of cells, but very little endogenous heparin circulates in the blood. Heparin may be administered for rapid induction of hypocoagulability. The drug protamine has direct antiheparin activity.

The coumarin drugs are given therapeutically to inhibit coagulation. These act by preventing normal vitamin K utilization, thus depressing hepatic synthesis of factors VII, IX, and X and prothrombin. Parenteral administration of vitamin K antagonizes the effect of coumarin compounds.

TESTS OF CLOTTING FUNCTIONS

The following tests of plasma clotting activity are in common use: whole blood clotting time; clotting time of plasma to which ionized calcium is added (recalcified clotting time); thrombin clotting time; one-stage prothrombin time; thromboplastin generation test; prothrombin consumption test; and partial thromboplastin time. The bleeding time, platelet count, tourniquet test, and clot retraction test are considered to measure platelet function. Fibrinogen can be measured directly with the result expressed in milligrams, and platelets can be enumerated in thousands per cubic millimeter. All the other tests of clotting function and individual factors rely on indirect means and inference.

For all tests requiring venous blood, the venepuncture should be accurate and atraumatic to avoid introducing tissue juices. Excessive stasis should be avoided. A two-syringe technique permits collection of free-flowing and uncontaminated blood by discarding the first few milliliters aspirated after entering the vein. After good flow is established in the first syringe, the tourniquet should be removed and the syringe detached from the needle. The second syringe can be any size and can contain anticoagulant solution or other additives if desired.

WHOLE BLOOD CLOTTING TIME

Among the oldest tests of coagulation is observation of the time required for shed blood to clot. Freely flowing venous blood must be used because "fingerprick" samples contain admixed tissue elements. For this reason, the coagulation time using a capillary tube has little to recommend it.

Instead, one milliliter of venous blood should be placed in each of several glass tubes of known diameter. At regular intervals, the first tube is tilted gently. As the tube is tilted, fluid blood runs down the side, and there is ample opportunity for surface activation to occur. When clotting occurs in the first tube, the second tube, hitherto undisturbed, is tilted at intervals until a clot forms and then the third tube is tilted.

The clotting time of the third tube is the time reported. This will vary not only with the degree of agitation and the amount of surface contact, but also with the temperature. If the tubes are kept at 37°C, clotting is somewhat enhanced and minimal abnormalities may be obscured. It is preferable to conduct the test at room temperature and in the room where the blood is drawn since transporting the tubes inevitably causes jiggling and temperature change.

Causes of Prolonged Clotting Time

Deficiencies of any factor in the intrinsic clotting scheme or in the common phase commencing with factor X may prolong the clotting time, as may fibrinogen deficiency or presence of a circulating anticoagulant. Excessively rapid fibrinolysis may make the blood appear incoagulable, although actually a clot forms and is promptly dissolved. Unfortunately, the clotting time is difficult to standardize and demonstrates only gross abnormalities of hemostasis. A prolonged clotting time indicates that a problem exists, but a normal clotting time does not ensure that hemostasis is normal.

RECALCIFIED CLOTTING TIME

Anticoagulants such as oxalate, citrate, and EDTA prevent coagulation by binding calcium ions needed at various stages of clotting. Once the blood is collected and the plasma separated, ionized calcium can be restored under controlled conditions. Measurement of the time required for clotting of recalcified plasma demonstrates the same general abnormalities as the whole blood clotting time, but is somewhat more sensitive. An additional advantage is that determination of recalcified clotting time can be performed at leisure in the laboratory rather than immediately after withdrawal of the needle from the vein.

PROTHROMBIN TIME

In this test, tissue extract and calcium are added to freshly drawn and separated citrated plasma, and the time in which this mixture clots is reported in seconds. The usual tissue added is prepared rabbit brain, but under appropriate circumstances, any one of a number of mammalian tissues may be used. The tissue extract bypasses the intrinsic clotting scheme so that only factors VII, X, and V, prothrombin, and fibrinogen affect the test results. The test does not specifically measure prothrombin and is, in fact, relatively insensitive to changes in prothrombin level. Alterations in factor VII affect the result most promptly, and changes in factor V are also significant. Since factor V is very labile, the test should be run as soon as possible after the blood is drawn; if storage up to four hours is necessary, the separated plasma should be refrigerated.

This test is frequently used to monitor the effects of coumarin compounds. Dicumerol depresses hepatic synthesis of factors VII, IX, and X and prothrombin; factor VII seems to indicate most rapidly the pharmacologic effects of Dicumerol. Relatively minor changes in the prothrombin time reflect considerable physiologic alteration, and the curve relating prothrombin time in seconds to "per cent prothrombin activity" is a hyperbole rather than a straight line.

Causes of Prolonged Prothrombin Time

The prothrombin time is prolonged if factor VII is deficient or with deficiency of any factor affecting the second or third stage of clotting, namely the events occurring after factor X has been activated. Deficiencies of the plasma thromboplastic factors XII, XI, IX, and VIII do not affect the prothrombin time. Because the clot forms in a short time, considerable technical skill is necessary to obtain consistently reproducible results, and if duplicate determinations do not agree closely, the results of both should be viewed with suspicion. Artefacts that affect the results include deterioration of the plasma, poor standardization or deterioration of the thromboplastin preparation, dirty glassware, and inability to judge the moment at which the clot appears.

Prothrombin Time with Snake Venom

A variation of the one-stage prothrombin time employs snake venom (Stypven) as the thromboplastic agent. This reacts directly with factor X, bypassing the earlier activating steps and also bypassing factor VII which is required only with tissue extracts.[25] If a patient has an abnormal prothrombin time and a normal viper venom time, the diagnosis is almost certainly factor VII deficiency. This clear-cut event is, however, extremely rare. Like the prothrombin time, the Stypven time is affected by the levels of factor V, prothrombin, and fibrinogen. Circulating anticoagulants, particularly those of the heparin type which antagonize thrombin, cause abnormal results in these and nearly all other clotting tests.

PARTIAL THROMBOPLASTIN TIME

Since the prothrombin time bypasses the intrinsic clotting system and the whole blood clotting time is insensitive to all but gross deficiencies of coagulation, there is need for a simple procedure to recognize mild to moderate deficiencies of the intrinsic clotting factors. In the partial thromboplastin time (PTT), a phospholipid with only moderate clot-promoting activity is added to the plasma. The phospholipid-plasma mixture normally clots in 60 to 90 seconds, as compared with the normal prothrombin time of 11 to 13 seconds.

If the phospholipid-plasma mixture is incubated with some physical or chemical agent which accelerates the *contact* phase, the PTT is shortened (to 30 to 40 seconds, ordinarily) and made somewhat more reproducible. This is called an activated PTT.

Since the process is more leisurely, minor deviations from normal can become apparent, and clotting is delayed by deficiencies of the factors in stage 1, as well as in stages 2 and 3. Factor VII, once again, is the "joker." A patient with factor VII deficiency will have a normal PTT and prolonged prothrombin time. Since variations in technique are widespread, the normal range for the PTT varies somewhat between laboratories, and results are usually expressed in seconds, "as compared with a normal of ... seconds."

Another use for the PTT is to demonstrate a circulating anticoagulant in plasma. Dilution of normal plasma with an equal volume of inactive fluid such as saline does not affect the PTT. If a mixture of patient's plasma and normal plasma has a PTT longer than that of normal plasma alone, it indicates that something in the patient's plasma has inhibited coagulation.

Diagnosis of Specific Deficiencies

Other information can be obtained from judiciously planned mixing experiments. When plasma is deficient in one or another clotting factor, addition of surprisingly small amounts of normal plasma can correct the abnormality. A presumptive diagnosis of certain deficiencies can be made by adding small amounts of the patient's plasma to samples of plasma known to be deficient in particular factors. For example, if a patient has a long PTT and his plasma corrects the PTT of plasma deficient in factor VIII but not in factor IX, a deficiency of factor IX can be inferred. Definitive diagnosis requires specific assay and in vivo correction studies as well as close scrutiny of the genetic pedigree, but a presumptive diagnosis may be sufficient for immediate treatment.

Artificially depleted substrates can be concocted if congenitally deficient plasmas are not available. For example, adsorption of normal plasma with barium sulfate or aluminum hydroxide removes factors VII, IX, X, and prothrombin. When plasma remains at room temperature for several hours, factors VIII and V deteriorate significantly. Normal serum contains factors XII, XI, IX, VII, and X, but contains no factor VIII, factor V, or fibrinogen, and only small amounts of prothrombin. By combining these depleted plasma fractions with serum in appropriate ways, suitable substrates can be found for testing a plasma's corrective abilities.

THROMBOPLASTIN GENERATION TEST

The thromboplastin generation test (TGT) permits fairly detailed analysis of a patient's clotting disorder. In this test, three preparations are made from the patient's blood: (1) native serum containing factors XII, XI, IX, VII, and X; (2) adsorbed plasma containing factors XII, XI, VIII, and V; and (3) a platelet suspension. When these three elements are combined with calcium, the mixture contains everything needed for coagulation except prothrombin. Incubation of the components permits thromboplastic activity to accumulate, and aliquots of the reaction mixture are added at intervals to normal plasma, where the reaction mixture behaves as exogenous thromboplastin. If thromboplastic activity is deficient, each component of the reaction mixture can be replaced by a normal component until the source of the defect is found.

Interpretation

If normal serum corrects the deficiency but substitution of normal adsorbed plasma has no effect, then the defect must lie in factor IX or X, the two elements found only in the serum sample. Similarly, correction by normal adsorbed plasma points to factor VIII or V. Correction by either serum or plasma points to factors XII and XI, which are exceedingly difficult to separate, and correction by neither suggests a circulating anticoagulant. Defective platelets can, of course, be demonstrated by replacement with normal platelets or a platelet substitute, but suspected platelet deficiency is usually diagnosed by other means. For this reason and also because preparation of the platelet suspension is time-consuming and rather tricky, platelet substitutes are frequently used, and only the patient's serum and plasma are tested.

Certain technical problems arise when the test is performed. Since some prothrombin frequently remains in the serum portion and fibrinogen is still present in the plasma, the incubation mixture may clot if residual prothrombin is converted to thrombin.

PROTHROMBIN CONSUMPTION TEST

This test indirectly measures thromboplastin generation and prothrombin response. When the intrinsic phase of coagulation converts prothrombin to thrombin, available prothrombin declines at a rate reflecting thromboplastic activity. Not all the prothrombin is utilized at the moment of clotting, and subsequent conversion of prothrombin to thrombin continues. The prothrombin consumption test measures the amount of prothrombin remaining unconverted after a specified time period. If plasma thromboplastin generation is deficient, more prothrombin will remain in the serum than normal.

When the test is performed, the blood sample is incubated two hours at 37°C. The serum and a supply of extrinsic thromboplastin are added to a prothrombin-free substrate of adsorbed normal plasma. The thromboplastin converts to thrombin whatever prothrombin is available, so the speed with which the plasma clots reflects the amount of residual prothrombin in the serum. A long clotting time means that little prothrombin was left, indicating ample thromboplastic activity in the original sample. A short clotting time in this test indicates defective conversion of prothrombin in the patient's blood sample.

Causes of Abnormal Prothrombin Consumption

The test mixture may clot more rapidly than normal if unneutralized thrombin remains in the serum. Excessive prothrombin may remain if starting levels of fibrinogen or factor V were low, even if thromboplastin generation is perfectly normal. Large deviations from normal, however, usually indicate genuine abnormality of the plasma clotting mechanism, pointing to defects of the plasma procoagulants, factors V and X, or even of platelets. The substrate plasma should, of course, be carefully screened to be sure the prothrombin has been removed.

THROMBIN TIME

Addition of bovine thrombin to plasma bypasses all of stages 1 and 2, and very rapidly converts fibrinogen to fibrin. To uncover abnormalities a somewhat dilute thrombin solution must be used. Under properly standardized conditions, a prolonged thrombin clotting time indicates deficiency of fibrinogen or the presence of an antithrombin inhibitor. Either heparin given therapeutically or a variety of abnormal endogenous substances will prolong the thrombin clotting time. Exogenous or endogenous inhibitors produce abnormalities in all other tests of clotting function, the tests relying on an indicator plasma as well as those measuring coagulation of the patient's own plasma. Patients with disorders involving abnormal fibrinolysis (see section on Complex Acquired Bleeding Disorders p. 372) often have circulating proteins which inhibit the thrombin clotting time, and which lengthen the thrombin time of admixed normal plasma.

Fibrinogen Deficiency

Fibrinogen deficiency affects those tests in which the patient's fibrin clot is the end-point, but the thromboplastin generation test would not be affected. In emergencies, the level of fibrinogen can be estimated by observing the speed with which a small amount of thrombin clots the patient's whole blood. When there is more time, the fibrinogen content of plasma can be measured directly and expressed in milligrams.

SPECIFIC ASSAYS

Assay procedures are available for all the known clotting factors, but only specialized laboratories consistently have the materials and trained personnel necessary to obtain reliable results. Even without specific assays, the procedures described above can provide sufficient information for diagnosis and treatment of many disorders.

TESTS OF PLATELET FUNCTION

As the complexity of platelet function becomes apparent, the number and variety of possible tests increases. The tests described below are time-honored and useful, but more descriptive than biochemical. Tests are now available to measure platelet adhesiveness, aggregation, ADP release, ADP response, and the action of "platelet factor 3." Although of great research interest, these tests are not in widespread clinical use because of their technical difficulty and incompletely understood medical correlations.

PLATELET COUNT

Platelets are counted directly, in thousands per cubic millimeter, under direct light or phase contrast microscopy. A number of techniques and diluting fluids are available, but the most satisfactory appear to be the Rees-Ecker fluid for light microscopy, in which blood is diluted 1:200, and the Brecher-Cronkite method of phase microscopy, in which the blood is diluted 1:100. The phase contrast method is ordinarily more accurate.

Technical Difficulties

Unfortunately, all methods of platelet enumeration suffer from the inherent characteristics of platelets themselves. They clump; they fragment; they adhere to the sides of blood vessels and of collecting implements. When blood is collected for platelet counts, tissue damage and manipulation of the blood should be kept to a minimum. For optimum results, duplicate counts should be performed on separate pipettes, individually diluted. Normal platelet counts range from 140,000 to 440,000 per cu mm with the Brecher-Cronkite method, and counts outside this range should be verified by examining the number of platelets present on direct smear. Electronic means of counting platelets, when available, offer the greatest accuracy.

Causes of Abnormal Platelet Counts

Low platelet counts occur in idiopathic thrombocytopenic purpura and in a number of systemic disorders, notably leukemias, aplastic anemia, "hypersplenism," septicemia, and exposure to certain physical or chemical agents. Bleeding rarely occurs until the platelet count is at or below 70,000 to 90,000/cu mm but, oddly enough, bleeding also complicates thrombocythemia, in which the platelet count may rise as high as one million.[30]

Patients with polycythemia very often have elevated platelet counts, and in chronic myelogenous leukemia the platelet count may rise parallel with the white count.

BLEEDING TIME

The bleeding time measures the time necessary for active bleeding from a clean, superficial wound to cease. The variables involved are vascular contractility and platelet aggregation, each of which serves to repair the capillary defect. To perform the test without interference from intrinsic and extrinsic coagulation systems, the incision must be made cleanly and swiftly, and accumulating blood must be removed from the surface before fibrin can develop to cover the vascular defect. Considerable skill is needed to produce uniform incisions and avoid introducing artefacts. Unavoidable are variations in skin thickness and in the degree to which patients cooperate by sitting still. Within the limits of the test requirements, the Duke method and Ivy method are in general use.

Duke Method

In the Duke method the cleansed earlobe is incised at its most dependent portion, and the blood is removed every thirty seconds until bleeding stops. The normal bleeding time ranges from two to six minutes, but considerable variation exists. Patients differ in the capillary supply to the earlobe, and it is difficult to induce a uniform degree of engorgement before making the incision. Occasional patients with normal bleeding times bleed very briskly when the incision is made and become upset when blood drips all over their shoulder.

Ivy Method

In the Ivy method of bleeding time determination, an incision is made on the inner surface of the forearm in an area with no visible superficial veins. A blood pressure cuff on the upper arm is inflated to 40 mm of mercury, enough to ensure capillary filling without interfering with venous return. As in the Duke method, the welling blood is removed on filter paper every 30 seconds until no blood appears on the paper. Normal values for the Ivy method range from three to seven minutes. If a small vein or venule is entered, the test is invalid. Additional problems include the variations of skin thickness encountered and the fact that children or uncooperative patients may be too frightened by the sight of blood to keep their arms still.

Causes of Prolonged Bleeding Time

The bleeding time is long when the platelet count is low and when platelet function is defective. Patients with von Willebrand's disease (vascular hemophilia) characteristically have long bleeding times and low levels of antihemophilic factor, but patients with other plasma deficiencies have normal bleeding times. Even patients with severe hemophilia and patients with congenital absence of fibrinogen have normal bleeding times. Acute acquired afibrinogenemia, however, is often accompanied by thrombocytopenia which lengthens the bleeding time. Episodes of disseminated intravascular clotting consume platelets as well as plasma factors and fibrinogen, and the bleeding time may be abnormal. A patient with a normal bleeding time may bleed excessively from acquired injuries, because the bleeding time tests only the response to superficial injury of limited extent. Within the limits of the technique, a well standardized bleeding time procedure is a highly reliable screen for both quantitative and qualitative platelet disorders.[17]

Secondary Bleeding Time

The secondary bleeding time may be useful in diagnosing suspected bleeding disorders. In this test, a shallow incision 10 mm long is made on the forearm and is left undisturbed for 24 hours after bleeding ceases. After 24 hours the scab is removed with as little trauma as possible and the time required for the reopened cut to stop bleeding is recorded as the secondary bleeding time. This test evaluates the intrinsic clotting scheme, for removing the scab does not activate tissue factors or induce platelet adherence or vascular contraction. Presumably hemostasis occurs when fibrin occludes the exposed defects in the vessel walls. The secondary bleeding time is prolonged in patients with hemophilia, deficiencies of other intrinsic clotting factors, or factor XIII (fibrin stabilizing factor) deficiency.

TOURNIQUET TEST

This test measures both platelet function and capillary fragility and is specific for neither. A well-fitting blood pressure cuff on the upper arm is inflated to a point midway between the systolic and diastolic blood pressure. The volar surface of the forearm should be carefully inspected for blemishes or bruises before the test is begun. The pressure is maintained steadily for 5 to 10 minutes, and then the cuff is removed. In many normal individuals a small crop of petechiae will appear just beneath the lower edge of the cuff. A positive tourniquet test consists of petechiae on the volar surface of the forearm, appearing within five minutes after the pressure is released. The number of petechiae on the hand and arm may be estimated as 0 to 4+ with 0 or ± considered normal, or petechiae may be counted in a measured area the size of a quarter. Normal individuals may have 0 to 10 petechiae; between 10 and 20 is equivocal; and more than 20 indicates abnormal hemostatic function.

Causes of Abnormal Tourniquet Test

The test is positive in primary and secondary thrombocytopenia and in disorders of platelet function. Additionally, diseases of the blood vessels and connective tissue may cause increased capillary fragility as occurs, for example, in scurvy and certain protein disorders. Some, but by no means all, patients with Henoch-Schoenlein's (allergic) purpura may have a positive tourniquet test. Senile degeneration of the connective tissue may cause a positive test.

CLOT RETRACTION

This simple procedure consists of observing the degree to which a clot shrinks and expresses serum. In a laboratory the test tube containing whole blood is left at 37°C, but a clot can also be observed at room temperature at a patient's bedside. At 37°C, clot retraction begins in 30 minutes, and at four hours there should be a well-defined red clot surrounded by abundant clear serum. At room temperature complete retraction may require 12 hours. Occasionally dried blood causes the clot to adhere to the test tube, and serum cannot be seen until the clot is gently loosened.

Causes of Abnormal Clot Retraction

When platelet function or number is decreased, clot retraction is impaired. Rapid fibrinolysis may dissolve the clot, leaving a fluid mixture of serum and cells which superficially resembles a totally unretracted clot, but closer examination easily distinguishes the two. If the hematocrit is high, the plasma and fibrinogen content are decreased in proportion to the total red cell mass. Thus the clot may appear to retract poorly, owing to the large number of red cells suspended in a relatively sparse fibrin mesh.

Methods of measuring clot retraction by comparing the volume of serum expressed against an "expected normal" contribute little to the test's essentially qualitative value. A better index of clot constitution can be gained from thromboelastography, which measures the tensile strength of the clot. Thromboelastography is valuable in research but is not widely used in clinical practice.

CLINICAL DISORDERS OF HEMOSTASIS

The clinical discussion, like the physiologic discussion, of hemostasis can conveniently be divided into disorders of vascular function, defective coagulative (fibrin-forming) function, and deficient platelet activity. Unfortunately, as in all systems of classification, the clinical realities tend to be more complex than the categories.

VASCULAR DISORDERS

If vascular permeability is increased or contractility is decreased, a purpuric tendency may result. Purpura is extravasation of blood into the skin and mucous membranes, as distinct from blood flow to the outside or into body cavities and soft tissue. In purely vascular disorders, tests of clotting function and platelet function are normal and often the signs and symptoms of some causative disease are apparent. Purpuric manifestations may be secondary to a variety of infections (notably meningococcemia and Rocky Mountain spotted fever); to drug reactions; to tissue changes resulting from chronic renal, cardiac, or hepatic disease; or to the presence of abnormal proteins in conditions like multiple myeloma, macroglobulinemia, and amyloidosis.

In vitamin C deficiency the vascular walls undergo changes which permit widespread bleeding from small vessels, and the tourniquet test is often positive. Even in the absence of frank scurvy, assay for plasma ascorbic acid levels may occasionally suggest vitamin C deficiency to be the cause of unexplained purpura.

Allergic Purpura

This term refers to a variety of clinical events subsumed under many names such as rheumatic purpura, Schoenlein's purpura, and Henoch-Schoenlein's purpura or disease. There may be joint symptoms, abdominal pain, bleeding into the urinary tract, urticaria, or fever or combinations of these, with or without petechiae and easy bruisability. Alteration of the vascular endothelium appears to be the common element, and various chemical, physical, and vegetable agents have been implicated as the allergen. In some cases, no agent can be incriminated. Diagnosis depends largely upon excluding other diseases and keeping this entity in mind. A positive tourniquet test and the existence of eosinophilia are helpful when present, but both findings are inconstant. Platelets are not reduced, which distinguishes this condition from allergic reactions which cause thrombocytopenic purpura.

Hereditary Telangiectasia

This vascular disorder produces gross hemorrhage rather than submucous or subcutaneous extravasation. Vascular malformations, often quite small, occur on the face, hands and feet, and mucous membranes. The condition is apparently due to an autosomal dominant gene. Though small, the malformations may bleed profusely, and there is no effective treatment save blood replacement and surgical removal of accessible lesions. All tests of clotting function are normal, and the only laboratory findings are those of blood-loss anemia.

Von Willebrand's Disease (Vascular Hemophilia)

This condition is discussed here because the word *vascular* appears in its name and because it does not readily fit into any other category. Also called von Willebrand's disease, it is transmitted in an apparently dominant, autosomal fashion, although there is some evidence that more than one gene may be involved.[4] The bleeding tendency is lifelong, with hemorrhage especially from the gums, nose, and female genitalia, and following surgical procedures, but characteristically, the bleeding is less severe than in other genetically determined bleeding disorders.

The characteristic laboratory findings include prolonged bleeding time and low levels of antihemophilic factor (factor VIII). Unfortunately, neither finding is constant even in the same patient at different times. Plasma factor VIII is depressed but not absent. There is also a platelet defect, in which the platelets lack normal adhesiveness, but clot retraction and the tourniquet test are normal. The prolonged bleeding time can be corrected by transfusing normal plasma and by administering plasma congenitally lacking in factor VIII. Patients with von Willebrand's disease can produce their own factor VIII within 12 to 24 hours after receiving normal or hemophilic plasma, but plasma from patients with von Willebrand's disease does not help patients with classical hemophilia. Despite its name, the disease is probably not primarily a vascular disorder, though some workers believe there is deficiency of a normally present plasma factor that promotes vascular reactivity. Others consider it to be a primary platelet disorder, and still others believe that some step or factor in factor VIII manufacture is missing.

PLATELET DISORDERS

Any condition in which there are fewer platelets than 70,000/cu mm is, by definition, thrombocytopenia. A quantitative platelet deficiency is frequently accompanied by such bleeding manifestations as easy bruising and diffuse oozing from operative sites or from seemingly minor injuries. Thrombocytopenia may result from depressed platelet synthesis or increased destruction. If some disease, drug, or environmental agent can be implicated in depressing the platelet count, the condition is called secondary thrombocytopenia; if no etiology can be invoked, the term idiopathic is used.

The essential laboratory findings are similar in all cases and consist of decreased platelet count, prolonged bleeding time, poor clot retraction, a positive tourniquet test, and somewhat impaired prothrombin utilization. Following severe bleeding, the signs and symptoms of acute or chronic blood loss are superimposed. Bone marrow findings vary, depending on what produced the problem. Thus with increased destruction of circulating platelets, the marrow may contain normal or increased numbers of megakaryocytes; in bone marrow depression, the megakaryocytes will be sparse and other hematopoietic elements may also be depressed.

Idiopathic Thrombocytopenia

This condition usually affects young adults, though neither infants nor the elderly are completely spared. In addition to the laboratory findings cited above, several specific phenomena may accompany idiopathic thrombocytopenia (ITP). Fresh platelets transfused into patients with ITP are rapidly destroyed, though in some cases the transfusion may shorten the bleeding time. Some circulating factor seems to cause the destruction, since plasma from a patient with ITP rapidly induces thrombocytopenia if transfused into a normal individual. In addition, globulins from ITP patients inhibit in vitro reactivity of normal platelets.[10] The spleen plays an important but poorly understood role in ITP. Some patients with ITP have improved platelet counts following splenectomy, even though their plasma still contains the platelet-depressing substance. Splenectomy does not benefit every patient with ITP. Autoimmune mechanisms are probably involved, because the patients in whom steroids induce a remission are those most often benefitted by splenectomy, and when both steroids and splenectomy are unavailing, immunosuppresive drugs have sometimes been beneficial.[8,24] Abnormal megakaryocyte morphology is noted in some, but not all, patients with ITP. This could result from the same circulating antiplatelet factor implicated in platelet destruction, or could imply some other cause or several causes of the disease. Eventually the single category of idiopathic thrombocytopenic purpura may be divided into several different entities as our understanding increases.

Secondary Thrombocytopenias

Drugs. Certain drugs and physical agents, such as irradiation and the immunosuppressive drugs, consistently cause thrombocytopenia in any recipient who receives an adequate dose. An impressive list of other drugs cause thrombocytopenia on an apparently idiosyncratic basis. Quinine compounds, antibiotics, and salicylates are among the more prominent offenders, but the mechanism is not understood. In the case of Sedormid, a distinct antibody against the drug-platelet complex has been identified[1] but in most other drug-induced thrombocytopenias the responsible mechanism is not known.

Antibodies. Platelets share certain antigens with white cells and other cells, notably the antigens of the HL-A system, and possess unique antigens as well. Immunocompetent patients who receive frequent transfusions, especially of platelet concentrates, may develop HL-A antibodies which cause isoimmune destruction of subsequently transfused incompatible platelets. Platelets from HL-A compatible donors survive normally.[16] Antibody specificity has not been proven in the humoral factor associated with idiopathic thrombocytopenic purpura, but some form of autoimmunity is probably involved.

Several rare but dramatic conditions result from antibodies against the platelet antigen Pl^A1, which 98 per cent of the general population possesses. Analogous to hemolytic disease of the newborn is isoimmune neonatal thrombocytopenia, in which the Pl^A1-negative mother transmits the antibody transplacentally to the Pl^A1-positive fetus.[2] A more obscure disorder is post-transfusion purpura (PTP), in which the patient, who is Pl^A1-positive, approximately a week after a seemingly uneventful transfusion, develops an anti-Pl^A1 antibody. This produces profound thrombocytopenia which gradually improves as the antibody disappears. Although only 10 cases have been reported,[9] the condition is important because of the myriad immunologic puzzles it poses.

Decreased Synthesis. Diseases of the hematopoietic system, especially acute leukemias, may have thrombocytopenia as one manifestation. Other diseases affecting the bone marrow, such as metastatic malignant neoplasms and the lipid storage diseases, may inhibit platelet production. In pernicious anemia, thrombocytopoiesis may be impaired, but no specific deficiency has been demonstrated.

Loss from Bleeding. Although prompt thrombocytosis follows acute hemorrhage, the body has little mobilizable platelet reserve, and platelet loss from copious bleeding cannot be rapidly compensated. Following massive hemorrhage, when more than 10 units of bank blood are given in a few hours, severe thrombocytopenia may occur. Restoration of the platelet count may require three to four days, during which time significant bleeding may occur. When large volumes of bank blood have been given for replacement and bleeding is subsiding, fresh blood or platelet-rich plasma will prevent thrombocytopenia. Since fresh platelets will not, by themselves, stanch the flow from a large bleeding site, the most effective time to administer fresh platelets is immediately following repair of the primary defect.[27]

Hypersplenism. The spleen, which contains a labyrinth of reticuloendothelial elements, has repeatedly been implicated in platelet destruction as well as red cell destruction. Quite probably, the peculiarities of circulation and the enormous reticuloendothelial surface cause the destruction, rather than some platelet-destroying function intrinsic to the spleen. For whatever reason, conditions in which the spleen is enlarged are often accompanied by thrombocytopenia, and splenectomy is often followed by prompt increase in platelet count. Splenomegaly, however, is not a conspicuous feature of ITP.

Functional Defects. Both congenital and acquired defects may prevent platelets from normally initiating the temporary hemostatic plug or undergoing viscous metamorphosis. The term *thrombasthenia* is used to describe the hereditary defect of platelet aggregation, while variants of the term *thrombocytopathy* are often used to describe defective chemical release mechanisms.

Acquired functional disorders are much more common than constitutional disorders. Aspirin markedly inhibits ADP release,[37] often producing clinically significant hemorrhagic tendencies.[32] This may be due to acetylation of platelet peptides,[20] since sodium salicylate does not have this effect. Chronic renal disease results in numerous platelet malfunctions, apparently due to the presence of circulating, dialyzable agents other than urea itself,[19] although there is evidence that urea alone decreases platelet adhesiveness.[13] Dialysis, not platelet transfusion, is the treatment of choice.[29] Chronic liver disease and other dysproteinemias also interfere with platelet-mediated hemostasis, and treatment must be directed at the underlying disease.

DISORDERS OF BLOOD COAGULATION

Defects in fibrin formation cause dramatic clinical findings and have received considerable publicity, but they occur far less frequently in clinical practice than disorders of platelet function. Coagulation disorders can be divided into congenital and acquired. Through studies on patients congenitally deficient in single clotting factors, present theories of clotting process have evolved. Acquired disorders usually affect more than one factor and constitute a theoretical and clinical test of our present understanding.

Deficiencies

FACTORS VIII AND IX. Congenital absence of each of the clotting factors has been documented, but most are clinical rarities of great theoretical interest. The most common congenital deficiency affects factor VIII (antihemophilic factor), and causes classical hemophilia, "the disease of kings," which is transmitted as a sex-linked recessive trait. Similar to classical hemophilia is deficiency of factor IX (Christmas factor, or PTC). The inheritance, clinical manifestations, and laboratory findings are the same in the two diseases, but since different factors are missing, the plasma of either will correct the deficiency in the other. Factor IX deficiency, also called Christmas disease or hemophilia B, is approximately one-fifth as common as factor VIII deficiency. Each is characterized by repeated episodes of severe hemorrhage into joints, soft tissues and body cavities, and massive bleeding after injuries. A spectrum of deficiency exists, and patients are classified as severely, moderately, or mildly affected, depending upon the amount of the factor present. Patients with levels of 20 per cent or more of normal rarely have bleeding manifestations.

LABORATORY FINDINGS. The laboratory findings for both conditions are characteristic. The partial thromboplastin time is markedly prolonged but the prothrombin time, which bypasses the plasma thromboplastin phase, is normal. Although the whole blood clotting time is prolonged in most of the severe cases, patients with significant disease may have a normal clotting time. Bleeding time is normal, as are the platelet count and all other tests of hemostasis except those which measure intrinsic thromboplastin generation. Definitive diagnosis can be made by assaying the deficient factor. The ability of remarkably small volumes of plasma to correct defective coagulation is used for assay procedures, and small aliquots of the plasma under test are combined with plasma known to be deficient in any suspected factor.

TREATMENT. Treatment is administration of the missing factor. At present no long-acting preparations are available, and there is no prophylactic therapy given while the patient is asymptomatic. When bleeding occurs, the missing factor must be given intravenously. Commercially prepared concentrates of factor VIII and of the *liver factors* (factor II, VII, IX, and X) are available and have greatly facilitated treatment of life-threatening hemorrhage. Because they are made from large plasma pools, they carry considerable hepatitis risk. For less serious bleeds, many centers prefer to use less concentrated single-donor products.

Factor XI. Deficiency of factor XI (PTA) is rare, causing a bleeding tendency that tends to be less severe than that of either factor IX or factor VIII deficiency. Since the deficiency affects the plasma phase of coagulation, the laboratory findings are similar to those in factor VIII and factor IX deficiency, and the specific defect can be diagnosed if factor XI-deficient plasma is available. This defect appears to reside on an autosomal gene and can occur in either sex.

Factor XII. Deficiency of factor XII very seldom causes clinical symptoms. In factor XII-deficient individuals, the partial thromboplastin time, whole blood clotting time, prothrombin utilization, and thromboplastin generation test will be abnormal, but the patient himself is normal. In the absence of symptoms, the incidence of the condition is difficult to estimate.

Fibrinogen. Plasma fibrinogen levels below 100 mg per 100 ml usually create a bleeding tendency. The deficiency may be congenital or may result from any one of a number of pathologic conditions. Since all clotting mechanisms culminate in conversion of fibrinogen to fibrin, all clotting tests are abnormal if the patient's plasma is used for the end-point. Thus, whole blood clotting time, partial thromboplastin time, and prothrombin time are abnormal. No clot develops when bovine thrombin is added to the patient's blood or plasma, and the prothrombin utilization test is invalidated since, in the absence of clotting, there is no serum. The bleeding time, which depends upon vascular integrity and platelet function, is normal, as is the tourniquet test. Without a clot, of course, clot retraction cannot be evaluated. The thromboplastin generation test is normal, since the incubation mixture is added to a fibrinogen-containing substrate. Definitive diagnosis is made by demonstrating low levels of fibrinogen by direct measurement. Under emergency conditions, adding thrombin to the patient's blood can strongly suggest the correct diagnosis in 30 seconds.

CONGENITAL AFIBRINOGENEMIA. Congenital absence or partial deficiency of fibrinogen is transmitted by an autosomal recessive gene. Surprisingly, the lifelong bleeding diathesis may be less troublesome clinically than that of classical hemophilia, but episodes of massive hemorrhage may occur. Treatment is administration of fibrinogen preparations and, if needed, whole blood. Until recently, fibrinogen was the only clotting factor in commercially available preparations, and it has long been used for the treatment of congenital and acquired afibrinogenemia.

ACQUIRED HYPOFIBRINOGENEMIA. Under certain conditions, plasma fibrinogen may rapidly disappear, producing a generalized, severe bleeding problem. Fibrinogen is not the only element affected, and several mechanisms may contribute to the complex process. It appears that, at times, there may be widespread formation of small intravascular clots, possibly following dissemination of thromboplastin-containing tissue juices such as those from lung or placenta. With widespread intravascular clotting, all hemostatic elements are consumed, including fibrinogen, the plasma procoagulants, and platelets. (See Complex Acquired Bleeding Disorders, p. 372.)

Disorders of Vitamin K Metabolism

The Coumarin Drugs. The most common single cause of coagulation disorders is administration of anticoagulants. Drugs of the coumarin group inhibit vitamin K activity, thereby affecting hepatic production of factors VII, IX, and X and prothrombin. The drugs are given for the control of thromboembolic disease and may produce a significant bleeding tendency. Therapeutic dose levels are frequently monitored with the one-stage prothrombin time. Changes in the prothrombin time probably reflect changing levels of factors VII and X more sensitively than variation of prothrombin level. The prothrombin time is prolonged whenever the vitamin K-dependent factors are reduced, including conditions of impaired vitamin K absorption or diminished hepatic function.

Other Causes. Common bile duct obstruction and malabsorption syndromes prevent adequate absorption of fat-soluble vitamin K, but the defect can be corrected by parenteral administration of the vitamin. If the liver is severely damaged, additional vitamin K will not improve the clotting defect. Hemorrhagic disease of the newborn also results from impaired vitamin K absorption and is readily corrected by administration—to the mother—of vitamin K injections, timed so that the vitamin crosses the placenta to the infant shortly before birth. Another cause of clinical bleeding and prolonged prothrombin time is the ingestion of large doses of coumarin drugs. This may be accidental, but a surprising number of cases occur following deliberate consumption of doses sufficient to produce a bleeding tendency.

Endogenous Anticoagulants

Patients with congenital deficiencies of single clotting factors may, following transfusion therapy, develop inhibitors against the infused substance. These inhibitors may be transient or long-lasting and cause understandable dismay in the patient and his therapists. Occasionally a previously normal man or woman develops, usually late in life, an inhibitor to factor VIII.[30] The patient then is seen with all the signs and symptoms of classical hemophilia, to the great surprise of those who expect to diagnose hemophilia only in young boys. The cause of this phenomenon is unknown. Patients with certain dysproteinemias, notably lupus erythematosus and multiple myeloma, may develop an antagonist which in some manner prevents the interaction of factors X and V and prothrombin. These patients may have a positive serologic test for syphilis and functional platelet disorders as well.

Circulating anticoagulants are diagnosed by studying the interaction of patient's plasma with normal plasma. Once the site of abnormality has been identified, normal and abnormal plasmas can be mixed and the test repeated on the combined plasma. If the defect is due to deficiency of a clotting factor, small amounts of normal plasma will correct it. If the defect is due to an inhibitor, normal plasma will not correct the abnormality, and addition of the patient's plasma to previously normal plasma results in prolongation of the clotting tests.

COMPLEX ACQUIRED BLEEDING DISORDERS

Sometimes physiologic mechanisms intended to be protective work to the individual patient's severe disadvantage. Complex biochemical interactions result in fibrin formation, necessary to prevent excessive hemorrhage, and only slightly less complex interactions produce fibrin dissolution, necessary to prevent excessive fibrin accumulation. Inappropriate activity of either system or unbalanced activity of both can produce generalized bleeding disorders characterized by multiple abnormal findings.

Normal Equilibrium

The action of thrombin appears to be critical in these states of excessive coagulation/fibrinolysis.[11] Thrombin not only clots fibrinogen, it activates platelets, it has an autocatalytic effect on the intrinsic coagulation system, and it can directly activate plasmin, the potent protease which dissolves fibrin. Vascular endothelium and its interaction with platelets also have important roles.[36] Vascular injury leads to factor XII activation, which not only instigates clotting, but also eventuates in plasmin production. Endothelial elements, alone and in conjunction with platelets, promote both coagulation activity and plasmin production. Normal hemostasis and fibrinolysis depend on normal circulation, normal hepatic function, normal reticuloendothelial function, and adequate localization of the coagulation process to a discrete site.

Intravascular Coagulation

In the complex acquired bleeding disorders, a simplified description of events is as follows. Widespread, rather than local, activation of coagulation mechanisms develop, due to circulating thromboplastic materials, endothelial damage, infectious or immunologic processes, pH derangement, neoplastic disease, and so forth. Fibrin may or may not be deposited rather widely, and platelet aggregation and trapping occur, both where fibrin is formed and at sites of endothelial change. This widespread coagulation depletes available clotting factors and circulating platelets, whether or not visible fibrin deposition can be discerned.

Fibrinolysis

The same stimuli that activate clotting also activate plasminogen to plasmin, as does the deposition of fibrin. Plasmin digests more than just fibrin. It partially digests fibrinogen, producing polypeptide fragments which clot either slowly or not at all. The combined effect of plasmin and thrombin upon fibrinogen results in degradation products (split products) which not only are unclottable themselves, but which inhibit coagulation of undigested fibrinogen. These degradation products also impair the normal hemostatic activity of platelets.

Clinical Findings

The result of these interactions is depletion of most clotting factors, depletion of platelets with impairment of those that remain, release of circulating fragments which inhibit clotting, and acceleration of lytic destruction of whatever fibrin may evolve. The patient, not surprisingly, develops a severe bleeding diathesis, even though the initiating event was hypercoagulability. The names given to this unfortunate series of events include *consumption coagulopathy, defibrination syndrome,* and *disseminated intravascular coagulation* or *DIC.*

Laboratory Studies

Complete unravelling of DIC situations may be impossible in clinical emergencies. The laboratory diagnosis will vary with the availability of specialized techniques, but basic information necessary for presumptive diagnosis is within the capability of nearly all laboratories. The preliminary findings are prolongation of prothrombin time, of partial thromboplastin time, and of bleeding time, with depletion of platelets. Mixing equal parts of patient plasma and normal plasma in the partial thromboplastin time reveals that the patient's blood inhibits coagulation of normal blood. The next phase is to evaluate stage 3 of the clotting process. Fibrinogen, if assayed, will be found seriously depleted. Simpler and more immediately useful is the thrombin-clotting time. By adding exogenous thrombin to the patient's plasma, one can roughly infer the amount of fibrinogen present from the appearance of the clot and the speed of clot formation. If the patient's plasma prolongs the thrombin clotting time of normal plasma, the presence of circulating stage 3 inhibitors is proved. This, combined with demonstration of thrombocytopenia, is highly suggestive of DIC.

More detailed investigations can document the presence of fibrinogen degradation products. The tests most widely used employ immunologic reactions of fibrinogen and its degradation products with antifibrinogen antibodies. This can be done by latex agglutination, immunodiffusion, or hemagglutination inhibition, of which the last is probably the most sensitive and specific, but is technically the most difficult.[35] Increased fibrinolytic activity can sometimes be demonstrated rather quickly by observing the effect of epsilon amino caproic acid (EACA, a chemical with antiplasmin activity) on the thrombin clotting time of dilute plasma.[15] This procedure is much more rapid than the euglobulin lysis or dilute blood lysis tests, which also demonstrate increased fibrinolysis but require several hours unless activity is extremely marked.

Fibrinogen Split Products

Fibrinogen degradation products (FDP), presumably deriving from fibrinolytic activity beyond that needed for physiologic fibrin removal, can be found circulating in patients without overt bleeding disorders. The more sensitive the test method, the more patients who will have positive results, but significant levels of FDP occur in many patients with advanced cirrhosis.[34,35] Low levels of plasminogen and prolonged thrombin clotting times in these patients suggest that a low grade fibrinolytic process may accompany cirrhosis without producing clinical bleeding. FDP levels may be elevated in pre-eclampsia,[6] and, to a lesser extent, in normal pregnancy[7] and in women taking oral contraceptives.[35]

BIBLIOGRAPHY

1. ACKROYD, J.F.: Platelet agglutinins and lysins in the pathogenesis of thrombocytopenic purpura, with a note on platelet groups. Br. Med. Bull. 11:28, 1955.
2. ADNER, M.M., FISCH, G.R., STAROBIN, S.G., AND ASTER, R.H.: Use of "compatible" platelet transfusions in treatment of congenital isoimmune thrombocytopenic purpura. N. Engl. J. Med. 280:244, 1969.

3. BACHMAN, F.: The paradoxes of disseminated intravascular coagulation. Hosp. Pract. 6:113, 1971.
4. BARROW, E.M., AND GRAHAM, J.B.: "Von Willebrand's disease," *In* Moore, C.V., and Brown, E.B. (eds.): Progress in Hematology, Grune & Stratton, New York, 1964, vol. 6.
5. BECKER, G.A., AND ASTER, R.H.: Platelet transfusion therapy. Med. Clin. North Am. 56:81, 1972.
6. BIRMINGHAM ECLAMPSIA STUDY GROUP: Intravascular coagulation and abnormal lung-scans in pre-eclampsia and eclampsia. Lancet 2:889, 1971.
7. BONNAR, J., DAVIDSON, J.F., PIDGEON, C.F., ET AL.: Fibrin degradation products through-out normal pregnancy. Br. Med. J. 3:137, 1969.
8. BOURONCLE, B.A., AND DOAN, C.A.: Treatment of refractory idiopathic thrombocyto-penic purpura. J.A.M.A. 297:2049, 1969.
9. CIMO, P.L., AND ASTER, R.H.: Post-transfusion purpura. N. Engl. J. Med. 287:290, 1972.
10. CLANCY, R., JENKINS, E., AND FIRKIN, B.: Qualitative platelet abnormalities in idiopathic thrombocytopenic purpura. N. Engl. J. Med. 286:622, 1972.
11. DEYKIN, D.: The clinical challenge of disseminated intravascular coagulation. N. Engl. J. Med. 283:36, 1970.
12. EBBE, S.: "Origin, production, and life-span of blood platelets," *In* Johnson, S.A. (ed.): The Circulating Platelet, Academic Press, New York, 1971.
13. EKNOYAN, G., WACKSMAN, S.J., GLUECK, H.I., AND WILL, J.J.: Platelet function in renal failure. N. Engl. J. Med. 280:677, 1969.
14. FREIMAN, D.G.: "Disorders of the circulation: Thrombosis, embolism, infarction," *In* Brunson, J.G., and Gall, E.A. (eds.): Concepts of Disease, Macmillan Co., New York, 1971.
15. GIDDINGS, J.C., AND BLOOM, A.L.: A study of two methods for estimating plasma fibrinogen and the effect of epsilon aminocaproic acid and protamine. J. Clin. Pathol. 24:467, 1971.
16. GRUMET, F.C., AND YANKEE, R.A.: Long-term platelet support of patients with aplastic anemia. Ann. Intern. Med. 73:1, 1970.
17. HARKER, L.A., AND SLICHTER, S.J.: The bleeding time as a screening test for evaluation of platelet function. N. Engl. J. Med. 287:155, 1972.
18. HARRINGTON, W.J., MINNICH, V., HOLLINSWORTH, J.W., AND MOORE, C.V.: Demonstra-tion of a thrombocytopenic factor in the blood of patients with thrombocytopenic pur-pura. J. Lab. Clin. Med. 38:1, 1951.
19. HOROWITZ, H.I.: Uremic toxins and platelet function. Arch. Intern. Med. 126:823, 1970.
20. KRANE, S.M.: Action of salicylates. N. Engl. J. Med. 286:317, 1972.
21. KWAAN, H.C.: Disorders of fibrinolysis. Med. Clin. North Am. 56:163, 1972.
22. KWAAN, H.C.: Disseminated intravascular coagulation. Med. Clin. North Am. 56:177, 1972.
23. LANGDELL, R.D.: "Coagulation and hemostasis," *In* Davidsohn, I., and Henry, J.B. (eds.): Todd-Sanford Clinical Diagnosis by Laboratory Methods, ed. 14. W.B. Saunders Co., Philadelphia, 1969.
24. LAROS, R.K., AND PENNER, J.A.: "Refractory" thrombocytopenic purpura treated suc-cessfully with cyclophosphamide. J.A.M.A. 215:445, 1971.
25. MACFARLANE, R.G.: The coagulant action of Russell's viper venom; the use of antivenom in defining its reaction with a serum factor. Br. J. Haematol. 7:496, 1961.
26. MURPHY, E.A., AND SALZMAN, E.W.: The diagnosis of VonWillebrand's disease. Blood 39:284, 1972.
27. OBERMAN, H.A.: The indications for transfusion of freshly drawn blood. J.A.M.A. 199:93, 1967.
28. POOL, J.G., AND SHANNON, A.E.: Production of high-potency concentrates of antihemo-philic globulin in a closed-bag system: assay in vitro and in vivo. N. Engl. J. Med. 273:1443, 1965.
29. RABINER, S.F.: Bleeding in uremia. Med.Clin. N.Am. 56:221, 1972.
30. RATNOFF, O.D.: The blood clotting mechanism and its disorders. D.M.1-49, Nov., 1965.

31. ROBBOY, S.J., LEWIS, E.J., SCHUR, P.H., AND COLMAN, R.W.: Circulating anticoagulants to Factor VIII. Am. J. Med. 49:742, 1970.
32. ROSSI, E.C.: The function of platelets in hemostasis. Med. Clin. North Am. 56:25, 1972.
33. ROSSI, E.C., AND GREEN, D.: Disorders of platelet function. Med. Clin. North Am. 56:35, 1972.
34. SACK, E.S., AND BURASCHI, J.: Fibrinogen degradation products, (letter). N. Engl. J. Med. 284:1441, 1971.
35. THOMAS, D.P., NIEWIAROWSKI, S., MYERS, A.R. ET AL.: A comparative study of four methods for detecting fibrinogen degradation products in patients with various diseases. N. Engl. J. Med. 283:663, 1970.
36. WALSH, P.N.: The role of platelets in the contact phase of blood coagulation. Br. J. Haematol. 22:237, 1972.
37. WEISS, H.S., ALEDORT, L.M., AND KOCHWA, S.: The effect of salicylates on the hemostatic properties of platelets in man. J. Clin. Invest. 47:2169, 1968.
38. WRIGHT, I.S.: The nomenclature of blood clotting factors. J.A.M.A. 180:733, 1962.

CHAPTER 16

The Endocrine Glands

PITUITARY GLAND

Secretions of the pituitary gland control most of the other endocrine glands and directly affect various somatic tissues. The pituitary has two morphologically and embryologically distinct parts: the anterior glandular part or adenohypophysis; and the posterior part, of neural origin, called the neurohypophysis. The two parts jointly occupy the sella turcica, but the functions and control of each part are separate.

ADENOHYPOPHYSIS

Cell Types and Hormones

The adenohypophysis secretes at least six hormones, several of which have more than one name. These are growth hormone (somatotropin); thyroid-stimulating hormone (TSH, thyrotropin); follicle-stimulating hormone (FSH); luteinizing hormone (LH, interstitial cell-stimulating hormone); luteotropic hormone (LTH, prolactin); and adrenal cortical-stimulating hormone (corticotropin, adrenal corticotropic hormone, ACTH).

Four major cell types, named for their affinity for tissue stains, comprise the anterior pituitary: acidophils, basophils, chromophobes, and amphophils. Although morphologic changes in various diseases suggest individual functions for individual cells, it is not certain which cells produce which hormones. Acidophils appear to be associated with growth hormone, and basophils with ACTH and thyrotropin. Basophilic cells of slightly different appearance may secrete the gonadotropic hormones FSH and LH. The origin of prolactin is undetermined.

Several other substances are associated with the pituitary, although their sites of origin and biologic nature are unclear. These are the melanocyte-stimulating hormone, and exophthalmos-producing factor which is not the same as thyrotropin alone. Long-acting thyroid stimulator (LATS), a substance associated with hyperthyroidism, may not be pituitary in origin. Present in the blood of hyperthyroid patients even after hypophysectomy,[1] it has many properties characteristic of gamma globulin, although an immune origin has not been demonstrated.

Corticotropin. Corticotropin (ACTH, adrenal cortical-stimulating hormone) has been intensively studied. Its primary action is upon the adrenal cortex, but it has extra-adrenal effects on fat, carbohydrate, and amino acid metabolism.[10] Under its influence, glucocorticoids and adrenal estrogens and androgens enter the blood stream. Minimal aldosterone secretion may follow ACTH stimulation, but the pituitary does not exert primary control over the mineral corticoids. ACTH secretion is, itself, controlled by hypothalamic response to the blood level of hydrocortisone. Hypothalamic secretions, elaborated in response to varying levels of circulating hormones, affect the production of other tropic hormones in addition to ACTH. Both bioassay and immunoassay procedures measure ACTH levels.

Somatotropin. Growth hormone exerts an imperfectly understood influence on the body as a whole. The results of somatotropic stimulation include increased amino acid transport and protein synthesis; mobilization of free fatty acids; and retention of calcium, phosphorus, sodium, potassium, and nitrogen. Approximately 4 to 10 mg of growth hormone are found at all ages in the pituitary,[10] which is believed to produce and store somatotropin. The very small amounts of circulating hormone are measured by immunoassay and radioimmunoassay procedures. Blood levels follow a diurnal pattern, and basal levels can best be determined early in the morning.[44]

Thyrotropin. Thyroid-stimulating hormone promotes all synthesizing functions of the thyroid gland, resulting in increased gland weight and increased levels of circulating thyroid hormones. It is the change in these circulating levels that regulates TSH production, probably through hypothalamic mediation. Thyrotropin may independently affect connective tissue, but isolation of TSH from such associated proteins as exophthalmos-producing factor is so difficult that its extrathyroidal activity cannot be fully characterized. TSH is measured by bioassay.

Gonadotropins. Production of the gonadotropins—follicle-stimulating hormone, luteinizing hormone, and luteotropic hormone—is apparently under hypothalamic control. In the female, follicle-stimulating hormone promotes maturation of the ovarian follicle. The maturing follicle produces estrogens, and as the level of circulating estrogen rises, luteinizing hormone is produced. Through combined LH and FSH activity, the ovum matures and the follicle ruptures. The secretory activity of the corpus luteum requires adequate levels of both luteinizing hormone and luteotropic hormone. The luteotropic hormone is also called prolactin because it initiates and sustains lactation, but successful milk secretion also requires the actions of estrogens, progesterone, growth hormone, and adrenal cortical hormones. In males, follicle-stimulating hormone promotes spermatogenesis, while luteinizing hormone stimulates the interstitial cells to secrete androgens. Both FSH and LH levels in the blood and urine can be measured by relatively uncomplicated bioassay, and by immunoassay procedures.

Diseases of the Anterior Pituitary

Pituitary abnormalities may be due to overproduction or underproduction of any or all of the adenohypophyseal hormones. Overproduction is almost always associated with gross or microscopic evidence of tumor. Underproduction usually follows hypophyseal destruction from disease or from operative procedures. In rare cases, there may be underproduction of isolated hormones, usually the gonadotropins, with no histologic or anatomic evidence of pituitary disease. Since the hypothalamus is so important to pituitary control, it is likely that isolated hormonal defects have their origin in individual loci of the hypothalamus.

Somatotropin Deficiency. The most dramatic pituitary dysfunctions are disorders of growth hormone. Pituitary dwarfism occurs when postnatal supplies of somatotropin are inadequate; most such children have had normal intrauterine development. Craniopharyngioma causes approximately one third of these cases,[10] while the remainder are of unknown cause. Associated with retarded skeletal growth is retarded sexual maturation, although intelligence is usually normal. Despite reduced levels of thyroid and adrenal hormones, the patient is generally healthy, and there is no evidence of hypometabolism. Low fasting blood sugar is fairly common, but symptomatic hypoglycemia is unusual.

DIFFERENTIAL DIAGNOSIS. Pituitary dwarfism must sometimes be distinguished from so-called "primordial dwarfism," hypothyroidism, and gonadal aplasia. In primordial dwarfism, hormone production is normal, but the somatic tissues do not respond normally. Despite small stature, bone age and sexual development are usually normal, and thyroid and adrenal secretions are not diminished. In hypothyroidism, as in pituitary dwarfism, bone age and sexual development are retarded, but other clinical features point to childhood hypothyroidism, namely mental retardation, bradycardia, hypothermia, coarsening of skin and hair, and abnormal calcification of teeth and bones. Gonadal disorders, notably the XO chromosomal condition, may be associated with short stature and failure of sexual maturation, but other physical abnormalities are often present, and the nuclear sex pattern is abnormal.

Somatotropin Excess. Overproduction of growth hormone occurs in eosinophilic or mixed adenomas. If overproduction precedes epiphyseal closure, striking long bone enlargement produces gigantism. If the epiphyseal plates have fused, the facial and acral bones enlarge, producing the characteristic acromegalic appearance—enlarged facial features, protruding jaw, broad hands and feet, and enlargement of tongue and viscera. Advanced acromegaly is readily recognized, but frequently progression is gradual and many years elapse before the diagnosis is made.

LABORATORY FINDINGS. Laboratory changes include altered carbohydrate metabolism, with diabetic glucose tolerance curve or frank diabetes mellitus; elevated BMR; increased glomerular and renal tubular function; elevated serum levels of alkaline phosphatase and inorganic phosphorus; and increased serum levels of growth hormone when assay is performed.[37] Visual field defects are common if the pituitary tumor compresses the optic chiasm, and x-ray examination may show generalized osteoporosis as well as increased new bone formation.

Corticotropin Excess. The pituitary basophilic cells apparently produce ACTH, and increased levels of ACTH are frequently associated with basophilic adenomas. Autopsy series on patients with adrenal hyperfunction reveal that approximately one-fourth have pituitary tumors. Patients who have undergone bilateral adrenalectomy for treatment of Cushing's disease may subsequently develop basophil or chromophobe adenomas, but Addison's disease, in which ACTH production is also high, is not often associated with pituitary tumors.

Serum ACTH is measured by bioassay and immunoassay. Existence of an ACTH-producing tumor may be suggested if administration of a potent glucocorticoid, such as dexamethasone, fails to suppress ACTH production, or if corticosteroid excretion does not fall after the suppressor drug is given. Excessive steroid production, unresponsive to suppressor drugs, can occur with either pituitary or adrenal gland tumors, so both glands must be evaluated. X-ray examination of both areas may be helpful in the differential diagnosis. Certain nonpituitary tumors, notably those of the lung and pancreas, may secrete an ACTH-like substance and produce hyperadrenalism.

Other Hormones. Other pituitary hormones may be present in excess, but ACTH and somatotropin are by far the most common. Excess prolactin has been invoked to explain lactorrhea in women with acromegaly, and lactorrhea associated with amenorrhea may be the presenting symptoms of pituitary tumor.[17] Thyrotropin disorders are extremely rare. Most hyperthyroidism appears to arise from intrathyroid abnormalities.

Panhypopituitarism. Generalized hypopituitarism may occur when more than three quarters of the gland is destroyed by surgical ablation, tumor, or non-neoplastic destruction. The first deficiency to appear clinically is of gonadotropin, followed by somatotropin (noticeable only in children), thyrotropin, and lastly corticotropin. Non-neoplastic destruction is nearly always due to infarction, often following hemorrhagic shock, as in Sheehan's syndrome in which hypopituitarism follows obstetric bleeding. Such infections as tuberculosis and syphilis formerly caused pituitary destruction, but are now very rare. Very rarely hemochromatosis, Hand-Schuller-Christian disease, or noninfectious giant cell granuloma may destroy the gland, while some patients with hypopituitarism are found at autopsy to have diffuse fibrosis of unknown cause.

DIFFERENTIAL DIAGNOSIS. Hypopituitarism must be distinguished from other conditions of hypometabolism, loss of gonadal function, and anemia. When pituitary infarction follows obstetric shock, lactation does not occur, the menses do not resume, and there is gradually progressive disability. In long-standing hypopituitarism, there is genital atrophy, generalized depigmentation, sparsity of body hair, and evidence of thyroid and adrenal hypofunction. Cachexia is uncommon, distinguishing hypopituitarism from anorexia nervosa. The skin is waxy with fine wrinkles and diminished sweating.

Diagnosis rests on evaluation of hormonal levels. Urinary gonadotropins are low, a finding especially significant in older individuals, since normal young adults may have variably low gonadotropin excretion. Urinary excretion of 17-ketosteroids and 17-OH steroids is low, but the levels rise following three or four days of ACTH stimulation. After adrenal function has been established, pituitary failure is documented by administering the adrenal blocking agent metyrapone, which normally causes ACTH stimulation and marked increase in urinary steroids. All the tests of thyroid function are low, including BMR, ^{131}I uptake, circulating thyroxine, and the like, but after several days of TSH stimulation, thyroid function returns to normal.

END-ORGAN FAILURE. Pituitary failure results in endocrine hypofunction, but the target organs can be stimulated to normal function by exogenous tropic hormones. It may be difficult to distinguish between severe primary hypothyroidism and long-standing hypopituitarism since, in both cases, there are hypometabolism and decreased adrenal and genital function. The thyroid gland, after prolonged absence of TSH stimulation, may atrophy so severely that the TSH stimulation test remains negative. In such cases, the thyroid gland is usually extremely small, while primary causes of hypothyroidism frequently produce a normal-sized or enlarged gland. This difference in size is not, unfortunately, of universal occurrence. Anorexia nervosa may present another difficult diagnostic problem, since amenorrhea and loss of thyroid and adrenal function can occur with this as well as other types of chronic malnutrition. Hypopituitarism, however, is usually characterized by a better nutritional state, loss of body hair, and loss of pigmentation. In chronic malnutrition, urinary steroid excretion tends to be higher than in hypopituitarism.

INDIRECT TESTS. As specific hormonal tests become available, indirect tests of pituitary function are less important. Hypoglycemia, insulin hyperreactivity, anemia, hyponatremia, and increased water retention are nonspecific findings of inconstant occurrence and should not be considered diagnostic. Such tests as insulin tolerance and water tolerance may be dangerous for the patient, and they provide less information than direct hormonal evaluation.

NEUROHYPOPHYSIS

The posterior, neural portion of the pituitary is a storehouse rather than a producer of hormones. The neurohypophyseal hormones originate in the hypothalamus and travel down the neurohypophyseal tract to the pituitary pars nervosa. Two hormones are involved: vasopressin, also called antidiuretic hormone (ADH); and oxytocin. Their structures are remarkably similar, but the difference of one amino acid confers different properties on each.[12]

Functions of ADH

The two names of one hormone—vasopressin and antidiuretic hormone—signal its two actions: It stimulates vascular smooth muscle contraction, and it affects renal fluid excretion. The pressor effect occurs to a mild degree in anesthetized patients, but it is probably of little physiologic significance. Highly significant, however, is the antidiuretic effect. Diabetes insipidus, the clinical condition caused by neurohypophyseal insufficiency, is a dramatic example of physiologic derangement.

Antidiuretic hormone directly affects the distal convoluted tubule of the nephron. Emerging from the loop of Henle, urine is markedly hypotonic relative to the plasma in adjacent capillaries. ADH permits water to diffuse through the distal tubular epithelium, going from the dilute fluid in the tubule to the relatively concentrated medium of plasma. Without ADH, water cannot traverse the epithelium, so that large quantities of dilute urine are excreted. Changes in plasma osmolality appear to regulate ADH production, although changes in blood volume may also play a part. Nicotine, morphine, and ether promote ADH secretion, while alcohol produces diuresis by inhibiting ADH production.

Function of Oxytocin

Oxytocin also has two effects: It promotes uterine contraction and stimulates milk ejection. Neither the mechanism of oxytocic effects nor the interrelationships between ADH secretion and oxytocin release are clearly understood. Patients with diabetes insipidus have normal labor and successful lactation. Isolated deficiency or excess of oxytocin has not been reported, but oxytocin deficiency occurs in patients with panhypopituitarism, especially with postpartum pituitary necrosis.

Diabetes Insipidus

Diabetes insipidus may follow neoplastic and, occasionally, traumatic or granulomatous destruction of the fibers connecting the hypothalamus with the neurohypophysis. Hypothalamic disease, with or without apparent histologic change, may cause ADH deficiency. The presenting symptom is enormous urine output, characteristically 7 to 11 liters daily, but even more in many cases. The urine is pale and dilute, with a specific gravity of less than 1.005. Patients with diabetes insipidus consume enormous amounts of water or else rapidly become dehydrated, since urine output continues despite diminished fluid intake. The basal metabolic rate is sometimes elevated. X-ray examination, electroencephalogram, chemical or bacteriologic studies, or visual field determination may, in some cases of pituitary destruction, reveal abnormalities diagnostic of the primary disease.

Differential Diagnosis. Before diabetes insipidus is conclusively proved, two points must be confirmed. The kidneys must be capable of response to ADH, and the patient must be incapable of producing ADH after appropriate stimulation. To be excluded are psychogenic polydipsia, nephrogenic diabetes insipidus, and acquired renal damage. In hyperparathyroidism or vitamin D intoxication, hypercalcemia may cause ADH-resistant polyuria, but this is readily diagnosed by serum electrolyte studies. Administration of exogenous ADH has no effect on patients with nephrogenic (vasopressin-resistant) diabetes insipidus. Exogenous ADH causes a marked but short-lived increase in urine osmolality, both in true diabetes insipidus and in psychogenic polydipsia. The differential diagnosis is made by demonstrating secretory response, or lack of it, to changes in plasma osmolality.

Water Deprivation Test. In the water deprivation test, water is withheld until 2% to 5% of the body weight is lost. This usually requires 6 to 12 hours, during which time the patient must be constantly watched, for patients with psychogenic polydipsia may display extreme cunning in obtaining illicit fluids, while patients with diabetes insipidus may collapse from dehydration. Carefully monitored stimulation by hypertonic sodium chloride or nicotine may also be used to alter plasma osmolality. However the change is produced, increased plasma osmolality causes decreased urine volume and increased urine concentration in a patient with an intact neurohypophyseal system and responsive kidneys. The patient with diabetes insipidus continues massive urine excretion, although the specific gravity may rise slightly.

Inappropriate ADH Secretion

The observation that certain patients have expanded total body water and continuing low serum osmolality has suggested that ADH can be secreted independent of any volumetric or osmometric stimulus.[3] Bronchogenic carcinoma has been shown to elaborate a material indistinguishable from ADH, and many other intrathoracic lesions and intracranial abnormalities produce similar clinical findings. Excessive ADH activity leads to water retention, with dilutional hyponatremia, This stimulates increased glomerular filtration and sodium excretion[63] resulting in net sodium loss and a urine significantly hyperosmolar to the serum.

ADRENAL CORTEX

The adrenal gland, like the pituitary, consists of two functionally and embryologically distinct portions. The cortex is of mesodermal origin and secretes hormones essential to maintain life. The medulla derives from the ectoderm, and its secretions, though important for normal existence, are not vital.

STEROIDS AND THEIR STRUCTURES

The cortical hormones have as their basic structure the cyclopentanoperhydrophenanthrene ring, a 17-carbon structure. Specific hormones derive their functions and characteristic chemical and physical

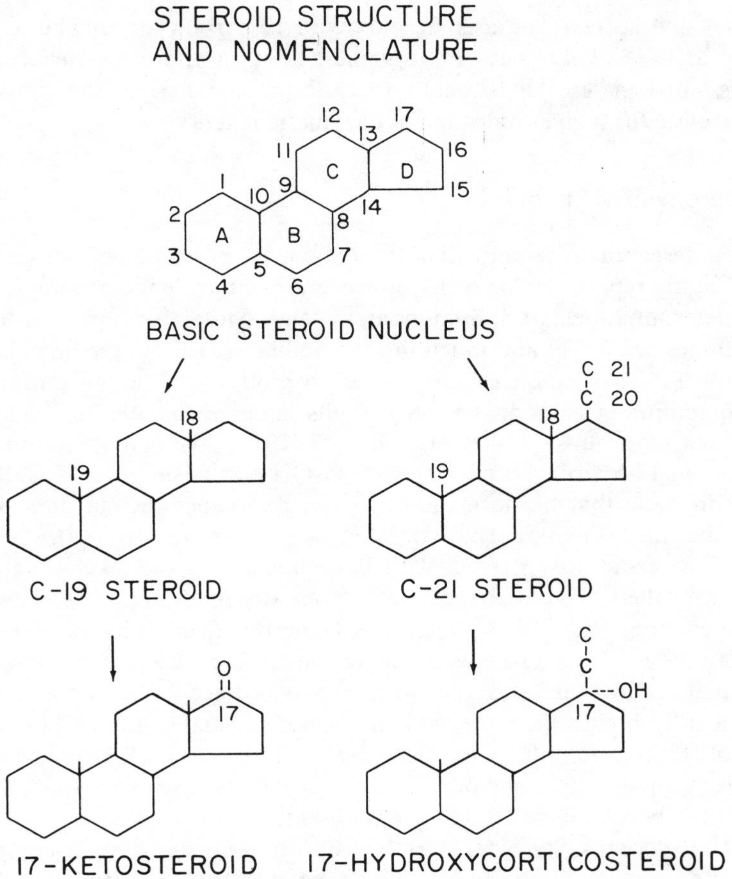

Figure 20. Structure and nomenclature of principal steroids in the adrenal cortex. (Redrawn from Lauler, D.P., Williams, G.H., and Thorn, G.W., *In* Wintrobe, M.M. et al. [eds.]: Harrison's Principles of Internal Medicine, ed. 6. McGraw-Hill Book Co., 1970. Used by permission of McGraw-Hill Book Co.)

properties from additional groups present on several of the carbon atoms. Although innumerable active and intermediate compounds are known, the major adrenal cortical products can be grouped fairly simply (Fig. 20).

Zones of Production. The outer and middle zones of the adrenal cortex produce hormones with 21 carbon atoms. Those with a hydroxyl group at position 17 are called 17-hydroxycorticosteroids or glucocorticoids, since one of their significant effects is on glucose metabolism. Twenty-one-carbon corticoids without the OH group at C-17 principally affect mineral metabolism and are called mineralocorticoids. The inner zone of the cortex produces steroids with 19 carbon atoms and a ketone group at C-17. These have androgenic activity and are produced in both males and females. All adrenal cortical hormones derive from cholesterol and acetate through a multitude of enzymatic reactions.

Measurement of Steroids

In research work and detailed diagnostic procedures, bioassays can yield highly reproducible results; however, in clinical endocrinology, chemical determinations and immunoassay and competitive protein-binding techniques are useful and much more readily available. Screening chemical procedures are done on urinary excretion products, although serum levels are sometimes measured. Urinary steroids can conveniently be divided into three major groups: 17-ketosteroids (17-KS), 17-ketogenic steroids (17-KGS) and 17-hydroxycorticosteroids (17-OH corticosteroids, 17-OHCS). It is unfortunate that the terms are so similar, because the substances measured are quite different. These differences are presented in Figure 21.

17-Ketosteroids. Steroids with 19 carbon atoms and a ketone group at C-17 are called 17-ketosteroids and are usually measured by the Zimmerman reaction. Not all 17-ketosteroids derive from adrenal hormones. Among the excreted 17-ketosteroids in the mature male are metabolites of testicular androgens, and the normal 17-ketosteroid levels for men are significantly higher than for women. In normal males, the 24-hour excretion of 17-ketosteroids is 7 to 25 mg, with a mean of 15 mg. Normal females excrete 5 to 15 mg of 17-ketosteroids daily, with a mean of 10 mg.[35] Prior to puberty, this sex difference is absent.

17-Ketogenic Steroids. A rather similar term describes a completely different group of compounds. The term 17-ketogenic steroid refers to compounds having 21 carbon atoms and a hydroxyl group at C-17. This hydroxyl group can be converted to a ketone group by oxidation, which also removes the side chain of C-20 and C-21 regardless of its nature. The group of compounds capable of oxidation to 17-KS includes several glucocorticoid derivatives, as well as pregnanetriol. These compounds are sometimes called *Norymberski steroids,* after the method used for their determination. In both men and women, normal excretion of 17-ketogenic steroids is 5 to 20 mg in 24 hours. The original urinary 17-ketosteroids must be either inactivated or measured separately before the 17-ketogenic steroids are studied.

17-Hydroxycorticosteroids. A third group of urinary compounds is called the 17-hydroxycorticosteroids, a misleading term since not every 21-carbon compound with a 17-hydroxyl group is included. The steroids

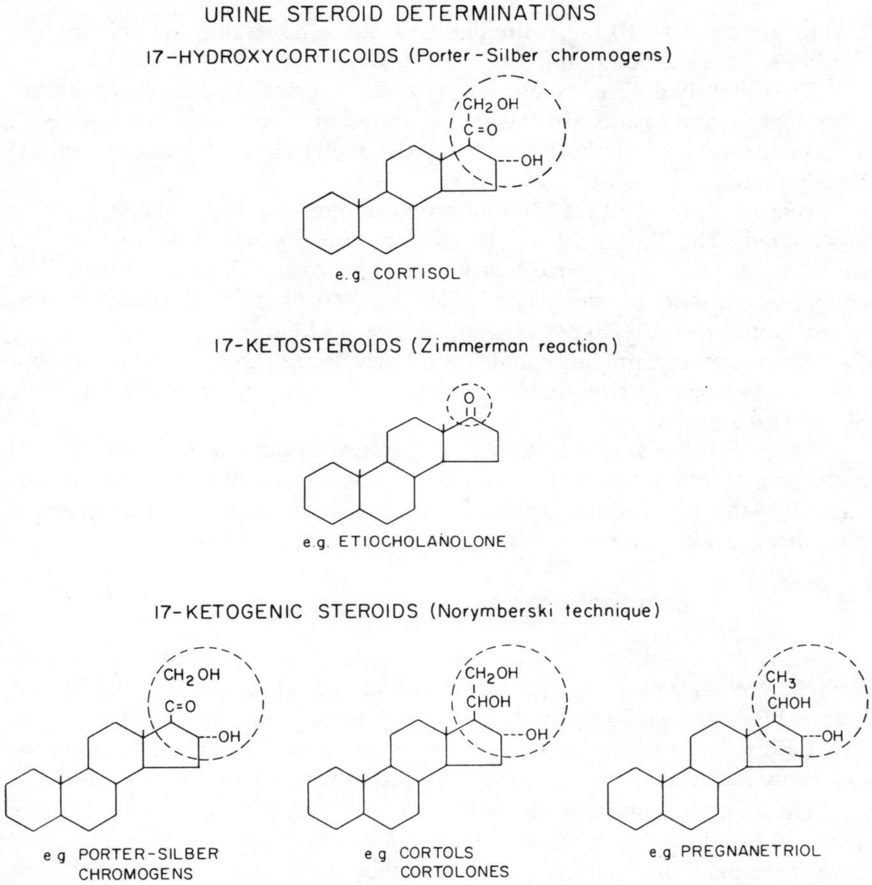
URINE STEROID DETERMINATIONS
17-HYDROXYCORTICOIDS (Porter-Silber chromogens)
CH2 OH
C=O
OH
e.g. CORTISOL
17-KETOSTEROIDS (Zimmerman reaction)
O
e.g. ETIOCHOLANOLONE
17-KETOGENIC STEROIDS (Norymberski technique)
CH2 OH
C=O
OH
e.g PORTER-SILBER CHROMOGENS
CH2OH
CHOH
OH
e.g CORTOLS CORTOLONES
CH3
CHOH
OH
e.g. PREGNANETRIOL

Figure 21. Reactive groups that participate in urinary steroid determinations. (Redrawn from Lauler, D.P., Williams, G.H., and Thorn, G.W., *In* Wintrobe, M.M. et al. [eds.]: Harrison's Principles of Internal Medicine, ed. 6. McGraw-Hill Book Co., 1970. Used by permission of McGraw-Hill Book Co.)

included are those with 21 carbons and a dihydroxyacetone side chain. This combination of hydroxyl groups at C-17 and C-21, and a ketone group at C-20 reacts with phenylhydrazine to form a yellow compound. This is the Porter-Silber reaction, and these steroids are often called *Porter-Silber chromogens.* Included in this group are aldosterone and several metabolites of glucocorticoids. Owing to its high potency, aldosterone contributes little to the total quantity of urinary 17-OH corticosteroids, even in conditions of excess. The normal 24-hour excretion of Porter-Silber chromogens is 1 to 10 mg, with slight variation depending on the method used to extract the compounds.

Two slightly different methods are used for extracting the Porter-Silber chromogens, and results are usually expressed in terms of the method used. The Glenn-Nelson method gives slightly higher normal values than the Reddy method.

It is worth noting that 17-OH corticosteroids and 17-ketogenic steroids are related. The Porter-Silber chromogens are, in fact, 17-ketogenic steroids, since their 17-hydroxyl group can be oxidized to a ketone. The compounds commonly designated 17-hydroxycorticosteroids normally contribute approximately 40 per cent of the total 17-ketogenic steroids.

Aldosterone. Circulating aldosterone levels are rarely measured except in exacting research situations. Normal values are said to be 5 to 15 mcg per 100 ml.[35]

Other Products. In addition to the groups of compounds described, a multitude of other products can be extracted from blood, urine, or the adrenal gland itself. Because of the exacting requirements for determination, these products are not used in routine clinical diagnosis.

INDIRECT TESTS OF ADRENAL FUNCTION

Clinicians evaluated adrenal cortical function long before steroids were isolated and purified. Adrenal hormones produce so many effects that many different derangements could be studied and manipulated. More specific information can now be obtained through steroid determinations, especially in tests using purified ACTH and other hormone preparations.

The classical indirect studies of adrenal function relate to glucose metabolism, fluid balance, and hematologic findings. These procedures have little diagnostic significance, now that hormonal measurements are. readily available. The Thorn test, in which circulating eosinophils decline to less than 50 per cent of their baseline level after ACTH administration, may be combined with other procedures employing ACTH. No indirect tests of androgenic function are needed, since history and physical examination testify to sexual changes, and determination of urinary 17-ketosteroids can now confirm the clinical impression.

DIRECT TESTS OF STEROID PRODUCTION

ACTH Stimulation

The Thorn test was the first of the more specific tests of adrenal function, but it remains an inferential procedure. Direct measurement of steroid output following ACTH stimulation is more reliable. To provide maximum information, this test should include four or five daily doses of 50 units of ACTH with measurement, in each 24 hours, of 17-ketosteroid and 17-hydroxycorticosteroid excretion. Of critical importance is the accurate collection and measurement of urinary output, and it may be advisable to monitor the adequacy of collection by measuring creatinine content of each 24-hour sample.

Normal Rise in 17-OHCS. Once complete collection is assured, changes in ketosteroid and hydroxysteroid excretion mirror adrenal response. In the patient with potentially normal adrenal glands and inadequate pituitary function, steroid output rises progressively over the five days of the test. On the last day, the 17-hydroxycorticosteroids should be five to ten times the starting level, while ketosteroids increase twofold to threefold. Patients with partial adrenal function respond to intensive stimulation with a mild rise in hydroxycorticoids but no significant change in the ketosteroids. If the 17-OHCS rise less than 2 mg in 24 hours, marked adrenal insufficiency can be inferred.

Tests of Pituitary-Adrenal Axis

Both the pituitary and the adrenal glands are important in regulating corticosteroid production. Glucocorticoid levels are controlled by ACTH secretion, and ACTH secretion depends, in turn, on the amount of adrenal hormones in the circulation. Two tests are available to measure the integrity of this "feed-back" mechanism. In the dexamethasone suppression test, the pituitary perceives high levels of circulating hormones, and it should respond by curtailing ACTH production causing subsequent diminished excretion of steroid metabolites. In the metyrapone test, hormone synthesis is blocked, and the pituitary tries to increase the levels of active hormone by producing more and more ACTH, thus provoking more and more synthesis of the inactive precursors.

Dexamethasone Suppression Test. Both dexamethasone and 9-alpha-fluorohydrocortisone are potent glucocorticoids, causing marked metabolic effect and pituitary suppression with little quantitative change in steroid excretion. Either drug could be used for this test, but 9-alpha-fluorohydrocortisone produces sodium retention, an undesirable side effect. Following baseline determination of 24-hour 17-hydroxycorticosteroid excretion, 0.5 mg of dexamethasone is given every six hours for two days. In patients with a normally responsive pituitary-adrenal axis, steroid production drops in response to decreased ACTH stimulation, usually to 2.5 mg or less per 24 hours, on the second day of medication.

INCREASED DEXAMETHASONE DOSAGE. Patients with Cushing's disease from any cause fail to show a drop in steroid excretion after the total dose of 4 mg. It is often possible to distinguish bilateral hyperplasia from adrenal tumor as the cause of adrenal hyperfunction by repeating the dexamethasone test with higher dosage. In patients with bilateral hyperplasia, administration of 2 mg of dexamethasone every six hours for eight doses usually produces a fall in 17-OH corticosteroid excretion to 50 per cent or less of the basal value, while patients with adenomas are unaffected by the total dose of 16 mg. Patients with Cushing's disease associated with pituitary gland tumors may have suppressed steroid excretion after the larger, but not the smaller, dose of dexamethasone.[35]

RAPID DEXAMETHASONE TEST. To avoid the disadvantages of prolonged medication and the pitfalls of repeated 24-hour urine collections, a rapid screening test of dexamethasone suppression has been introduced. In this simplified version, 1 mg of oral dexamethasone is given at midnight, and in the morning a five-hour urine sample is collected. The total 17-OH corticosteroids and the creatinine content in the five-hour sample are determined, and the ratio of steroid to creatinine excretion is calculated as

$$\frac{\text{mg 17-OHCS}}{\text{mg creatinine}} \times 1000.$$ Good separation can be obtained between normal

individuals and patients with Cushing's disease. The mean normal excretion of 17-OHCS after the single suppressing dose is 0.1 mg, with a mean steroid-creatinine ratio of 0.6. The mean values for patients with Cushing's disease are 3.2 mg of 17-OHCS total, and a steroid-creatinine ratio of 20.4.[61]

Metyrapone Test. This test measures the ability of the pituitary gland to correct declining levels of circulating cortisol. Metyrapone (SU 4885) inhibits certain enzymes required to convert 17-OH precursors into cortisol. When the drug is given, cortisol levels decline, while precursor products accumulate. If the pituitary is normally responsive, increasing ACTH levels cause acceleration of efforts at synthesis and further accumulation of the 17-OH precursors. Urine is collected in 24-hour aliquots during and for one day after oral administration of 500 or 750 mg of metyrapone every four hours for 24 hours. The 24-hour excretion of 17-hydroxycorticosteroids on the last day of collection should be at least double the baseline excretion. The result will be abnormal if the adrenals cannot respond to stimulation, so this test should be done only if the ACTH stimulation test gives normal results. Chlorpromazine interferes with the normal response to metyrapone and should not be given during the testing period.[23]

EVALUATION OF ADRENAL DISORDERS

Tests of adrenal cortical function are used to evaluate the four major groups of adrenal dysfunction: Cushing's syndrome (excess of glucocorticoids), hyperaldosteronism, adrenal virilism, and Addison's disease (adrenal hypofunction).

Cushing's Syndrome

The commonest cause of glucocorticoid excess is adrenal hyperplasia, with adenoma and carcinoma together accounting for approximately one fourth of the total number of cases. Bilateral hyperplasia apparently results from increased ACTH stimulation or possibly from inherent end-organ hypersensitivity. In some cases, pituitary tumors are found; in others the defect is ascribed to hypothalamic dysfunction without anatomic changes. Certain nonendocrine tumors, notably small cell carcinomas of the lung, secrete substances with ACTH-like activity.

Usual Findings. Cushing's syndrome, of whatever origin, is characterized by elevated urine and plasma levels of 17-OH corticosteroids, and usually by increased 17-ketosteroids as well. The normal diurnal cycle, with lower steroid production at night, is usually diminished or absent. Patients have eosinopenia of less than 100 per cubic millimeter, mild neutrophilia, and a variable degree of lymphopenia. Serum uric acid levels are low, and increased uric acid is excreted in the urine. The glucose tolerance curve is abnormal, and overt diabetes is a fairly common related finding. Abnormalities of serum electrolytes are not always present although potassium and chloride levels may be low.

Response to Medications. Hyperplasia is characterized by hyper-reactivity to exogenous ACTH, with double or triple the normal rise in urinary 17-OH corticosteroids and 17-ketosteroids. When hyperplasia is due to hypothalamic dysfunction or pituitary tumor, dexamethasone suppression is sluggish, and doses of 2 mg every six hours may be needed to produce even moderate suppression. Apparently the 0.5 mg dose is too small to contrast with the already high levels of circulating hormone. ACTH-producing carcinomas of nonpituitary origin secrete ACTH independent of circulating hormone level, and the resultant steroid overproduction is not altered by dexamethasone or metyrapone. Patients with hypothalamic dysfunction, on the other hand, respond dramatically to metyrapone; when cortisol production is blocked, ACTH is produced in still greater amounts, and the hyperplastic gland enthusiastically responds with accelerated hydroxysteroid production.

Differential Findings. Adenomas may be difficult to evaluate. Some remain amenable to ACTH, while others, although not carcinomas, nevertheless behave autonomously. Adenomas responsive to changes in ACTH frequently react to exogenous ACTH by increasing 17-OH steroid production much more than 17-ketosteroid production. ACTH-sensitive, or partially autonomous, adenomas respond to dexamethasone suppression as do hyperplastic glands: high doses are needed to induce suppression. The pituitary-adrenal axis is, however, distorted; metyrapone produces relatively little effect in these patients. This could, perhaps, be due to reduced pituitary ACTH-producing capacity following prolonged steroid elevation, but patients with bilateral hyperplasia have a striking response to metyrapone. The highest combined levels of 17-hydroxycorticosteroids and 17-ketosteroids occur in adrenal carcinoma. Neither ACTH stimulation nor dexamethasone suppression alters steroid excretion, and the remaining potentially responsive glandular tissue frequently atrophies. Autonomous benign adenomas cannot be distinguished from carcinomas by laboratory tests.

Hyperaldosteronism

The syndrome of hyperaldosteronism is a relative newcomer to lists of adrenal malfunctions. Primary hyperaldosteronism is usually due to a relatively small and usually benign adenoma producing only the mineralocorticoid, so that 17-hydroxycorticosteroid and 17-ketosteroid levels are normal. In some cases of cortical hyperplasia, there is increased secretion of all the cortical steroids, with the mineral effect of the glucocorticoids enhancing the effect of aldosterone. Secondary hyperaldosteronism results when continuing stimulation promotes adrenal secretion, producing excessive potassium loss and other physiologic concomitants of hormonal effect, without altering the underlying problem. Accelerated hypertension and states of persistent edema may produce this picture.

Physiology. This potent hormone promotes the exchange of sodium for potassium in the distal convoluted tubule, resulting in sodium retention and potassium excretion. Sodium retention increases extracellular fluid (ECF) volume through passive transfer of water. ECF volume changes regulate aldosterone secretion through the renin-angiotensin system, whereby a perceived drop in ECF causes the kidney to secrete renin, which activates angiotensin, which directly stimulates the adrenal to secrete aldosterone. The cycle is normally completed when aldosterone-induced sodium retention repletes the ECF, causing renin production to cease. Very subtle volume changes alter renin activity levels. The stimulus of upright posture produces sufficient shifts in fluid compartments to serve as a renin-inducer; renin measurements before and after posture change, combined with serial determinations of blood and urinary electrolytes, permit excellent assessment of this complicated interrelationship.

In primary hyperaldosteronism, autonomous hormone production permanently depresses renin activity. Most patients have persistent diastolic hypertension, for reasons which are not fully clear, but do not manifest edema. Since early hyperaldosteronism need not manifest pronounced hypokalemia,[8] it has been suggested that much "essential" hypertension may actually be due to excessive aldosterone secretion. Studies of renin activity and potassium metabolism have not been conclusive.[65]

In secondary hyperaldosteronism, the adrenal responds appropriately to renin stimulation, but the renin levels remain inappropriately high. Accelerated hypertension is a common cause, and persistent edema, as from cirrhosis or nephrotic syndrome, also increases aldosterone production. The stimulus to excess renin production in these conditions presumably arises from alterations in renal arterial dynamics, causing a physiologically perceived hypovolemia, regardless of the actual whole-body state of fluid volume.

Laboratory Findings. Low serum potassium characterizes both primary and secondary hyperaldosteronism. Serum sodium tends to be high in the primary form, and in severe cases increased bicarbonate levels and metabolic alkalosis compound the problem. In addition to excessive urinary potassium, there is usually impaired urinary concentrating ability and neutral or alkaline urine. Patients with primary aldosteronism have low levels of renin activity, which fails to increase in the upright position. Persistently high renin activity occurs in secondary aldosteronism, and serum sodium levels tend to be lower than in the primary form.

Electrolyte Responses. Although aldosterone is not easily measured, its physiologic effects on urinary sodium and potassium are readily observed. In a patient with suspected hyperaldosteronism, dietary manipulation can give valuable information. After measurement of sodium and potassium excreted while the patient eats a relatively normal diet of 80 to 100 mEq sodium and 100 mEq potassium daily, the sodium intake can be reduced to 10 mEq per day, while the potassium intake remains unchanged. The normal individual will respond to sodium depletion by increasing aldosterone production, resulting in increased potassium excretion over a five-day period. Sodium excretion falls with sodium restriction. In the patient with autonomous overproduction of aldosterone, there may be little change in hormone secretion. Indeed, potassium excretion tends to fall during sodium restriction, for the tubular urine contains less sodium to be exchanged for potassium.

Salt Loading. After a period of restricted sodium intake, a high sodium regimen (200 mEq per day) can be instituted, again with constant potassium intake. The normal individual promptly suppresses aldosterone secretion, and urinary potassium falls significantly during five days of salt loading. In the patient with primary hyperaldosteronism, the excess sodium is excreted adequately, so that an increased sodium load traverses the distal tubule. This accentuates the tendency toward potassium exchange, and potassium excretion increases over the baseline level. Patients with secondary hyperaldosteronism also react abnormally to a salt load administered after sodium deprivation. These patients reabsorb the excess sodium, resulting in accentuated hypernatremia and edema and in diminished sodium excretion. Because the sodium is reabsorbed in the proximal tubule, the sodium load in the distal tubule is too small to affect potassium excretion to a significant degree; therefore, in secondary hyperaldosteronism, increased potassium excretion does not occur, and urinary sodium excretion is abnormally low.

Serum levels of sodium and potassium should be monitored throughout the test, especially since symptoms of severe hypokalemia may complicate the salt-loading portion of the procedure. Whenever urinary electrolytes are measured, the values should be checked against the serum values, to avoid misinterpretation of abnormal results.

Adrenal Virilism

The clinical signs of adrenal virilism vary with age and sex. There is inappropriate appearance of masculine traits in prepubertal children of either sex; virilization in mature females; and less easily recognized accentuation of the male secondary sex characteristics in mature men. There are two forms of adrenal virilism with two different etiologies.

Defective Synthesis. Congenital adrenal virilism is due to any of several inborn enzymatic defects in cortisol synthesis. As glucocorticoids are normally synthesized, many preliminary products are 19-carbon steroids with androgenic properties. If normal cortisol production is blocked by enzyme deficiencies, ACTH secretion continues at a high level, producing glandular hyperplasia which results in continuing high levels of the precursor substances. A number of different genetically determined defects have been implicated.

Despite the inborn nature of the disease, symptoms may become manifest at any time, although most cases are recognized at birth or in early childhood. The effect of massive doses of androgenically active steroids in utero is masculinization of the female infant who may appear to be a pseudohermaphrodite; or production, in the male infant, of macrogenitosomia. If aldosterone production is impaired along with cortisol synthesis, there may be sodium loss and potassium retention in the so-called salt-losing type of adrenal virilism.

LABORATORY FINDINGS. Laboratory findings in adrenal virilism include, preeminently, increased levels of plasma and urine 17-ketosteroids, decreased 17-hydroxysteroids, and high levels of circulating ACTH. The most common defect, that of inadequate C_{21}-hydroxylation, produces high levels of pregnanetriol, a 21-carbon steroid. This compound is measured in the 17-ketogenic steroids, so in these cases there will be high levels of 17-ketogenic steroids but low 17-hydroxysteroids.

In most patients with congenital adrenal hyperplasia, the gland remains sensitive to ACTH stimulation. Exogenous ACTH further elevates the already high levels of 17-ketosteroids, but 17-hydroxycorticosteroids do not rise. A rare form of the syndrome arises from a defect of 11 β-hydroxylation, and 17-OH precursors of cortisol accumulate, analogous to the situation when normal individuals receive metyrapone. In this form, 17-hydroxycorticosteroids are elevated, and there is increased mineralocorticoid activity and hypertension.

Tumors. Occasional cases of adrenal virilism in adults are due to late manifestations of congenital enzyme defects. More often, however, they are due to hyperplasia or tumor. Benign androgenic hyperplasia in which 17-ketosteroids are elevated but 17-hydroxycorticosteroids are normal is rare. Adrenal virilization is usually due to carcinoma, and usually there are increased 17-hydroxycorticosteroids in addition to the high levels of 17-ketosteroids.

Addison's Disease

The clinical findings of chronic adrenal hypofunction are the reverse of those in Cushing's syndrome. There is weight loss, hypotension, nausea and vomiting, and hyponatremia with elevated serum potassium. Weakness is a constant finding, hypoglycemia may occur, and there is increased sensitivity to insulin. Characteristically, the basal metabolic rate is low in patients with Addison's disease, but other tests of thyroid function are normal if the pituitary gland is intact.

Laboratory Findings. When chronic adrenal hypofunction is suspected, the initial test will be determination of 24-hour 17-ketosteroid and 17-hydroxycorticosteroid excretion. These may be in the low-normal range or frankly low: 3 to 6 mg/24 hours and 0 to 2 mg/24 hours, respectively. The diagnosis of primary adrenal insufficiency is confirmed by failure of the adrenal glands to respond to ACTH stimulation. In some cases of partial insufficiency, an initial small rise in steroid excretion is followed by falling levels, despite continuing ACTH stimulation. This may represent exhaustion of the maximally stimulated gland. High plasma levels of ACTH are found with primary adrenal deficiency.

Secondary adrenal hypofunction occurs when ACTH production is deficient. When ACTH deficiency has been of short duration, the adrenals maintain their responsiveness to exogenous stimulation, and by the fourth or fifth day of ACTH administration, urine 17-hydroxycorticosteroid levels may rise by as much as tenfold. The rise in 17-ketosteroids is also prompt.

Secondary Adrenal Atrophy. Prolonged ACTH deficiency causes severe adrenal atrophy and is ordinarily iatrogenic, due to prolonged steroid medication. Following prolonged steroid medication, the glands may take from several weeks to several months to recover their function and reactivity. Prolonged stimulation causes gradual rise in steroid excretion, 17-hydroxycorticosteroids generally rising first. Once adrenal reactivity has been established, pituitary response can then be tested. Pituitary responsiveness to changes in circulating cortisol returns later than adrenal sensitivity, once exogenous therapy is discontinued.

ADRENAL MEDULLA

The adrenal medulla, although entirely surrounded by cortex, has no functional or histologic resemblance to the cortex. The principal cell type is the chromaffin cell, which bears within its cytoplasmic granules the two hormones of the adrenal medulla. These are the two catecholamines, epinephrine and norepinephrine, both mediating the "fight or flight" reflexes, but producing slightly different physiologic effects. Chemically, their only difference is that epinephrine has a methyl group that norepinephrine lacks.

HORMONE SYNTHESIS AND DEGRADATION

Epinephrine is the major medullary hormone. Of total secreted and stored hormone, approximately 80 per cent is epinephrine. Norepinephrine, however, predominates in the urine, much of it deriving from postganglionic synapses of the autonomic nervous system. The synthesis and degradation of the two compounds are similar, and most clinical laboratories do not distinguish between the two hormones. Catecholamine synthesis starts with the amino acid phenylalanine, which is oxidized to tyrosine. Subsequent oxidative and other reactions produce norepinephrine, to which a methyl group is added in epinephrine synthesis. For both substances, the degradative end products are acids, usually studied in terms of 3-methoxy-4-hydroxy mandelic acid, also called vanilmandelic acid (VMA). The enzyme monoamine oxidase is required for VMA production.

Epinephrine and Norepinephrine _ epinephrine + NorEp._

Catecholamine secretion is stimulated by cholinergic nerve impulses and by such stimuli as physiologic or psychologic stress, hypoxia, hemorrhage, and a number of drugs, among them reserpine, histamine, and nicotine. The two hormones have disparate cardiovascular effects: norepinephrine constricts vascular smooth muscle, slows the heart rate, and raises both systolic and diastolic blood pressure, while epinephrine increases heart rate and cardiac output, and produces only systolic hypertension. Both increase the metabolic rate, raise the blood sugar, and cause elevated plasma fatty-acid levels. Despite their widespread and dramatic physiologic effects, the medullary catecholamines are not essential for life. Bilateral adrenalectomy may, in fact, alter urinary catecholamine excretion very little, since urinary levels derive largely from norepinephrine synthesized at sympathetic nerve endings.

PHEOCHROMOCYTOMA

The adrenal medulla is much simpler to discuss than the adrenal cortex. Only one condition is clinically significant—the tumor, pheochromocytoma. This may be either benign or malignant; distinction, difficult even after histologic examination, is impossible by laboratory testing. Characteristically, pheochromocytoma is seen with intermittent or sustained hypertension, although the generalized symptoms of nervousness, weight loss, palpitations, headache, and paroxysmal sweating may first bring the patient to medical attention. Since many other conditions may cause hypertension, with or without the additional symptoms, the diagnosis of pheochromocytoma rests on demonstrating increased adrenomedullary secretion. Urinary and plasma catecholamines are measured fluorometrically after careful absorption, elution and oxidation. The normal quantities in plasma are small, less than 1 mcg per L.[41] Urinary catecholamine excretion is less than 100 mcg per 24 hours, although the metabolites metanephrine and normetanephrine are excreted in larger quantities and constitute a fairly accurate index of physiologically active amines.[2] The quantities are so small and the procedure so exacting that catecholamines are ordinarily measured only in reference laboratories.

VMA Excretion

Urinary vanilmandelic acid (VMA) is frequently measured to indicate catecholamine production. Both VMA and catecholamine measurement require a 24-hour urine specimen kept at pH of 3.0 or below by collection in 6N hydrochloric acid. Normal values for 24-hour VMA excretion depend somewhat upon the method used, one method giving a range of 1.8 to 10.8 mg; another widely used method has a range of 0.7 to 6.8 mg. The findings in pheochromocytoma do not overlap either normal range, ranging from 15 to 90 mg in 24 hours in one series.[58] Elevated VMA levels may occasionally occur in retinoblastoma, carotid body tumor, malignant carcinoid, and acrodynia. Urinary VMA is frequently high in the presence of neuroblastoma and ganglioneuroma, which secrete dopa, an oxidation product of tyrosine. Mild elevations may occur with childbirth, surgical or traumatic stress, and burns.[58]

Artefacts. Certain chemicals distort the tests for both catecholamines and VMA, and it is customary to forbid dietary intake of potential interfering substances, such as coffee, tea, bananas, and anything containing vanilla. Sunderman[58] states, however, that the VMA elevation induced by ingestion of four bananas does not exceed the upper limits of normal, and newer methods of VMA measurement are not affected by dietary intake. Insulin may increase catecholamine excretion, but therapeutic doses do not affect VMA levels. Insulin shock therapy, however, is followed by rising VMA excretion. Monoamine oxidase inhibitors naturally depress VMA excretion, since that enzyme is necessary to degrade catecholamines. Oral chlorpromazine may cause a moderately low level, and slight decrease may follow morphine or Pentothal administration. Intramuscular reserpine causes a moderate rise in VMA levels.[58]

Pressor Tests

Classical diagnostic procedures for pheochromocytoma employ manipulation of blood pressure. In patients with initial pressure below 170 over 110 mm Hg, the histamine test is used. Intravenous injection of 0.01 to 0.025 mg histamine causes a prompt, dramatic rise in blood pressure if pheochromocytoma is present. Often this is preceded by a cold pressor test since general vasomotor instability may mimic a positive result. The diastolic pressure rise after histamine injection should be at least 50 mm Hg higher than the elevation provoked by immersion of one hand in cold water. To reverse a possibly disastrous hypertensive response, antihypertensive agents should be immediately available. Urine collected after the test should contain increased catecholamines or their metabolites.

Phentolamine (Regitine) promptly antagonizes the hypertension induced by excess catecholamine. This drug is an antidote for untoward responses to the histamine test, and it can also be used diagnostically in patients with baseline blood pressure above 170 over 110 mm Hg. In hypertensive patients with pheochromocytoma, intravenous phentolamine provokes a systolic drop of at least 35 mm and a diastolic drop of 25 mm or more.

THYROID GLAND

INTRODUCTORY PHYSIOLOGY

The thyroid gland synthesizes its hormones from iodine and the essential amino acid tyrosine. Most of the body's iodine enters through the alimentary tract as iodide (I^-), but under certain circumstances, the lungs and skin may be portals of entry. Of the iodine that enters the body, approximately one-third enters the thyroid gland and the remaining two-thirds leaves the body in urine.

Synthesis of Thyroid Hormones

In the thyroid gland, enzymes oxidize iodide to organic iodine, which is incorporated into monoiodotyrosine and diiodotyrosine. These one and two-iodine-containing compounds are building blocks for the active thyroid hormones thyroxine, which has four iodine molecules, and triiodothyronine which has three. These synthesizing steps occur in the intrafollicular colloid, mediated by enzymes from epithelial cells which line the follicle. A single complex molecule, thyroglobulin, is the principal constituent of follicular colloid, and hormonal synthesis occurs within the thyroglobulin molecule.

The thyroid hormones, once formed, are loosely bound to thyroglobulin, and can be cleaved enzymatically and liberated into the blood stream. In the blood the hormones are bound fairly tightly to thyroid-binding globulin and other serum proteins.

The pituitary hormone thyrotropin (thyroid-stimulating hormone, TSH) stimulates all stages of hormonal synthesis including uptake of circulating iodide, synthesis of new hormone, and release of formed hormone. The level of circulating hormone, by a feed-back mechanism, regulates the level of thyrotropic activity, although the metabolic activity of adrenal and gonadal hormones exerts some influence on TSH production.

Effects of Thyroid Hormones

Control of oxygen consumption is the most conspicuous biologic effect of the thyroid hormones, a physiologic variable measured in simplest fashion by the basal metabolic rate. Thyroid hormones also influence carbohydrate and protein metabolism, the mobilization of electrolytes, and the conversion of carotene to vitamin A. Although the mechanism is not known, thyroid hormones are essential for development of the central nervous system and the thyroid-deficient infant suffers irreversible mental damage. The thyroid-deficient adult may have slowed deep tendon reflexes and diffuse psychomotor retardation, but these changes are reversible with hormone replacement therapy.

Factors That Decrease Thyroid Activity

Genetically determined enzyme deficiencies may interfere with iodine metabolism at any step, causing congenital goiter. Much more frequently, depressed thyroid function results from external causes. Exogenous thyroid hormone suppresses hormone production by depressing TSH levels. Drugs of the thiocyanate and perchlorate groups interfere with iodide concentration, while thiourea and thiouracil prevent incorporation of thyroidal iodine into organic compounds. The antithyroid effects of iodine are not fully understood, but probably include inhibition both of iodine binding and of hormonal release, while radioactive iodine selectively irradiates hormonally active tissue, owing to its concentration in the actively functioning gland.

TESTS OF THYROID FUNCTION

The Basal Metabolic Rate

The oldest and least specific test of thyroid function is the basal metabolic rate (BMR). This measurement of oxygen consumption is expressed as kilocalories expended per square meter of body surface per hour, with the fasted patient in a condition of mental and physical repose. In clinical use, the results are expressed as percent of the expected normal, with suitable corrections made for the individual patient's height, weight, age, and sex. As more specific tests have become available, the BMR, a general test subject to many artefactual alterations, has lost its primary usefulness. Although insufficient, by itself, for the diagnosis of thyroid disease, it remains useful for evaluating patients under treatment with drugs which might invalidate the more specific tests.

To be useful at all, the BMR must be accuratey performed by skilled operators who can obtain good patient cooperation. The normal range for the BMR is generally considered to fall between − 10 per cent and + 10 per cent of the expected normal, while values from − 15 per cent to + 15 per cent are considered by many to be essentially normal.

The Elevated BMR. Hyperthyroidism always causes a high BMR, sometimes as high as 80 to 100 per cent above the expected normal. Such marked hyperthyroidism usually presents no diagnostic difficulties, and the BMR is unnecessary to diagnose severe cases. In less marked hyperthyroid states, the differential diagnosis is more difficult, and unfortunately the BMR cannot differentiate between mild hyperthyroidism and emotional disturbance or low grade infection as the cause of hypermetabolism.

The greatest problem in performing a valid BMR test is maintaining the patient in a genuinely basal condition. Apprehension, discomfort, smoking, eating, or recent exertion elevate the metabolic rate. For this reason, some workers use mild sedation to obtain relaxation or actual sleep while performing the test. Technical errors, notably failure to detect leaks in the spirometer, may falsely elevate the net reading. A classic but infrequent cause of spurious elevation is oxygen leak intrinsic to the patient— namely, a perforated eardrum.

NONTHYROID CONDITIONS THAT ELEVATE THE BMR. Genuine elevation of the metabolic rate occurs in many conditions unrelated to the thyroid. Of these, the most frequent is emotional distress. Also significant is temperature elevation of any cause, and each Fahrenheit degree of fever produces a 7 to 9 per cent elevation of metabolic rate. Significant elevations of the BMR occur in leukemia, particularly chronic myelocytic and the acute leukemias. Dyspnea and hyperpnea of any origin increase oxygen consumption; thus, severe pulmonary or cardiovascular disease or acidosis will produce a high BMR reading. Patients with either polycythemia or severe anemia may have a high BMR, as do many patients with advanced malignant disease. Acromegaly, diabetes insipidus, and Cushing's disease are endocrine disorders in which the metabolic rate is increased, and rapid anabolism due to convalescence from wasting disease or simply normal growth will increase oxygen consumption. Pheochromocytoma is often associated with a high BMR. Paget's disease of bone, congestive heart failure, amyotrophic lateral sclerosis, and some cases of hypertension are associated with high basal metabolic rates, and any condition associated with tremor or simple shivering accelerates metabolism.

The Decreased BMR. Artefactual depression of the BMR rarely occurs, since emotional or physical effects can only alter the patient's condition above the basal state. The most common technical artefact causing low BMR readings is exhaustion of the soda lime, which must be changed regularly to absorb expired CO_2.

Genuine hypometabolism is often due to hypothyroidism, but other pathophysiologic states must be considered. Undernutrition and inanition from any cause will lower the metabolic rate, especially hypopituitarism, Addison's disease, and anorexia nervosa. A low BMR often occurs in patients with nephrotic syndrome, for reasons that are not entirely clear. Although this may be due to urinary loss of protein-bound thyroid hormones, the administration of thyroid hormones does not alter the metabolic rate or clinical condition. Patients in shock due to cardiovascular collapse have a low basal metabolic rate but are not ordinarily subjected to BMR determination.

Serum Lipids

Thyroid hormones affect the synthesis, degradation, and intermediate metabolism of adipose tissue and circulating lipids, and abnormalities of endocrine function are reflected in altered lipid levels. In hyperthyroidism, degradation and excretion increase more than synthesis, resulting in low circulating levels of cholesterol, phospholipids, and triglycerides; hypothyroidism slows catabolism more than it affects synthesis, and hypercholesterolemia and hypertriglyceridemia reliably accompany myxedema. This produces a predominantly pre-beta lipoprotein pattern when lipids are partitioned,[32] and increased cholesterol levels may be the earliest indicator of impending hypothyroidism.[20]

Thyroid Hormonal Iodine

The thyroid gland is the only organ that actively metabolizes iodine, and virtually all circulating endogenous iodine is in thyroid-derived compounds. Thyroxine (T_4), containing four iodine moieties, is the principal circulating hormone. Like many metabolically active compounds, an inactive form travels through the blood bound to specific carrier proteins, but hormonal activity results from the tiny amount free at the target site. Measurements of circulating iodine include both bound and unbound hormone, but cannot distinguish between the large amount attached to protein and the quantitatively tiny free fraction. Inorganic iodides contribute nothing to hormonal function but elevate the measurable iodine, thereby invalidating the physiologic significance of the test.

Protein-Bound Iodine Tests for protein-bound iodine (PBI), or the functionally similar though more accurate butanol-extractable iodine (BEI), exclude these inorganic contaminants and measure organic iodine. Unfortunately, iodine-containing organic compounds like x-ray contrast media, vaginal suppositories, amebicides, and some skin preparations elevate the protein-bound iodine level to a variable and unpredictable degree. If exposure to these compounds can reliably be excluded, the normal protein-bound iodine level of 3.5 to 8.0 mcg per 100 ml accurately reflects bound thyroxine.

T₄-by-Column. Far fewer organic contaminants affect the results of column chromatographic iodine techniques. When contamination is present, the column technique signals this fact, unlike the PBI or BEI, which give only a single figure for all the iodine measured. The T_4-by-column test appears, at present, to be the most accurate way to measure circulating thyroxine.

ELUTION In the T_4-by-column procedures, thyroxine is cleared from serum proteins by alkalinizing the serum, which is then passed through an ion exchange resin column. The resin particles trap thyroxine and all sorts of other constituents—proteins, inorganic iodine, and exogenous organic iodine compounds. These unwanted compounds are removed with wash solutions of suitable chemical composition and pH. Thyroxine requires a notably high acid concentration for elution from the resin, so the critical elutions are performed last, with 50 per cent acetic acid. This effluent is analyzed for iodine. Two or more elutions are performed to secure complete iodine removal and also to signal contamination by nonthyroxine iodine. The proportion of thyroxine iodine eluted into the first and second effluents remains fairly constant in uncontaminated serums, despite differences in absolute concentration. The expected ratio of iodine in the first and second eluates may be 10 to 1. If the second eluate from a serum sample contains 20 per cent of the total iodine, a substance other than thyroxine is assumed to be contributing to total iodine.

CONTAMINANTS. Exogenous contaminants are far fewer for the column technique than for BEI or PBI. Most of the amebicides, vaginal preparations, and contrast media used for urography, bronchography and alimentary tract procedures cause no trouble. A few compounds used in cholecystography add contamination for as long as a year. The T_4 results are also affected by exogenous thyroid preparations. Patients taking thyroxine or thyroid extract may have high levels of circulating thyroxine iodine with hypermetabolism. Patients on triiodothyronine (T_3) have very low levels of T_4 while clinically euthyroid, because the metabolically active triiodine compound does not register on the T_4 test. The test cannot, therefore, be used to monitor appropriate dose levels for exogenous T_3 or T_4. The results of iodine or other antithyroid therapy can, however, be monitored by T_4 testing, since the test accurately reflects the amount of circulating hormone that the patient produces.

Normal values for T_4-by-column vary slightly with the specific manufacturer's reagents. Each laboratory must determine its own normal range, and patient results should be compared against this value. The T_4 iodine is consistently slightly lower than the PBI and BEI.

ABNORMALITIES NOT DUE TO THYROID CHANGES. The diagnostic significance of elevated or decreased T_4-by-column results is the same as that for uncontaminated PBI or BEI. High values for thyroxine iodine, if not due to hyperthyroidism, nearly always result from increased levels of thyroid-binding globulin (TBG). Normal pregnancy and treatment with estrogens or other antiovulatory drugs cause increased production of carrier protein, and these patients tend to be euthyroid. Early hepatitis sometimes leads to high T_4 values.

Low T_4 values, if not due to hypothyroidism, may mean decreased levels of thyroid-binding globulin or else displacement of thyroxine by other compounds which attach to TBG. Diphenylhydantoin (Dilantin) and high doses of salicylates displace T_4 from binding sites, leading to low T_4 results but not to hypothyroidism.[66] Decreased plasma levels of TBG occur in nephrosis, chronic liver disease, some cases of pancreatic malabsorption, and treatment with androgens or anabolic steroids. Mercurial diuretics, which interfere with the PBI test procedure although not with thyroid function, do not affect T_4 results.

Free Thyroxine

From the foregoing, it is apparent that the amount of metabolically active free thyroxine is highly significant. This constitutes about 0.05 per cent of the total circulating thyroxine.[47] Since the normal for total thyroxine iodine is in the range of 5 mcg per 100 ml, the absolute amount of free thyroxine is tiny indeed. An analytic procedure using dialysis and radioimmunoassay has been developed,[57] but it is not in wide clinical use. The normal values are in nanogram units. Without actually measuring free thyroxine, one can estimate the functional level by a calculation called the free thyroxine index.[7] Since T_4-by-column indicates the total circulating thyroxine, and the resin T_3 test (see below) measures the level of transport protein available, the product of these two values gives some indication of how much thyroxine is unbound.

Free Thyroxine Index. In an euthyroid individual, increased TBG levels are followed by increased thyroxine production to fill the available binding sites. Otherwise there would be disproportionate binding, and functional hypothyroidism would result because insufficient thyroxine was available to the tissues. Conversely, decreased thyroxine production accompanies diminished TBG, to avoid oversupply of unbound hormone at the site of end organ stimulation. Increased TBG levels give a low value on T_3 tests. Thus if a high level of circulating thyroxine (T_4-by-column) is due to some condition producing increased TBG, multiplying the high T_4 value by the low T_3 gives a normal ratio. If, however, the amount of TBG is normal and excessive thyroxine really is present, the T_3 results will be high or high-normal, the T_4 value will also be high, and the numerical product will be above the normal range. The same situation obtains in evaluating low results. If thyroxine production is deficient (low T_4) while TBG levels are normal, the T_3 values are low, and the numerical product will indicate hypothyroidism. If TBG is reduced, the T_3 value will be high. In this case the absolute amount of circulating T_4 will be low, but the high T_3 value multiplied by low T_4 gives a normal numerical product, indicating clinical euthyroidism.

Calculating the index obviously depends on the normal range for both determinations; the product cannot be expressed in objective units. If a laboratory reports 25 to 35 per cent as the normal resin T_3 uptake, and 2.9 to 6.4 mcg/100 ml as normal T_4 iodine, then the range of normal for the product would be 72.5 to 224, or 0.72 to 2.24 if the product is divided by 100. Values falling outside this range indicate abnormality of the active hormone level. Frequently the nature of nonthyroid influences on these laboratory results is clinically obvious, but using the ratio may help to place seeming abnormal values into proper perspective. Its greater value is to signal that abnormality genuinely exists despite normal values for one test.

Radioactive Iodine Within the Body

The body metabolizes all the isotopes of iodine in identical fashion, so that introduction of radioactive isotopes provides a convenient marker for studying iodine physiology. The isotope most frequently used is ^{131}I, which has a half-life of eight days, and is considered adequately safe for all patients except pregnant women.

Since radioactive iodine is absorbed and metabolized exactly as is stable iodine, the rate of its metabolism accurately reflects the state of iodine kinetics. Direct proportionality can be assumed, however, only if the total iodine pool is of normal size for the individual being tested. If the iodine pool is expanded, as following ingestion of iodinated medications or contrast media, then the administered dose of radioactive iodine occupies an abnormally small proportion of the total body iodine and only a small percentage will appear to be metabolized. Similarly, the radioactive iodine will appear to be metabolized very rapidly if the total body iodine pool is small, since the administered dose occupies an excessively large proportion of the total supply.

Epithyroid Uptake. In this test, a known dose of radioactive iodine is given either by mouth or intravenously. The rate at which radioactivity increases over the thyroid gland reflects the speed with which the gland traps iodine. The remainder of the administered dose is excreted in the urine.

There are several variants of this procedure, depending upon the timing of the subsequent counts. Radioactivity over the thyroid can be measured as soon as 10 minutes after intravenous administration of a tracer dose. Following oral administration, significant uptake occurs within one hour. This follows a rather characteristic curve over the subsequent 24 hours.

Perhaps the most commonly used test of thyroidal radioactive iodine uptake employs an epithyroid count one hour and then 24 hours after oral ingestion of a tracer dose. In hyperthyroid patients, the whole process of uptake, hormonal synthesis, and subsequent release of formed hormone may be so rapid that in 24 hours much of the labelled iodine has already left the gland. If the one-hour count is high, it may be desirable to do a six-hour count to catch peak activity before thyroidal radioactivity declines. In normal individuals, the epithyroid count made 24 hours after an oral dose of ^{131}I ranges between 15 and 45 per cent of the administered radioactivity.

ARTEFACTS THAT LOWER ^{131}I UPTAKE. The most common factitious cause of depressed radioactive iodine uptake is intake of exogenous iodine, which enlarges the body's total iodine pool. Depression of radioactive iodine uptake may occur before the PBI is affected, so a careful history must accompany the procedure. In addition to the obvious sources of exogenous iodine, such as cough preparations and x-ray media, there may be absorption of iodine through the skin from suntan lotions or nail polish. Enriched breakfast cereals, amebicides, vaginal and anal suppositories, and some vitamin-mineral preparations may be unsuspected offenders in enlarging the iodine pool.

If the administered iodine dose is not absorbed, as in severe diarrhea or intestinal malabsorption syndromes, the thyroidal uptake may appear low even though the gland is functioning normally. Rapid diuresis during the test period may deplete the supply of available iodine, causing an apparently low percentage of iodine uptake. Drugs that depress thyroid function will, of course, depress the radioactive iodine uptake, and ACTH and corticosteroids may have this effect, as may phenylbutazone, arsenicals, and cobalt and other heavy metals. Administration of thiouracils may cause a high six-hour uptake, but the overall uptake at 24 hours is lower than normal.

ARTEFACTS THAT ELEVATE ^{131}I UPTAKE. The converse of the above conditions may cause a seemingly high uptake in euthyroid individuals. Hypoiodinism, with resultant failure to dilute the tracer dose, causes a large percentage of the administered dose to appear in the thyroid. Renal failure, with decreased excretion of the administered dose over the 24 hours of the test, may permit excessive amounts of the tracer radioactivity to enter the gland. Because different artefacts have different effects, more than one test of thyroid function is usually advisable.

Thyroid Stimulation Test. The thyroid gland may have impaired ^{131}I uptake because of intrinsic disease or because it is insufficiently stimulated by the pituitary. Thyroidal responsiveness can be measured following administration of thyroid-stimulating hormone (TSH) which is available commercially. In normal individuals, ^{131}I uptake increases within 8 to 10 hours after TSH is given. Subsequently, the serum level of protein-bound iodine rises, and the thyroid gland itself increases in weight.[18] This latter change is not easily measured, but the increase in iodine uptake and serum hormone level constitutes a valuable diagnostic test. Different workers suggest different dose schedules for this test. Although 5 to 10 USP units of thyrotropin usually provoke increased activity, some workers prefer to stimulate the gland maximally, giving injections of TSH for three to five days before measuring the stimulated uptake.[18] If the initially low uptake is due to inadequate pituitary stimulation of an intrinsically normal thyroid, TSH administration should increase ^{131}I uptake by at least 10 per cent, and the PBI should rise 1.5 micrograms per 100 ml or more. The rise in ^{131}I uptake is measured in absolute units; that is, a rise from 15 per cent uptake in 24 hours to 25 per cent uptake in 24 hours constitutes a 10 per cent increase. The rise is not measured as a 10 per cent increment of the baseline value. Failure of TSH to increase ^{131}I uptake indicates primary end-organ failure.

CLINICAL APPLICATIONS. TSH stimulation of thyroid function is most dramatic in patients with low-normal ^{131}I uptake—in the range of 15 per cent. Individuals with considerably higher 24-hour uptakes have a relatively small increment following stimulation, but these patients would not ordinarily need the test. The thyroid stimulation test can be used even if a patient is receiving thyroid replacement therapy, but inorganic iodine not only invalidates ^{131}I uptake results, but may antagonize TSH stimulation.

Besides distinguishing primary from secondary hypothyroidism, the TSH test can suggest the level of glandular activity. Patients with a decreased volume of functioning thyroid following subtotal thyroidectomy, irradiation therapy, or thyroiditis may have normal or low-normal ^{131}I uptake, but fail to respond to thyrotropin stimulation. Such patients, with low "thyroid reserve," need prolonged observation in order that incipient myxedema may be forestalled.

Thyroid Suppression Test. The interrelationship of thyroid and pituitary is used in investigating high thyroidal iodine uptake. In normal individuals, administration of thyroid hormone causes lessened ^{131}I uptake, since the increased level of circulating hormone depresses TSH production. If the thyroid-pituitary axis functions normally, ^{131}I uptake after thyroid medication should be less than 20 per cent in 24 hours. Patients with

Graves' disease have little or no suppression due, perhaps in part, to the effect of the long-acting thyroid stimulator. Unfortunately, some patients with nontoxic goiters have inadequate thyroid suppression, and some euthyroid patients have suppression failure for as long as five years after successful therapy for Graves' disease.[53]

Synthesis of ^{131}I-Labelled Hormones. Radioactive iodine is used in several tests of hormonal synthesis, the two most common being the 24-hour conversion ratio and the PB[131]I. These tests can be useful in diagnosing thyroid hyperfunction, but are of no value in hypothyroidism or in assessing treatment of hyperthyroidism or hypothyroidism.

CONVERSION RATIO. The conversion ratio compares total plasma radioactivity with protein-bound radioactivity at a specific time following administration of the isotope. This interval is usually 24 hours; timing is important in this test, for eventually all of the ^{131}I is converted into hormone. Of the total circulating ^{131}I, only 20 to 50 per cent is normally incorporated into protein-bound hormone within 24 hours. Patients with thyroid hyperfunction ordinarily convert more than 50 per cent of the plasma ^{131}I into bound hormone in that time. In this test, both iodine uptake and hormonal synthesis are measured. The usual problems of interpreting isotope uptake apply to this test, and cardiovascular and renal function are especially important. If urinary loss is less than usual, a high percentage of nonhormonal circulating isotope will be present at 24 hours, causing the conversion ratio to appear low.

PROTEIN-BOUND [131]I. The protein-bound [131]I (PB[131]I) level is expressed as per cent of administered dose per liter of plasma. Timing is less important for this test, since the level of isotope in the circulating hormone continues to rise for several days. The test sample is ordinarily drawn 48 or 72 hours after the isotope is administered, and values above 0.4 per cent indicate hyperthyroidism. Values between 0.2 and 0.4 per cent are considered suspicious. This test is useful in distinguishing the high PBI due to nontoxic goiter from that due to hyperthyroidism. If thyroid volume is diminished, as with partial ablation or thyroiditis, the PB[131]I will be high, since the labelled iodine leaves the gland very rapidly even though the total output of hormone may not be abnormally large.

Resin T_3 Uptake

In the circulating blood, thyroid hormone exists principally as thyroxine, which is bound to thyroid-binding globulin (TBG). The amount of circulating TBG is independent of the amount of thyroid hormone it is carrying, so the degree to which thyroid-binding globulin is saturated indirectly indicates the level of circulating hormone.

In the T_3 uptake test (Fig. 22), a known amount of ^{131}I-labelled triiodo-

Principle of T₃ Uptake Test

EUTHYROID

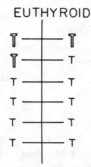

Thyroid-binding globulin(TBG), with 12 available binding sites, 9 of which are occupied by endogenous thyroxine (T)

When 10 units of radioactive thyroxine (T) are added, 3 attach to the TBG and 7 are left over.

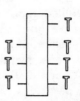

Indicator substance picks up the left-over radioactive hormone, which can easily be measured.

HYPOTHYROID

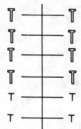

Thyroid-binding globulin with 12 available binding sites, only 4 of which are carrying endogenous hormone.

When 10 units of radioactive thyroxine are added, 8 attach to the TBG and only 2 are left over.

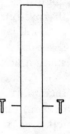

Indicator substance picks up the 2 left-over radioactive units. The radioactivity of the indicator in hypothyroidism is much less than if normal amounts of thyroid hormone were present.

HYPERTHYROID

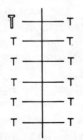

hyroid-binding globulin with 12 available binding sites, 11 of which are occupied by ndogenous hormone.

When 10 units of radioactive thyroxine are added, only one can attach to the TBG, and 9 are left over.

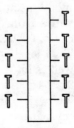

Indicator substance picks up the 9 left-over radioactive units. The radioactivity of the indicator in hyperthyroidism is much greater than if normal amounts of thyroid hormone were present.

Figure 22. Schematic depiction of the principle of the T₃ uptake test.

thyronine (T_3) is added to a sample of blood. Unoccupied sites on the thyroid-binding globulin will combine with the added labelled hormone. The left-over labelled hormone remains free and unbound in the plasma. Variations of the test use different methods to measure the unbound labelled T_3. As the test was originally performed, labelled T_3 was added to fluid whole blood. Whatever hormone was left, after the TBG sites were filled, then attached itself to the red cells. The amount of left-over radioactive hormone could be measured by separating plasma from cells and determining red cell radioactivity. A later modification employs plasma alone, avoiding the problem of variable hematocrits. In this technique, labelled T_3 is added to plasma in the presence of finely divided resin particles or a sponge. The resin or sponge adsorbs the left-over hormone, and the radioactivity of the separated material reflects the amount of hormone that could not attach to binding sites.

Interpretation. Both tests are interpreted in the same way. If large quantities of endogenous hormone are present, nearly all the available thyroid-binding sites are occupied and few sites will be free to bind the test dose of labelled hormone. Therefore, a large amount will attach to the secondary binding substance, be this resin or red cells. If there is only a small amount of circulating hormone, many binding sites will be available to combine with the labelled hormone, so relatively little will remain for the secondary binding substance. Thus, in hyperthyroid conditions, the red cell or resin uptake is high; that is, a large amount of administered hormone is left over from the nearly saturated TBG. In hypothyroidism, the red cell or resin uptake is low because the nearly empty TBG attaches most of the labelled dose, and little radioactivity attaches to the secondary site.

This test is useful for patients on iodine-containing medications, since iodine-containing material does not affect the results. The patient is spared exposure to radioisotopes since the radioactive material is added to the blood sample. Unfortunately, the quantity of thyroid-binding globulin varies from individual to individual, and this may affect the results. For example, normal T_3 uptake could occur in a hyperthyroid patient if his TBG level were sufficiently high to accommodate the added tracer dose as well as his own hormone.

Artefacts Affecting T_3 Uptake. The T_3 uptake does not always correlate well with abnormal results of other tests, possibly because the level of thyroid-binding globulin is somewhat variable. Certain conditions are known to alter the level of TBG and introduce artefacts into the test's usefulness. Thyroid-binding globulin is elevated in pregnancy, in patients taking estrogens and contraceptive hormone combinations, and in patients with estrogen-secreting tumors. In these conditions, resin T_3 uptake is correspondingly lowered to seemingly hypothyroid levels, despite normal thyroid function. Conversely, androgen administration may decrease the amount of thyroid-binding protein. Conditions that depress the plasma proteins are associated with high T_3 uptakes because the amount of TBG is reduced. Thus, high values are found in nephrotic syndrome and severe liver disease. Dilantin and salicylate, which compete with thyroxine for TBG sites, may cause a seemingly high T_3 uptake.[66]

Thyroid Antibodies

Antibodies to three types of thyroid antigens have been noted in patients with various thyroid diseases. Of these, two are essentially research tools, while tests for the third are clinically useful and readily available. Most patients with Hashimoto's thyroiditis (Hashimoto's struma, struma lymphomatosa, chronic lymphocytic thyroiditis) and some with primary myxedema have antibodies to human thyroglobulin, and it is highly probable that these diseases have an autoimmune basis. Thyroglobulin antibodies can be demonstrated quite simply, since they cause agglutination. Tanned red cells or latex particles can be coated with thyroglobulin. When these coated particles are mixed with a serum that contains the antibody, readily visible agglutination occurs. The tanned cell technique is the more sensitive, while the latex particle test is suitable as a screening technique.

The other two antibodies react with the epithelium of thyroid follicles and with an unidentified component of colloid. These may acquire greater clinical significance as they are more fully studied.

Clinical Application. Antibody tests are useful in the differential diagnosis of thyroid enlargement, with antibody usually present in Hashimoto's thyroiditis and absent in cases of nodular colloid goiter or carcinoma. The distinctions are by no means clear-cut, since up to 8 per cent of normal individuals may possess thyroglobulin antibodies,[56] and up to 20 per cent of patients with "simple" hypothyroidism may also have detectible antibody.[30] It may be that in some thyrotoxic patients, high antibody titers may be associated with widespread, progressive thyroiditis which subsequently terminates in hypothyroidism.

DIAGNOSIS OF THYROIDAL ABNORMALITIES

Thyroid disease can profitably be divided into five clinical categories: simple goiter, hypothyroidism, hyperthyroidism, thyroiditis, and neoplasms. These categories are not mutually exclusive, since transitions occur from any one to any of several others. Usual diagnostic findings in a variety of thyroid disorders are listed in Table 19.

Table 19.   Results of Thyroid Function Tests in Various Clinical Situations

Diagnostic and Clinical Status	24-hr^131 I uptake, %	Serum PBI,* μg/100 ml	Serum T4† μg/100 ml	BMR, % normal standard	Resin T3,‡ uptake, % normal control
Euthyroidism:					
Normal values	15-50	4-8	4-11	-15-+15	85-115
Pregnancy	Normal/high	High	High	+20-+25	Low
Iodide deficiency	High	Normal/low	Normal/low	Normal/low	Normal
Iodide therapy, 3.0 mg/day	Low	High	Normal	Normal	Normal
Thyroid, USP, >120 mg/day	Low	Normal/high	Normal/high	Normal/high	Normal/high
L-Thyroxine, >0.4 mg/day	Low	Normal/high	Normal/high	Normal/high	Normal/high
L-Triiodothyronine, >0.1 mg/day	Low	Low	Low	Normal/high	Normal/high
Congestive heart failure	Variable	Normal/low	Normal/low	Variable	Normal/high
Hyperthyroidism:					
Untreated	50-100	7-20	11-20	High	115-160
Pregnancy	High	High	High	High	Normal/high
Iodide therapy, >2.0 mg/day	Low	>20	5-15	High/normal	High/normal
Antithyroid drug therapy (euthyroid)	Variable	Normal	Normal	Normal	Normal
Thyroiditis (acute):	Low	Normal/high	Normal/high	Normal/high	Normal/high
Myxedema (primary):					
Untreated	0-15	0-4	0-4	-20--50	Low‡
Thyroid USP, 120 mg/day (euthyroid)	Low	Normal¶	Normal¶	Normal	Normal
L-Thyroxine, 0.4 mg/day-euthyroid	Low	Normal/high	Normal/high	Normal	Normal/high
L-Triiodothyronine, 0.1 mg/day (euthyroid)	Low	Low	Low	Normal	Normal

* The presence in serum of trace quantities of mercurial salts will render low values for the PBI and BEI factitiously low by the usual methods. Normal values for the serum butanol-extractable iodine (BEI) and the serum T4 by column are 3.2 to 6.5 μg%.

† Serum T4 designates values obtained by the binding displacement method of Murphy and Pattee (J. Clin. Endoc. 26: 247, 1966).

‡ The Resin-T3 values listed here are for the resin sponge method (Triosorb, Abbott) expressed as a per cent of a standard control serum. This test is also expressed as an absolute per cent uptake with normal values ranging from 25 to 35 per cent (See JAMA 202: 135, 1967). The Resin-T3 test is not generally diagnostic of hypothyroidism because of excessive overlap of values in the low normal range with those in hypothyroidism.

¶ The PBI and serum T4 values may be lower than normal in patients receiving some lots of desiccated thyroid, USP, or thyroglobulin (Proloid). (Modified from Selenkow, H.A., and Ingbar, S.H., *In* Wintrobe, M.M. et al. [eds.]: Harrison's Principles of Internal Medicine, ed. 6. McGraw-Hill Book Co., 1970. Used by permission of McGraw-Hill Book Co.)

Simple Goiter

Simple, or nontoxic, goiter implies an enlarged gland whose function may be normal or depressed. In most cases, enlargement is due to persistent or intermittent TSH stimulation, resulting from persistent or intermittent deficiency of circulating thyroxine. The end result of hypothyroidism or euthyroidism depends on how successfully the gland responds to stimulation.

A euthyroid patient with a so-called simple goiter should have a normal BMR, normal PBI, and normal T_3 uptake. The thyroidal ^{131}I uptake may be normal or, if the gland is especially large, increased. TSH stimulation frequently causes relatively little response since the gland is already functioning at or near capacity. Simple goiter is not associated with circulating thyroid antibodies. Some patients with simple goiter gradually become hypothyroid; a few become hyperthyroid after a long course of multinodular goiter.

Hypothyroidism

Hypothyroidism can occur at any stage of life, from fetus to late adulthood, and may be due to primary thyroidal dysfunction, inadequate pituitary function, or such exogenous factors as drugs or thyroidectomy. In hypothyroidism, the BMR, PBI, or T_4 and epithyroid ^{131}I uptake are depressed, as is red cell or resin T_3 uptake. If the hypothyroidism is due to defective hormonal synthesis, as in severe iodine deficiency or certain congenital disorders, high TSH levels may cause a normal or high epithyroid iodine uptake. Occasionally, thyroid antibody titers are elevated in this condition, suggesting the possibility of autoimmune origin.

Certain tests have particular areas of usefulness. The thyroid stimulation test may differentiate primary thyroidal dysfunction from pituitary insufficiency as the cause of hypothyroidism. Patients with hypothyroidism occasionally resemble patients with nephrosis who also have edema, blunted sensorium, high cholesterol, and a low PBI. The epithyroid ^{131}I uptake may help to make this distinction, being normal in nephrosis. Serum creatine kinase and LDH levels may be increased in hypothyroidism, apparently reflecting myocardial alterations, since it is the cardiac LDH isoenzyme that increases.[53]

Hyperthyroidism

Hyperthyroidism may manifest itself in symptoms referable to many organs or systems, notably the cardiovascular system and gastrointestinal tract. The full-blown picture of Graves' disease is not difficult to diagnose, but in many patients, one or several symptoms may throw the classical syndrome out of balance. When hyperthyroidism is a possible diagnosis, elevation of the PBI or T_4, high thyroidal iodine uptake, and high red cell or resin T_3 uptake are reliable indicators. The BMR is elevated, but this may not be helpful, since many conditions in the differential diagnosis will also cause a high BMR. Thyrotropin stimulation alters very little the thyroidal iodine uptake, because hyperthyroidism, like toxic adenoma, may be associated with autonomous activity of the target gland. This autonomy remains unaltered by administration of exogenous thyroid hormones which normally depress TSH levels and reduce the ^{131}I uptake. Thyroid antibodies may occur, but their diagnostic significance is limited. Additional findings in hyperthyroid patients may include low serum cholesterol, and creatinuria.

Thyroiditis

Thyroiditis of the lymphocytic type (Hashimoto's struma) causes the highest thyroglobulin antibody titers. A characteristic finding early in the disease is a low or normal PBI associated with an elevated ^{131}I uptake. This occurs when iodinated protein escapes from the gland into the blood where it affects the PBI test. Because it is not hormonally active, however, the pituitary responds with increased TSH production, which results in a high RAI uptake. Ultimately, however, the gland becomes unable to respond, and ^{131}I uptake diminishes to hypothyroid levels if the disease progresses. In some patients, the ^{131}I uptake is higher than normal at six hours, but declines to normal or even subnormal levels by the 24-hour reading. The abnormal iodinated protein is not butanol extractable so that in the early stage of Hashimoto's thyroiditis, the BEI or column-T_4 determination will be abnormally lower than the PBI.

Tumors

Neoplasms of the thyroid gland include adenomas and carcinoma of varying histological types. Characteristically, adenomas secrete hormones and may cause hyperthyroidism. Hyperfunctioning, or toxic, adenomas are most readily diagnosed by isotopic scanning procedures, in which the adenomas appear as localized areas of increased radioactivity, sometimes surrounded by areas of depressed function. Thyroid carcinomas, on the other hand, usually cause no endocrine disorder although many well-differentiated tumors concentrate iodine and secrete hormone. History and physical examination may suggest the diagnosis, especially if there is a history of radiation to the neck in childhood. Nodular goiter and Hashimoto's thyroiditis are part of the differential diagnosis, and antibody determinations may be helpful in these cases. In cancer of the thyroid, the BMR, T$_4$, and tests employing radioactive iodine are usually normal. A localized area of decreased isotope concentration in a scan may suggest an area of malignant change, but it is hardly diagnostic. The diagnosis of thyroid carcinoma cannot be made or excluded by laboratory examination alone.

PARATHYROID GLANDS

The parathyroid glands, which may vary in number from two to ten, produce only one hormone. Parathyroid hormone, or parathormone, regulates calcium and phosphorus metabolism, but its specific activity has been the topic of endless debate and experimentation. Through its effect on plasma calcium concentration, parathormone influences neuromuscular function in all organs and affects a wide spectrum of body functions.

PARATHORMONE EFFECTS

Present concepts suggest that parathormone has at least two specific effects, and it is probably fruitless to argue over which is primary. The hormone mobilizes calcium directly from bone into the blood; it also suppresses renal tubular resorption of phosphate, promoting active urinary excretion of phosphate. Because the serum levels of calcium and inorganic phosphorus are inversely proportional, the two effects are interrelated. The end result is elevation of serum calcium and depression of serum inorganic phosphorus. Parathormone production appears to be regulated by the level of serum calcium, with no influence from tropic hormones.

Serum Calcium and Phosphorus

The normal concentration of serum calcium is 9 to 11 mg per 100 ml, also expressed as 4.5 to 5.5 milliequivalents per liter. Approximately half is bound to the serum proteins, so abnormal protein levels may distort the results of a calcium determination, despite normal ion concentration. The proportion of ionized and bound calcium can be calculated when the total calcium and total protein are known. The normal value for serum inorganic phosphorus is 2.5 to 4 mg per 100 ml in adults, and 4 to 5 mg per 100 ml in children.

HYPOPARATHYROIDISM

The commonest cause of parathyroid insufficiency is removal of the parathyroid glands by operation, either intentionally in parathyroidectomy or inadvertently in thyroidectomy. Inflammation, trauma, or other destructive processes are less likely to disrupt endocrine function because the glands are widely separated in the neck, and the undisturbed glands can compensate for loss of one or several others. Idiopathic hypofunction can occur in childhood or maturity, causing destruction, scarring, and atrophy which may have an autoimmune basis. Because the symptoms are prompt and dramatic and because physicians are alert to the possibility, acute hypoparathyroidism is readily diagnosed after operations on the neck. Chronic hypoparathyroidism presents a more difficult diagnostic problem. Symptoms in either form arise from low serum concentration of ionized calcium. Nonparathyroid causes of persistently low serum calcium include rickets, osteomalacia, severe steatorrhea, and renal failure.

Tetany

Tetany, a condition of increased neuromuscular irritability, may occur when the serum calcium drops to 7.5 mg per 100 ml or lower. Tetany sometimes occurs in patients with alkalosis or hyperventilation, but in these conditions the normal total calcium level in the serum eliminates hypoparathyroidism as a possible cause. Neuromuscular irritability may be manifest as cramps of the skeletal muscles or as laryngospasm, hypermotility of the gastrointestinal tract, or convulsive disorders. Chronic hypoparathyroidism may also present with central nervous system disorders, lenticular cataracts, and trophic disorders of the hair, nails, and skin.

Laboratory Findings

The diagnosis of hypoparathyroidism depends upon demonstrating consistent depression of serum calcium below 7.5 mg per 100 ml, with elevation of serum phosphate to 4 to 6 mg per 100 ml. The serum magnesium level may be reduced from the normal of 2.0 or 2.5 mg per 100 ml to 1.5 to 1.8 mg per 100 ml. Urinary calcium is usually absent, and addition of Sulkowitch reagent to the urine sample produces no turbidity. Phosphaturia is difficult to evaluate because it varies with dietary intake; even without parathormone activity, increased intake of phosphate results in increased excretion.

Excretion Tests. The Ellsworth-Howard test provides a fairly reliable index of parathyroid function, comparing unmodified phosphate excretion against excretion stimulated by exogenous parathormone. A standard dose of parathyroid extract is given, and phosphate excretion is measured at hourly intervals for three to five hours. In normal individuals, phosphate excretion rises fivefold or sixfold; in patients with hypoparathyroidism, the elevation may be tenfold or greater. Certain patients whose symptoms suggest hypoparathyroidism have a rise no greater than twofold. This condition is known as pseudohypoparathyroidism, due probably to faulty renal response to parathormone rather than to hormonal insufficiency.

Other tests of calcium or phosphorus balance require the strict supervision and standardization of a metabolic ward. Nonparathyroid causes of hypocalcemia include excessive fecal calcium loss in intestinal malabsorption syndromes and also phosphate retention due to renal disease. Distinction from hypoparathyroidism usually causes no difficulty. Vitamin D deficiency or rickets of renal origin also causes hypocalcemia along with more obvious signs of the primary disease.

HYPERPARATHYROIDISM

Excessive parathormone activity may be due to hyperplastic enlargement of all the glands or to adenomatous enlargement of only one or two. Sometimes hyperplasia is idiopathic, but frequently diseases of other organs cause changes in mineral metabolism that induce increased parathormone secretion. Since primary hyperparathyroidism damages kidneys, bones, lungs, and stomach, and diseases of each of these organs can induce secondary hyperparathyroidism, it may be difficult to distinguish cart from horse.

Clinical Symptoms

The symptoms of primary hyperparathyroidism develop insidiously, usually in adults and more often in females than in males. Increased calcium is mobilized from bone, and increased phosphorus is lost in the urine, leading to a variety of symptoms due to hypercalcemia, skeletal changes, and renal disease. The clinical symptoms almost always include weakness, anorexia, and vague aches and pains. Other nonspecific findings may include hyperextensibility of the joints, bradycardia, constipation, and anemia. The increased urinary solute load often produces polyuria, which is followed by polydipsia. Renal parenchymal damage and nephrolithiasis may impair the ability to concentrate urine above specific gravity of 1.022. In advanced hyperparathyroidism, widespread bone cysts may occur, often associated with osteoporosis, pathologic fractures, incomplete healing, and bizarre skeletal deformities. Some of the excessive circulating calcium may be deposited as ectopic calcification of kidneys, lungs, stomach, blood vessels, or myocardium. Less readily explained is the frequent occurrence of intractable peptic ulcer, pancreatitis, or deposition of corneal opacities (band keratitis).

Laboratory Findings

The laboratory findings in uncomplicated hyperparathyroidism are characteristic. The serum calcium is elevated above 12 mg per 100 ml and often much higher. The serum inorganic phosphorus is decreased below 2.5 mg per 100 ml. The urine contains large quantities of calcium and phosphorus, even if the diet is relatively low in phosphates. The serum alkaline phosphatase rises only with extensive skeletal involvement fairly late in the disease.

When hypercalcemia suggests hyperparathyroidism, several tests of mineral metabolism may provide moderate assistance. Intravenous infusion of calcium, which normally suppresses parathormone secretion and thus decreases urinary phosphate excretion, does not alter urinary phosphate levels in primary hyperparathyroidism. Unfortunately, other causes of hypercalcemia may produce similar results and, even in normal individuals, diurnal variation of phosphate excretion may be great enough to distort the test results.

Phosphate Reabsorption. Tubular reabsorption of phosphate can be measured directly, but the results are valid only if other urinary functions are demonstrated to be normal. The test itself is simple enough, requiring only collection of a timed urine specimen and a blood sample taken during the collecting period. The calculation compares relative serum and urine levels of creatinine and phosphorus, using the formula

$$TRP = \left(1 - \frac{UP \times SC}{UC \times SP}\right) \times 100,$$ where TRP is the tubular reabsorption

of phosphorus expressed as a percentage, U refers to urine concentration, S to serum concentration, C means creatinine and P means phosphorus. The normal TRP is 90 per cent or greater; in hyperparathyroidism, values are less than 85 per cent.

Differential Diagnosis

The difficulty in diagnosing hyperparathyroidism is in distinguishing it from other causes of hypercalcemia. The most common nonparathyroid

Table 10.   Summary of Chemical Features of Diseases
with Disturbed Plasma Calcium and Phosphate*

Disease	Serum			Urine	
	Calcium	Phosphate	Alkaline Phosphatase	Calcium	Phosphate
Hyperparathyroidism	Increased	Decreased	Normal or increased	Increased	Increased
Paget's disease	Normal	Normal	Increased	Normal	Normal
Hypoparathyroidism	Decreased	Increased	Normal	Decreased	Decreased
Renal insufficiency	Decreased	Increased	Normal or increased	Decreased	Decreased
Osteomalacia	Decreased or normal	Decreased	Increased	Decreased	Decreased
Senile osteoporosis	Normal	Normal	Normal	Normal	Normal
Multiple myeloma	Normal to increased	Normal	Normal	Normal to increased	Normal to decreased
Milk-alkali syndrome	Increased	Normal to increased	Normal	Normal to decreased	Normal to decreased
Vitamin D intoxication	Increased	Increased	Normal	Increased	Decreased
Metastatic carcinoma	Normal to increased	Normal	Normal to increased	Increased	Normal
Sarcoidosis	Increased	Normal to increased	Normal to increased	Increased	Decreased
Hyperventilation (alkalosis)	Normal	Normal	Normal	Normal	Normal

* From Bernstein, D.S., and Thorn, G.W., In Wintrobe, M.M. et al. (eds.): Harrison's Principles of Internal Medicine, ed. 6. McGraw-Hill Book Company, New York, 1970.

etiologies for hypercalcemia are malignant tumors, with or without apparent skeletal involvement; multiple myeloma; sarcoidosis; therapy with thiazide drugs; vitamin D intoxication; and milk-alkali syndrome. Calcium mobilization accompanying enforced inactivity (*acute bone atrophy*[24]) may also raise serum calcium to disturbing levels. A 10-day course of cortisone may assist in differential diagnosis, since serum calcium levels decline in patients with sarcoidosis, myeloma, and vitamin D overload, and are unresponsive when hyperparathyroidism exists. The hypercalcemia accompanying malignant tumors responds unpredictably.[24] Thiazide-induced hypercalcemia is usually mild[11] and recedes within a month after cessation of therapy. Increased serum protein levels elevate total circulating calcium at a rate of approximately 0.8 mg per 100 ml calcium for each 1 Gm per 100 ml of elevated albumia or globulin,[51] and serum protein studies should be a part of every hypercalcemia work-up. Parathormone can be measured directly by radioimmunoassay, but this may not be diagnostic when hypercalcemia results from the secretion of parathormone-like substance from solid malignant tumors.[54] Table 10 above outlines characteristic serum and urine alterations in many conditions affecting calcium and phosphorus metabolism.

Secondary Hyperparathyroidism

Secondary hyperparathyroidism is more common than primary hyperplasia or adenoma. The usual cause is advanced renal disease, in which phosphate retention causes reciprocal reduction of serum calcium. The low calcium level stimulates the parathyroids, which may overrespond and become hyperplastic. In such cases, both serum calcium and serum phosphate are elevated, and the skeletal, neuromuscular, and gastrointestinal complications of hyperparathyroidism are superimposed on the clinical picture of severe renal disease. The renal disease is usually well documented, and elevations of serum phosphates, urea, and creatinine are diagnostic. In the presence of demonstrated renal disease and elevated serum phosphate, an elevated or even high-normal calcium level indicates secondary hyperparathyroidism. Hyperparathyroidism may complicate renal disease without overt hypercalcemia and skeletal changes may be the first sign of its presence.

PANCREAS

Pancreatic endocrine function resides in the islets of Langerhans, which produce two different hormones. The beta cells produce insulin, the body's hypoglycemic agent, while the alpha cells produce glucagon, a hyperglycemic agent that promotes glycogenolysis. No significant clinical syndromes are known to involve glucagon, whose physiologic function is imperfectly understood.

DIABETES MELLITUS

Most significant of the pancreatic endocrine disorders is diabetes mellitus, which may be classified as pancreatic hypofunction, as contrasted with several relatively rare syndromes marked by hypoglycemia and insulin excess. Diabetes mellitus is a constitutional disease that produces abnormalities of carbohydrate metabolism and widespread vascular changes. Although heredity is known to influence the incidence of diabetes, the mode of inheritance and the relative roles of genetic and environmental factors remain to be clarified.

Diagnosis

The principal sign of diabetes mellitus is hyperglycemia. Whether this is due to inadequate insulin production, production of abnormal insulin products, presence of insulin antagonists, or defects in peripheral glucose utilization, the diagnosis remains the same. Full-blown diabetes mellitus is marked by the obvious and well-known symptoms of polyuria, polydipsia, and weight loss despite increased appetite. In such cases, demonstration of glucosuria and fasting hyperglycemia confirms the clinical impression. More difficult is accurate diagnosis of milder cases, or demonstration of a "prediabetic state" in relatives of diagnosed diabetics.

Urine Tests. Normally, the urine contains no glucose. The repeated presence of glucose in several urine samples indicates that either the renal threshold for glucose is low or that the blood levels exceed the normal renal threshold. If the defect is renal, normal blood sugar levels accompany the glucosuria.

Whenever "sugar" is found in the urine, further diagnostic measures are indicated. Many tests for urine sugar are not specific for glucose, and indicate only that some reducing substance is present. Copper sulfate methods, including Clinitest reagent tablets, become positive in the presence not only of glucose, but of other sugars, salicylate metabolites, homogentisic acid, and other metabolic end products. Specific tests for glucose are available, utilizing the enzyme glucose oxidase, often incorporated in a paper medium (Tes-Tape, Clinistix). For routine urinalysis a nonspecific test is probably preferable, since the presence of most reducing substances should be noted clinically. Once a reducing substance has been found, more specific tests should be used. In the majority of cases, the glucose oxidase test provides the answer, but occasionally some other cause will be found.

Blood Glucose Levels. Blood glucose is usually measured with the patient in a fasting state. The fasting blood sugar determination is most useful in diagnosing well-advanced cases of diabetes, in which fasting glucose levels may be as high as 500 mg per 100 ml, but the patient has surprisingly few other objective or subjective abnormalities. The normal fasting blood glucose ranges from 65 to 100 mg per 100 ml, depending upon the method used and the laboratory standards.

POSTPRANDIAL BLOOD GLUCOSE. Since carbohydrate metabolism is dynamic, observation of the patient's response to metabolic challenge may provide more valuable information than measurement of the fasting level. For this reason, the postprandial blood glucose level is a better screening test than the fasting level. The sample is drawn either one or two hours after the patient has eaten a meal of approximately 100 Gm of carbohydrate. Glucose values of 160 mg per 100 ml one hour after eating[31] have been considered diagnostic of diabetes, and values above 120 mg per 100 ml should probably be investigated.[14]

Glucose Tolerance Tests. To demonstrate diabetes more rigorously, the glucose tolerance test (GTT) is used. This test is unnecessary in patients with fasting blood glucose above 140 mg per 100 ml or postprandial levels above 180 mg per 100 ml. The patient should have had an adequate diet (minimum of 150 Gm of carbohydrate per day) for two or three days prior to testing, for inadequate diet by itself can diminish carbohydrate tolerance. Slightly different glucose loads are recommended by different groups. The Committee on Statistics of the American Diabetes Association recommends 40 Gm of glucose per square meter of body surface,[31] and their report provides a table for glucose dose based on height and weight. Other groups employ a standard dose of 100 Gm, or a dose of 1.75 Gm per kilogram "ideal body weight." The patient should fast for at least 8 hours, but no more than 16 hours, before beginning the test. Salicylates, nicotinic acid, and certain diuretics diminish glucose tolerance and should be omitted for three days before testing; oral contraceptives should be omitted for the entire cycle preceeding the test.[31]

Blood and urine samples are collected in the fasting state, and at intervals of one, two, and three hours after glucose ingestion. Results of urine testing do not affect the diagnosis, but give useful information about renal thresholds to the physician who must plan later therapy.

The diagnostic criteria for the glucose tolerance test vary somewhat with the dose employed and the standards agreed upon. In general, one-hour values at or above 160 or 170 mg per 100 ml whole blood (185 to 195 mg per 100 ml serum) and two-hour values at or above 120 mg per 100 ml whole blood (140 mg per 100 ml serum) are considered diagnostic. Another approach is to add the numerical values for the fasting, one-hour, two-hour, and three-hour specimens, and diabetes is diagnosed if the sum is 600 mg or more.

INTRAVENOUS GLUCOSE TOLERANCE TEST. The glucose tolerance curve may be virtually flat if gastrointestinal disease or enzymatic deficiencies prevent normal glucose absorption. To circumvent this, a 25 per cent solution of glucose may be given intravenously, 0.5 Gm per kg of ideal body weight, over two to four minutes. Following intravenous glucose infusion, the two-hour specimen provides the most diagnostic information, and failure to return to fasting level strongly suggests diabetes.

STEROID CHALLENGE. If the standard glucose tolerance test is equivocal, carbohydrate metabolism can be further challenged by giving adrenal cortical steroids prior to repeating the GTT. Such rigorous testing might be indicated in patients with suggestive vascular or neurological diseases or with a strong family history of diabetes, or in women whose pregnancies were marked by glycosuria and delivery of progressively larger infants. Cortisone increases blood glucose levels and may also decrease peripheral utilization.[50] Cortisone acetate 50 mg is given eight hours and again two hours before beginning the usual glucose tolerance procedure. Individuals whose two hour levels are 140 mg per 100 ml or above are often considered to be prediabetic and should be followed closely for development of overt diabetes.

DIFFERENTIAL DIAGNOSIS. In severe liver disease, abnormal glucose tolerance may simulate a diabetic response. The damaged liver does not produce glycogen from the excess circulating glucose, and then does not respond to declining blood glucose values with glycogenolysis. Prolonged or transient hyperglycemia may follow acute or chronic pancreatitis or pancreatectomy involving more than 90 per cent of the gland. If a glucose tolerance test is done during an attack of acute pancreatitis, it usually has a diabetic appearance. Hemochromatosis may produce sufficient pancreatic damage so that mild diabetes occurs ("bronze diabetes"). Acromegaly, Cushing's syndrome, thyrotoxicosis, and pheochromocytoma are other endocrine disorders that alter carbohydrate metabolism and may produce an abnormal GTT.[13]

Complications of Diabetes

Chronic Changes. Once diabetes has been diagnosed, treatment is usually monitored by repeated urinalysis for glucose and by periodic blood glucose determinations. Systemic changes due to microangiopathies, arteriosclerosis, and neuropathy cannot be monitored by laboratory examinations. Another indication for repeated urinalysis is the increased incidence of urinary tract infections in diabetics. If pyelonephritis occurs, urinalysis reveals proteinuria, pyuria, and bacteriuria, along with increased glycosuria and ketonuria. Progressive kidney damage due to diffuse glomerulosclerosis may cause progressive functional change, terminating in excretion of protein and casts, but nodular glomerulosclerosis (Kimmelstiehl-Wilson lesion) does not have a characteristic urinary profile.

Another chronic complication of diabetes is nerve root damage, which may increase spinal fluid protein levels to 50 to 100 mg per 100 ml, but does not cause pleocytosis.

Acute Ketoacidosis. Of the acute complications of diabetes, ketoacidosis is the one in which laboratory findings change most rapidly and most critically. At the beginning, blood glucose is elevated and there are ketones in the serum. When the body cannot meet its caloric requirements from circulating glucose, it mobilizes fat as an energy source, and the ketone bodies—acetoacetic acid, acetone, and beta-hydroxybutyric acid—are end products of this inefficient metabolic expedient. The normal serum ketone level is zero. Changes in the ketone level can be monitored by testing suitably diluted serum or plasma with Acetest powder. Large quantities of glucose and ketones appear in the urine, requiring excretion of cations to balance ketotic acids. Ketone bodies in the blood cause acidosis, and as the blood pH falls, respiration is increased. At pH of 7.2, Kussmaul respiration may become obvious; this reduces the body's CO_2 supply, but does not get rid of excess hydrogen ions.

LABORATORY FINDINGS. The results of diuresis, cation loss, and massive respiratory effort include: depletion of sodium, potassium, calcium, and other cations; pronounced drop in CO_2 combining power; progressive dehydration, with consequent fall in renal plasma flow and glomerular filtration rate; accentuated hyperglycemia because of diminishing renal clearance; temperature elevation due to dehydration; and leukocytosis of 15,000 to 30,000/cu mm, due simply to these physiologic derangements. If infection was the precipitating event, fever and leukocytosis will be even greater.

Potassium metabolism is especially sensitive to these changes. When hydrogen ions become more numerous in the blood, they enter the fixed cells in exchange for intracellular potassium which comes out into the plasma. The serum potassium level changes with influx of intracellular potassium and irretrievable loss through the kidneys, and the blood value at any given moment cannot reflect the massive depletion of whole-body supplies. Serum sodium determinations are affected by the same complex problems.

DIFFERENTIAL DIAGNOSIS. The differential diagnosis of diabetic ketoacidosis frequently must include hypoglycemic coma and salicylate intoxication. Blood glucose levels easily distinguish diabetic coma from insulin coma, and a still more rapid distinction may be obtained in doubtful cases by treating the patient with intravenous injection of 100 ml of a 50 per cent solution of glucose. If the problem is diabetic ketoacidosis, an additional 50 Gm of glucose will not aggravate the problem, but if the problem is hypoglycemia, dramatic improvement occurs. Further differentiating points are that hypoglycemia is usually of rapid onset and is characterized by shallow respiration rather than the deep Kussmaul respiration of diabetic coma. Salicylate intoxication may superficially resemble diabetic coma, since acidosis and Kussmaul respiration are frequently present, and reducing substances are present in the urine. Salicylate metabolites can readily be distinguished from urinary glucose by glucose oxidase testing, and the blood glucose, of course, is not elevated in salicylism.

HYPOGLYCEMIA

Symptomatic hypoglycemia usually results from functioning islet cell tumors, either benign or malignant, but sometimes occurs with early diabetes or with "functional" hyperinsulinism in which no histologic lesion is present. More rarely still, severe liver disease, pituitary or adrenal insufficiency, inborn enzymatic defects, or nonpancreatic tumors may cause spontaneous hypoglycemia. The diagnosis of hypoglycemia is made when low blood glucose levels accompany objective or subjective symptoms. Whipple's triad, originally applied to the diagnosis of islet cell tumors, documents hypoglycemia due to any cause: symptomatic attack, with blood glucose level less than 50 mg/100 ml and relief of symptoms by glucose administration.

Tolbutamide Test

Insulin-producing tumors occur most frequently in middle life and are usually benign. The distinction between benign and malignant may be difficult even after microscopic examination, and multiple tumors are common in either form. Characteristic findings in insulin-producing tumors are increasingly severe symptoms during prolonged fast, aggravation by exercise, and a positive tolbutamide test. In the tolbutamide test, blood samples drawn 15, 30, 45, 60, 90, 120, 150, and 180 minutes after intravenous administration of 1 Gm of tolbutamide are compared with the fasting glucose level. In normal individuals or in those with functional hyperinsulinism, blood glucose returns to at least 70 per cent of fasting level within three hours. Patients with insulinomas have continued, marked hypoglycemia, sometimes with neurologic symptoms that force the physician to administer glucose and terminate the test. If insulin assays are available, elevated plasma insulin activity can be shown to follow this stimulus. The tolbutamide test cannot be used if fasting glucose levels are below 50 mg/100 ml and false-positive results may occur in cases of severe liver disease, alcoholism, starvation, and occasional nonpancreatic tumors.

Effect of Fasting

Induction of a 24- to 72-hour fast may be helpful for diagnosis because, in functional hyperinsulinism, fasting produces little alteration in the glucose level, and exercise after a period of fasting causes blood glucose to rise. In patients with insulin-producing tumors, the blood glucose level falls progressively during the fast, and exercise may induce hypoglycemia if the fast itself has not produced symptoms.

Reactive Hypoglycemia

In reactive functional hyperinsulinism, rising blood sugar levels appear to stimulate excessive insulin secretion. Thus, after large amounts of carbohydrate are consumed, a normal mild hyperglycemia may be followed in two to four hours by signs and symptoms of hypoglycemia. An oral glucose tolerance test reveals the same pattern; glucose levels rise no higher than normal, but decline is excessive, and definite hypoglycemia occurs in two to four hours. A type of reactive hypoglycemia may occur in mild diabetes; in these cases, insulin secretion appears to be delayed. Blood sugar levels rise to diabetic levels, and then a delayed, overenthusiastic insulin response causes subsequent hypoglycemia.

NON-INSULIN-PRODUCING ISLET CELL ADENOMAS

Hormonal products of nonbeta islet cell tumors produce the Zollinger-Ellison (Z-E) syndrome of refractory, often atypically located gastric ulcers; intense gastric hyperacidity; and, often, watery diarrhea and malabsorption. These tumors which may be single or multiple produce enormous quantities of gastrin,[26,40] which stimulates enormous gastric acid production, which produces mucosal ulceration, impaired fat metabolism, and sometimes impaired vitamin B_{12} absorption,[55] each of which can lead to further symptoms. Surgical extirpation of the tumors may be difficult or impossible, but total gastrectomy prevents acid production and usually provides the best cure. After successful gastrectomy, extrapancreatic tumor nodules may disappear.[48]

Acid Secretion

Zollinger-Ellison syndrome should be considered when medical management fails to control peptic ulcer symptoms. Measurement of gastric acidity is the best diagnostic tool, but is not infallible. The diagnosis is suggested when overnight free acid secretion is 100 mEq or more, or if one-hour basal output exceeds 15 mEq, or if basal secretion is 60 per cent or more of maximally stimulated secretion. Serum gastrin can be measured by radioimmunoassay,[40] with Z-E patients having tenfold or greater elevations over normal range. This is not foolproof either, since gastrin secretion may be intermittent, and a single specimen may be unrevealing.

Other Syndromes

A histologically different nonbeta cell tumor produces a different clinical picture, characterized by massive watery diarrhea (up to 8 liters in 24 hours), hypokalemic alkalosis, and sometimes a diabetic glucose tolerance curve, but without gastric hyperacidity.[48] The hormonal product of this tumor has not been characterized. While complete tumor resection promptly relieves the symptoms, recurrences are not uncommon.

Pancreatic islet cell tumors are frequently part of the syndrome polyendocrine adenomatosis, with peptic ulceration present in more than half the cases. Demonstration of nonbeta cell adenomas should prompt careful examination for evidence of parathyroid, pituitary, adrenal, or thyroid adenomas in addition.

OVARIES

The ovaries contain three types of cells: germ cells, somatic cells of the cortex, and medullary cells which share a common origin with the adrenal cortex.[39] The germ cells have no endocrine function. Rather, they are influenced by pituitary and other hormones and propelled toward ovulation or involution. The cortical cells differentiate into the granulosa and theca cells of the ovarian follicle which produce estrogens and progestins, respectively. Medullary cells, usually scattered sparsely at the hilus, retain the capacity to produce androgens, usually in very small amounts.

HORMONES AND THEIR EFFECTS

The ovaries and the pituitary are linked in a reciprocal relationship. Critical levels of estrogen induce secretion of follicle-stimulating hormone (FSH) which in turn promotes estrogen production. Follicle-stimulating hormone and luteinizing hormone (LH) together induce ovulation, after which FSH and estrogen levels decline, while LH and progesterone secretion increase. Under the influence of LH, the ruptured follicle becomes the corpus luteum, and luteotropic hormone promotes continued elaboration of progesterone. Shortly before menstruation, progesterone secretion declines and there is a second, but lower, peak of estrogen production.

Progesterone and the estrogens are steroids, evolving by way of cholesterol from acetate fractions. The pathway is such that progesterone is a precursor of testosterone, which is a precursor of the estrogens. Many estrogen metabolites have been isolated; but the three principal substances, in order of diminishing potency, are estradiol, estrone, and estriol. In the maturing child, estrogens induce the secondary sex characteristics and closure of the epiphyses. Estrogen, in the female adult, thickens and cornifies the vaginal mucosa and produces uterine enlargement, salt and water retention, and mammary stimulation. Estrogen renders the endometrium sensitive to subsequent stimulation by progesterone. Progesterone has its major effect on the endometrium, which enters the secretory phase and becomes ready for implantation of the blastocyst if fertilization has occurred.

MEASURING OVARIAN SECRETION

Measurement of the ovarian hormones is difficult. Both bioassay and chemical methods are available, but the chemical methods are difficult and expensive, while the bioassay methods are time-consuming and, like all bioassays, rather difficult to standardize. Progesterone is usually measured as its principal excreted metabolite, pregnanediol. Both estrogen and pregnanediol determinations involve enzymic hydrolysis and chromatographic separation, followed by spectrophotometry.

A Note on Pregnanetriol. Pregnanediol should not be confused with pregnanetriol, despite the similarity of names. Pregnanetriol arises, not from progesterone, but from 17-hydroxyprogesterone, a precursor in adrenal corticoid synthesis, and elevated pregnanetriol levels occur in congenital adrenal cortical hyperplasia.

Progesterone Effects

Because direct hormonal measurement is somewhat difficult, ovarian function is commonly evaluated indirectly. In the adult, estrogenic function can be inferred from the degree of cornification of vaginal epithelial cells. Progesterone activity is evaluated by the presence or absence of secretory changes in an endometrial biopsy, taken at the appropriate phase of the menstrual cycle. Body temperature change also indicates progesterone activity; a sustained rise of one degree Fahrenheit in the basal temperature implies that ovulation has occurred.

HYPOFUNCTION

Ovarian hypofunction usually means estrogen deficiency, since an isolated deficiency of progesterone is rare. Combined deficiency of estrogen and progesterone results in menstrual irregularities and difficulty in conceiving. Estrogen deficiency may be due to primary ovarian insufficiency; or normal ovaries may be inadequately stimulated if pituitary gonadotropins are deficient. In the prepubertal child, primary or secondary ovarian hypofunction causes failure of sexual maturation and eunuchoid skeletal growth. Loss of ovarian function in a previously normal mature woman causes amenorrhea or oligomenorrhea, and this may subsequently be followed by regression of certain secondary sex characteristics. Actual masculinization does not occur unless androgen excess accompanies estrogen deficiency.

Secondary Insufficiency

Secondary ovarian insufficiency is diagnosed by demonstration of persistently low levels of pituitary gonadotropins. Since this may be due to tumor, infarction, infiltration, or idiopathic glandular failure, evaluation should include measurement of other pituitary functions, as well as evaluation of radiographic changes, visual fields, and other tests relating to potential disorders of the pituitary.

Primary Insufficiency

Primary ovarian insufficiency is nearly always associated with high levels of pituitary gonadotropins, once the age of normal puberty is attained. Primary insufficiency may be due to congenital hypoplasia or dysgenesis of the ovaries, scarring from infections, or changes from irradiation or surgery. In the normal menopause, pituitary gonadotropins reach high levels; and in the condition described as *premature climacteric,* there is a similar elevation of gonadotropin associated with diminished numbers of germinal follicles and diminished ovarian responsiveness.

Chromosomal Abnormality. In *gonadal dysgenesis* (Turner's syndrome), gonadotropin levels are high because there is no ovarian tissue to respond. In this condition, the individual has only 45 chromosomes instead of the normal complement of 46. The missing chromosome is the second sex chromosome—the patient has neither a Y chromosome which induces testicular development nor the second X chromosome of the female genotype. This condition can be recognized by the absence, from epithelial cells, of the Barr body, a tiny mass of chromatin material thought to represent the involuted, inactive second X chromosome.[64]

Systemic Disease. Ovarian hypofunction may be caused by certain systemic diseases such as chronic renal disease, advanced malignant disease, severe hypothyroidism, anorexia nervosa, or other conditions of generalized hypometabolism. In some cases, psychogenic factors appear to cause amenorrhea by depressing gonadotropin secretion. Depression of gonadotropin secretion may also occur in patients with androgenic adrenal hyperfunction. Apparently the high levels of androgen inhibit gonadotropin secretion.[39]

HYPERFUNCTION

Precocious Maturation

If the prepubertal ovary produces any hormones, it is hyperfunctioning. This leads to early appearance of female secondary sex characteristics and the occurrence of uterine bleeding. If hypothalamic disease is the cause of early maturation, cyclical gonadotropin and ovarian hormone production may lead to ovulation and fertility at a very early age. Such children demonstrate all the cyclic changes in hormone excretion, vaginal cornification, and endometrial morphology that occur in mature women. In many cases, no morphologic lesion is found in the hypothalamus and, except for early maturation (i.e., menarche before age 10) and short stature, the children prove to be normal. The children are short because the adult levels of estrogen cause the epiphyses to close very early.

In a very few cases, precocious puberty is due to granulosa-theca cell tumors of the ovary. These children have high urinary levels of estrogen, low levels of gonadotropin, and ordinarily a palpable ovarian mass.

Another cause for early feminization and estrogen excretion is ingestion of exogenous estrogens. This may occur when children swallow estrogen-containing pills or cosmetics belonging to adults, or it may be due to the presence of contaminating estrogenic compounds in other drugs.[37]

Ovarian Tumors

Relatively few ovarian tumors produce hormones. The most common hormonally active ovarian neoplasms are granulosa-theca cell tumors, which account for approximately 10 per cent of the solid ovarian tumors. These secrete estrogens which appear in the urine at very high levels. Frequently noted are other changes related to excessive estrogen production, such as irregular uterine bleeding, uterine and breast enlargement, and salt and water retention. Certain rare ovarian tumors, notably the arrhenoblastomas, produce androgens. Virilizing signs generally include hirsutism, acne, deepening of the voice, clitoral enlargement, involution of the breasts, and cessation of menses. Despite rather marked clinical virilization, urinary 17-ketosteroids may not be markedly elevated. Adrenal disease is a more common cause of significant 17-ketosteroid excess, especially congenital hyperplasia in children and virilizing adrenal carcinoma at all ages.

UTERINE BLEEDING

Functional uterine bleeding, an extremely common complaint, might be considered evidence of ovarian hyperfunction in the sense that excessive estrogen stimulates an endometrium insufficiently counterbalanced by progesterone. The precise defect may be difficult to pinpoint, since rather subtle upsets of the pituitary-ovary relationship can result in irregular uterine bleeding. Once coagulation disorders, pregnancy, and infection have been eliminated as causes, laboratory procedures offer little for diagnosis. Endometrial biopsy or curettage usually shows only changes due to estrogen stimulation, but curettage is advisable, especially in older women, to rule out endometrial carcinoma.

FEMALE INFERTILITY

Diagnostic regimens for involuntary infertility are beyond the scope of this discussion, but a few points should be considered. In addition to evaluation of the general health of each partner, certain specific laboratory procedures are indicated. Patency of the cervix, uterus, and fallopian tubes should be determined by insufflation or dye instillation.

Laboratory Findings

Evidence that ovulation and progesterone secretion have occurred is usually indirect. If the endometrium, at the onset of the menses, has a secretory pattern or if there has been a sustained rise in basal body temperature, it may be inferred that the hormonal cycle is normal. At the time of expected ovulation, it may be helpful to examine the cervical mucus for normally occurring changes in clarity, increased glucose content, tensile strength (ability to form a thread), and presence of a crystalline, fernlike pattern when the mucus dries on a glass slide. In some women, inadequate progesterone secretion is inferred from low urinary levels of pregnanediol and the demonstration of atypical secretory patterns in the postovulation endometrium. If ovulation has not occurred but gonadotropin levels are normal, suitable hormonal therapy sometimes induces ovulatory cycles. Repeated demonstration of low gonadotropin levels points to hypothalamic or pituitary disease, while excessively high levels of gonadotropin indicate failure of ovarian response. In patients with primary amenorrhea, cytologic examination for sex chromatin pattern is indicated despite outward evidence of feminine habitus.

Stein-Leventhal Syndrome

Many young women are first seen with secondary amenorrhea, mild hirsutism, and infertility problems. Certain such women have bilaterally enlarged cystic ovaries surrounded by a tough grayish-white capsule, a condition known as the Stein-Leventhal syndrome. These women have anovulatory cycles, normal or low levels of FSH, and LH levels which tend to be quite high, but fluctuate widely.[21] Suggested causes include the production of abnormal adrenal cortical hormones, production of increased quantities of testosterone by the ovarian stromal cells, inhibition of FSH production by prolonged estrogen production, and alterations in hypothalamic mechanisms. Ordinarily estrogen production is normal or high, and urinary 17-ketosteroids are within normal limits. Some women with the Stein-Leventhal syndrome, and certain others with idiopathic hirsutism, have been shown to excrete excessive 17-ketosteroid and 17-hydroxycorticosteroid after ACTH administration.[37] Additional support for adrenal hyperreactivity and possible hyperfunction as the etiology is the finding that certain such women succeed in conception when intrinsic ACTH production is partially suppressed by administration of small doses of glucocorticoids.

TESTES

The testes perform two functions: elaboration of the male hormones, predominantly testosterone; and the production of spermatozoa, the male gametes. The Leydig, or interstitial, cells secrete testosterone under the influence of the interstitial cell-stimulating hormone (ICSH, which is apparently the same as luteinizing hormone in females). Testosterone is a 19-carbon hormone but not a 17-ketosteroid. Its excreted metabolites, however, can be measured as 17-ketosteroids and constitute approximately one-third of the total 17-ketosteroid excretion in adult males. The remaining two-thirds derive from the adrenal and are present in both males and females. Testosterone stimulates the seminiferous tubules, but actual spermatogenesis is largely regulated by the pituitary gonadotropin called, in the female, follicle-stimulating hormone (FSH).

HORMONES AND THEIR FUNCTIONS

Interstitial cells are active during fetal development, secreting products that direct genital development toward the masculine habitus, but testicular function is largely dormant in the male from birth to puberty. An upsurge of pituitary gonadotropins heralds the onset of puberty and promotes secretion of testosterone, which initiates male secondary sex characteristics. Following puberty, abnormally diminished testosterone production is associated with high levels of pituitary gonadotropin, but the relationship between testes and pituitary is somewhat unclear. Some men with diminished spermatogenesis have elevated gonadotropin levels, despite normal excretion of testosterone metabolites.

Laboratory evaluation of testicular function rests upon measurement of androgen secretion and examination of the seminal fluid. Testosterone is measured when hypogonadism is suspected, and spermatogenesis is evaluated when a married couple desire children but have difficulty conceiving.

HYPOGONADISM

Hypogonadism cannot be suspected in an outwardly normal male child until after the age of expected puberty. Individuals vary so markedly that delayed maturation and hypogonadism are difficult to differentiate until after the patient is 19 or 20 years old. As with other endocrine defects, testosterone deficiency may be due to primary testicular failure or may be secondary to inadequate pituitary stimulation. The clinical findings of primary and secondary hypogonadism are the same: When first seen, the individual displays eunuchoid features of excessive growth of long bones, high-pitched voice, absence of male pattern of hair distribution, poor muscular development, and infantile external genitalia. These physical findings are not present in the mature male whose testes were damaged after puberty.

Primary Gonadal Insufficiency

In patients with primary testicular disorders, urinary gonadotropin levels are high after the age of expected puberty. One of the commoner causes of primary dysfunction is *Klinefelter's syndrome* in which there is a supernumerary X chromosome. These patients have a positive sex-chromatin pattern, despite male habitus. Primary testicular disorders in men with normal chromosomal complement are usually due to anatomic or developmental abnormalities demonstrable by testicular biopsy.

Secondary Gonadal Insufficiency. Patients with low gonadotropin levels may have complete or incomplete pituitary hypofunction. The gonadotropins suffer first when the pituitary is damaged, so that what appears to be an isolated defect in gonadotropin production is sometimes the first sign of progessive pituitary destruction. Demonstration of gonadotropin deficiency should prompt a careful search for the cause of pituitary disease: x-rays of the sella turcica and examination of visual fields to demonstrate tumor; serologic tests for syphilis; x-ray examination and immunologic evaluation for tuberculosis; and hematologic examination to rule out multiple myeloma. Gynecomastia cannot reliably be associated with estrogen levels or with changes in testosterone production and appears to require the presence of gonadotropins. Patients with pituitary failure do not develop gynecomastia despite the absence of testosterone.[46]

HYPERGONADISM

This condition becomes apparent most readily in young boys in whom secondary sex characteristics appear unexpectedly early. Gonadotropin levels are usually increased above preadolescent levels, sometimes due to demonstrable tumor in the region of the hypothalamus. In some boys, early maturation appears to be a hereditary constitutional syndrome without anatomic abnormalities.[9] Since testosterone is a potent androgen, there may be minimal change in 17-ketosteroid excretion in the early phases of precocious puberty. Subsequently, an adult pattern of 17-ketosteroid excretion develops, consistent with the developmental rather than chronologic age.

17-Ketosteroids

Early maturation with high levels of urinary 17-ketosteroids may be due to testicular tumors or, more commonly, to adrenal cortical hyperplasia. The 17-ketosteroid levels are especially high with congenital adrenal hyperplasia (adrenogenital syndrome) or tumors. In contrast to the full maturation produced by pituitary or constitutional precocious puberty, androgen overproduction does not stimulate spermatogenesis and the testes remain preadolescent in size. Urinary gonadotropins are virtually absent, presumably due to high levels of functioning hormones.

Tumors

Hormonally active testicular tumors are relatively rare even in adults.

Choriocarcinoma and those teratomas that contain chorionic elements may produce chorionic gonadotropin, which gives a positive reaction in a "pregnancy test." Patients with such tumors also have elevated levels of urinary estrogens. Tumors of the interstitial cells may produce androgen or estrogen or both. In prepubertal boys, interstitial cell tumors cause precocious development of male secondary sex characteristics, but androgen excess causes little clinical change in mature men. The rare estrogen-producing tumors are associated with gynecomastia and decrease of libido and testicular size.

SEMEN EXAMINATION

Evaluation of an infertile couple should include examination of the seminal fluid within one or two hours of ejaculation. Because rubber condoms may damage the spermatic morphology and motility and because coitus interruptus may cause the first portion of the ejaculate to be lost, masturbation is probably the best means of obtaining the specimen.

The ejaculate should be evaluated for quantity, viscosity, sperm count, and morphology and motility of the sperm. Normal volume is 3 to 5 ml; both smaller volumes (1 to 2 ml) and larger volumes (6 to 10 ml) are associated with lessened fertility for reasons not presently clear. The normal sperm count is approximately 60 to 250 million per ml, but documented impregnation has occurred with lower counts, and several authorities[38,67] mention 6 to 10 million per ml as the lowest possible limits at which conception is possible.

Motility and morphology must necessarily be evaluated subjectively. The combined effects of motility, morphology, and total sperm count influence fertility, and a high percentage of inactive or bizarre sperm is associated with decreased fertility. The viscosity of the seminal fluid may vary. The presence of a coagulum is very common shortly after ejaculation, but as this normally liquifies within a few minutes, failure to liquify should be considered abnormal.

Testicular biopsy may be indicated if the ejaculate contains no sperm at all, since there is always the possibility that an abnormality of the epididymis or vas deferens is preventing emission of normally produced sperm. Male infertility is difficult to evaluate and highly uncertain to treat. In primary spermatogenic arrest, FSH levels are persistently high, indicating that successful spermatogenesis exerts a negative feedback on FSH production.[22] The levels of LH cannot be reliably correlated with sperm production, and hormonal manipulation has not been successful in correcting abnormalities of spermatogenesis.

BIBLIOGRAPHY

1. ASTWOOD, E.B.: "Anterior pituitary hormones and related substances," *In* Goodman, L.S., and Gilman, A. (eds.): The Pharmacological Basis of Therapeutics, ed. 4. Macmillan Co., New York, 1970.
2. AXELROD, J., AND WEINSHILBOUM, R.: Catecholamines. N. Engl. J. Med. 287:237, 1972.
3. BARTTER, F.C., AND SCHWARTZ, W.B.: The syndrome of inappropriate secretion of antidiuretic hormone. Am. J. Med. 42:790, 1967.
4. BEIERWALTES, W.H.: Thyroiditis. Ann. N. Y. Acad. Sci. 124:586, 1965.
5. BERNSTEIN, D.S., AND THORN, G.W.: "Diseases of the parathyroid glands," *In* Wintrobe, M.M., Thorn, G.W., Adams, R.D. et al. (eds.): Harrison's Principles of Internal Medicine, ed. 6. McGraw-Hill Book Co., New York, 1970.
6. CIVANTOS, F., AND RYWLIN, A.M.: Carcinomas with trophoblastic differentiation and secretion of chorionic gonadotrophins. Cancer 29:789, 1972.
7. CLARK, F., AND HORN, D.B.: Assessment of thyroid function by the combined use of the serum protein-bound iodine and resin uptake of ^{131}I-triiodothyronine. J. Clin. Endocrinol. Metab. 25:39, 1965.
8. CONN, J.W., COHEN, E.L., ROVNER, D.R., AND NESBIT, R.M.: Normokalemic primary aldosteronism. J.A.M.A. 193:200, 1965.
9. CRIGLER, J.F., JR., ROSEMBERG, E., AND THORN, G.W.: "Diseases of the testes," *In* Wintrobe, M.M., Thorn, G.W., Adams, R.D. et al. (eds.): Harrison's Principles of Internal Medicine, ed. 6. McGraw-Hill Book Co., New York, 1970.
10. DAUGHADAY, W.H.: "The adenohypophysis," *In* Williams, R.H. (ed.): Textbook of Endocrinology, ed. 4. W.B. Saunders Co., Philadelphia, 1968.
11. DUARTE, C.G., WINNACKER, J.L., BECKER, K.L. ET AL.: Thiazide-induced hypercalcemia. N. Engl. J. Med. 284:828, 1971.
12. DUVIGNEAUD, V.: Trail of sulfur research: from insulin to oxytocin. Science 123:967, 1956.
13. EMMER, M., GORDEN, P., AND ROTH, J.: Diabetes in association with other endocrine disorders. Med. Clin. North Am. 55:1057, 1971.
14. FAJANS, S.S.: What is diabetes? Med. Clin. North Am. 55:793, 1971.
15. FELIG, P.: Pathophysiology of diabetes mellitus. Med. Clin. North Am. 55:821, 1971.
16. FITZGERALD, M.G., AND KEEN, H.: Diagnostic classification of diabetes. Br. Med. J. 2:1568, 1964.
17. FORBES, A.P., HENNEMAN, P.H., GRISWOLD, G.L., AND ALBRIGHT, F.: Syndrome characterized by galactorrhea, amenorrhea and low urinary FSH: comparison with acromegaly and normal lactation. J. Clin. Endocrinol. 14:265, 1954.
18. FORE, W., AND WYNN, J.: The thyrotropin stimulation test. Am. J. Med. 40:90, 1966.
19. FORSHAM, P.H.: "The adrenal cortex," *In* Williams, R.H. (ed.): Textbook of Endocrinology, ed. 4. W.B. Saunders Co., Philadelphia, 1968.
20. FOWLER, P.B.S., SWALE, J., AND ANDREWS, H.: Hypercholesterolemia in borderline hypothyroidism: stage of premyxoedema. Lancet 2:488, 1970.
21. FRANCHIMONT, P.: Human gonadotrophin secretion. J. R. Coll. Physic. London 6:283, 1972.
22. FRANCHIMONT, P., MILLET, D., VENDRELY, E. ET AL.: Relationship between spermatogenesis and serum gonadotropin levels in azoospermia and oligospermia. J. Clin. Endocrinol. Metab. 34:1003, 1972.
23. GOLD, E.M., DIRAIMONDO, V.C., AND FORSHAM, P.H.: Quantitation of pituitary corticotropin reserve in man by use of an adrenocortical 11-beta hydroxylase inhibitor (SU-4885). Metabolism 9:3, 1960.
24. GOLDSMITH, R.S.: Treatment of hypercalcemia. Med. Clin. North Am. 56:951, 1972.
25. GRAYSON, R.R.: Factors which influence the radioactive iodine thyroidal uptake test. Am. J. Med. 28:397, 1960.
26. GREGORY, R.A., GROSSMAN, M.I., TRACY, H.J., AND BENTLEY, P.H.: Nature of gastric secretagogue in Zollinger-Ellison tumors. Lancet 2:543, 1967.

27. GRIFFITHS, P.D.: Serum enzymes in diseases of the thyroid gland. J. Clin. Pathol. 18:660, 1965.
28. HARVEY, R.F.: Indices of thyroid function in thyrotoxicosis. Lancet 2:230, 1971.
29. HICKLER, R.B., AND THORN, G.W.: "Pheochromocytoma," *In* Wintrobe, M.M., Thorn, G.W., Adams, R.D. et al. (eds.): Harrison's Principles of Internal Medicine. ed. 6. McGraw-Hill Book Co., New York, 1970.
30. INGBAR, S.H., AND WOEBER, K.A.: "The thyroid gland," *In* Williams, R.H. (ed.): Textbook of Endocrinology, ed. 4. W.B. Saunders Co., Philadelphia, 1968.
31. KLIMT, C.R. ET AL.: Standardization of the oral glucose tolerance test. Report of the Committee on Statistics of the American Diabetes Association, June 14, 1968. Diabetes 18:299, 1969.
32. KOPPERS, L.E., AND PALUMBO, P.J.: Lipid disturbances in endocrine disorders. Med. Clin. North Am. 56:1013, 1972.
33. KRISS, J.P., PLESHAKOV, V., ROSENBLUM, A.L. ET AL.: Studies on the pathogenesis of the ophthalmopathy of Graves' disease. J. Clin. Endocrinol. 27:582, 1967.
34. LAULER, D.P.: Pre-operative diagnosis of primary aldosteronism. Am. J. Med. 41:855, 1966.
35. LAULER, D.P., WILLIAMS, G.H., AND THORN, G.W.: "Diseases of the adrenal cortex," *In* Wintrobe, M.M., Thorn, G.W., Adams, R.D. et al. (eds.): Harrison's Principles of Internal Medicine, ed. 6. McGraw-Hill Book Co., New York, 1970.
36. LEAF, A., AND COGGINS, C.H.: "The neurohypophysis," *In* Williams, R.H. (ed.): Textbook of Endocrinology, ed. 4. W.B. Saunders Co., Philadelphia, 1968.
37. LLOYD, C.W.: "The ovaries," *In* Williams, R.H. (ed.): Textbook of Endocrinology, ed. 4. W.B. Saunders Co., Philadelphia, 1968.
38. MACLEOD, J.: The semen examination. Clin. Obstet. Gynecol. 8:115, 1965.
39. MCARTHUR, J.W.: "Diseases of the ovary," *In* Wintrobe, M.M., Thorn, G.W., Adams, R.D. et al. (eds.): Harrison's Principles of Internal Medicine, ed. 6. McGraw-Hill Book Co., New York, 1970.
40. MCGUIGAN, J.E., AND TRUDEAU, W.L.: Immunochemical measurement of elevated levels of gastrin in the serum of patients with pancreatic tumors of the Zollinger-Ellison variety. N. Engl. J. Med. 278:1308, 1968.
41. MELMON, K.L.: "Catecholamines and the adrenal medulla," *In* Williams, R.H. (ed.): Textbook of Endocrinology, ed. 4. W.B. Saunders Co., Philadelphia, 1968.
42. MULROW, P.J.: The adrenal cortex. Annu. Rev. Physiol. 34:409, 1972.
43. NELSON, D.H., AND THORN, G.W.: "Diseases of the anterior lobe of the pituitary gland," *In* Wintrobe, M.M., Thorn, G.W., Adams, R.D. et al. (eds.): Harrison's Principles of Internal Medicine, ed. 6. McGraw-Hill Book Co., New York, 1970.
44. ONTJES, D.A., AND NEY, R.L.: Tests of anterior pituitary function. Metabolism 21:159, 1972.
45. O'SULLIVAN, J.B., AND MAHAN, C.M.: Prospective study of 352 young patients with chemical diabetes. N. Engl. J. Med. 278:1038, 1968.
46. PAULSEN, C.A.: "The testes," *In* Williams, R.H. (ed.): Textbook of Endocrinology, ed. 4. W.B. Saunders Co., Philadelphia, 1968.
47. PILEGGI, V.J., AND LEE, N.D.: Laboratory Aids in Thyroid Problems. Bio-Science Laboratories, Van Nuys, Calif., 1970.
48. PTAK, T., AND KIRSNER, J.B.: The Zollinger-Ellison syndrome, polyendocrine adenomatosis, and other endocrine associations with peptic ulcer. Adv. Intern. Med. 16:213, 1970.
49. RASMUSSEN, H.: "The parathyroids," *In* Williams, R.H. (ed.): Textbook of Endocrinology, ed. 4. W.B. Saunders Co., Philadelphia, 1968.
50. SAYERS, G., AND TRAVIS, R.H.: "Adrenocorticotropic hormone; adrenocortical steroids and their synthetic analogs," *In* Goodman, L.S., and Gilman, A. (eds.): The Pharmacological Basis of Therapeutics, ed. 4. Macmillan Co., New York, 1970.
51. SCHOLZ, D.A., PURNELL, D.C., GOLDSMITH, R.S. ET AL.: Diagnostic considerations in hypercalcemic syndromes. Med. Clin. North Am. 56:941, 1972.

52. SCHWARTZ, N.B., AND McCORMACK, C.E.: Reproduction: Gonadal function and its regulation. Annu. Rev. Physiol. 34:425, 1972.

53. SELENKOW, H.A., AND INGBAR, S.H.: "Diseases of the thyroid," In Wintrobe, M.M., Thorn, G.W., Adams, R.D. et al. (eds.): Harrison's Principles of Internal Medicine, ed. 6. McGraw-Hill Book Co., New York, 1970.

54. SHERWOOD, L.M., O'RIORDAN, J.L.H., AURBACH, G.D. ET AL.: Production of parathyroid hormone by nonparathyroid tumors. J. Clin. Endocrinol. Metab. 27:140, 1967.

55. SHIMODA, S.S., SAUNDERS, D.R., AND RUBIN, C.E.: The Zollinger-Ellison syndrome with steatorrhea. II. The mechanism of fat and vitamin B_{12} malabsorption. Gastroenterology 55:705, 1968.

56. SHULMAN, S.: Thyroid antigens and autoimmunity. Adv. Immunol. 14:85, 1971.

57. STERLING, K., AND BRENNER, M.A.: Free thyroxine in human serum: Simplified measurement with the aid of magnesium precipitation. J. Clin. Invest. 45:153, 1966.

58. SUNDERMAN, F.W., JR.: Measurements of vanilmandelic acid for the diagnosis of pheochromocytoma and neuroblastoma. Am. J. Clin. Pathol. 42:481, 1964.

59. TAIT, S.A.S., AND TAIT, J.F.: "Assay of aldosterone and metabolites," In Dorfman, R.I. (ed.): Methods in Hormone Research. Academic Press, New York, 1962.

60. THOMAS, J.E., ROOKE, E.D., AND KVALE, W.F.: The neurologist's experience with pheochromocytoma. J.A.M.A. 197:754, 1965.

61. TUCCI, J.R., JAGGER, P.I., LAULER, D.P., AND THORN, G.W.: Rapid dexamethasone suppression test for Cushing's syndrome. J.A.M.A. 199:379, 1967.

62. WAKIM, K.G.: Reassessment of the source, mode and locus of action of antidiuretic hormone. Am. J. Med. 42:394, 1967.

63. WELT, L.G.: "Disorders of fluids and electrolytes," In Wintrobe, M.M., Thorn, G.W., Adams, R.D. et al. (eds.): Harrison's Principles of Internal Medicine, ed. 6. McGraw-Hill Book Co., New York, 1970.

64. WILLIAMS, D.L., AND RUNYAN, J.W., JR.: Sex chromatin and chromosome analysis in the diagnosis of sex abnormalities. Ann. Intern. Med. 64:422, 1966.

65. WISENBAUGH, P.E., GARST, J.B., HULL, C. ET AL.: Renin, aldosterone, sodium, and hypertension. Am. J. Med. 52:175, 1972.

66. WOLFF, J., STANDAERT, M.E., AND RALL, J.E.: Thyroxine displacement from serum proteins and depression of serum protein-bound iodine by certain drugs. J. Clin. Invest. 40:1373, 1961.

67. ZORGNIOTTI, A.W., AND HOTCHKISS, R.S.: Male infertility. Clin. Obstet. Gynecol. 8:128, 1965.

CHAPTER 17

Pregnancy

Pregnancy deserves a chapter to itself since the condition is neither a disease nor a normal state. Although the etiology is straightforward, the physiologic changes are complex.

TESTS FOR THE EXISTENCE OF PREGNANCY

Fertilization occurs within several days of ovulation, at the mid-point of the menstrual cycle. The fertilized ovum floats down the fallopian tube into the uterus, where it implants on the welcoming secretory endometrium. Shortly after implantation, at the twenty-first to twenty-third day of the cycle, chorionic gonadotropin production begins.[15] Virtually all laboratory tests for the diagnosis of pregnancy measure the presence of chorionic gonadotropin, a hormone unique to the trophoblast.

Until the 1960's, pregnancy tests were bioassays, in which the presence of human chorionic gonadotropin (HCG) in serum or urine was demonstrated by its effect on animals. The earliest tests used mice and rabbits; subsequent tests used female rats or male frogs. These biologic tests have now been largely supplanted by immunologic tests which are more accurate, easier to perform, and do not require the laboratory to maintain animal facilities. In addition, the results are less subject to artefactual distortion by drugs the patient may be taking.[8]

PRINCIPLE OF IMMUNOLOGIC TESTS

The immunologic tests rely upon commercially available anti-human chorionic gonadotropin antibody (anti-HCG). The presence of HCG in serum or urine is documented by alteration in antibody activity, as shown by an indicator system. Red cells or latex particles are coated with human chorionic gonadotropin in such a concentration that unmistakable agglutination occurs upon contact with the antibody. When the test is performed, the patient's serum or urine is incubated with the antibody; HCG, if present, reacts with and thereby inactivates the antibody. The incubated antibody-sample mixture is then added to the indicator. If HCG was present in the sample, the antibody is inactivated, and the red cells or particles remain unagglutinated. If the sample does not contain HCG, the antibody remains active, and agglutination occurs (Fig. 23). Commercial testing kits include positive and negative control samples along with the vial of anti-HCG.

Results of Immunologic Testing

Immunologic tests have an accuracy rate of 95 to 99 per cent as compared with a range of 65 to 97 per cent accuracy with the rat ovarian hyperemia test.[8,19] Because the immunologic tests are sensitive to lower concentrations of HCG than the bioassays, the test becomes positive earlier in the pregnancy. Positives have been reported as early as 16 days after ovulation (two days after the first missed period), and most tests are reliable at three weeks after the first missed period. The tests with red cell indicators tend to be more sensitive than those which use latex particles. Since chorionic gonadotropin has some immunologic resemblance to the luteinizing hormone (LH) of the pituitary, some cross-reactivity occurs, and excessively sensitive tests would be subject to false positives from high levels of LH. Immunologic tests can be quantitated by diluting the urine or serum sample and comparing it with control dilutions of known potency.

Pregnancy tests should be performed on the first voided morning specimen, since this is the most concentrated urine. Although quantitative study of 24-hour samples is necessary to measure total hormonal excretion, the level in the first morning specimen parallels fairly closely the range of total excretion.

Value of Assay Procedures

Since immunologic assay is so much easier to perform than bioassay, serial determinations of HCG levels are simple and practical for studying women suspected of abnormal pregnancy or malignant trophoblastic disease. As a rule, less HCG is excreted in ectopic than in normal pregnancies. Only two thirds of women with ectopic pregnancy have positive pregnancy tests,[7] and in these, the titer is relatively low.

Abortion is followed by a prompt fall in HCG excretion. In women

PRINCIPLE OF AGGLUTINATION INHIBITION TESTS

rticles or red cells coated with
nan chorionic gonadotropin(HCG).

Antibody to HCG, produced by
injecting purified hormone into
rabbits or guinea pigs.

When antibody and antigen combine,
the particles are agglutinated.

POSITIVE PREGNANCY TEST

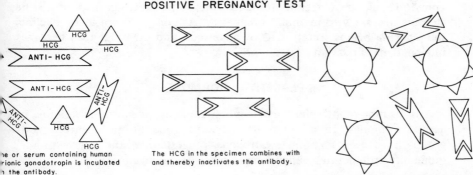

ne or serum containing human
rionic gonadotropin is incubated
n the antibody.

The HCG in the specimen combines with
and thereby inactivates the antibody.

The inactivated antibody cannot combine with
the HCG on the cells, so agglutination does
not occur.

NEGATIVE PREGNANCY TEST

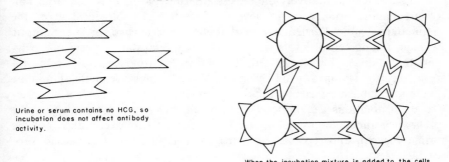

Urine or serum contains no HCG, so
incubation does not affect antibody
activity.

When the incubation mixture is added to the cells
or particles, the antibody is still active and
agglutination occurs.

Figure 23. Presence of chorionic gonadotropin is demonstrated when activity of an agglutinating antibody is inhibited. This principle of agglutination inhibition is used in many serologic tests.

with a previous history of abortion, serial determinations during the first trimester are especially useful during episodes of vaginal spotting. If the HCG level remains high during an episode of spotting, the pregnancy is likely to continue.[31] Since the range of values varies from one woman to another, a single determination provides little prognostic information, but repeated tests can establish the curve for any particular woman. In women with hydatidiform mole or choriocarcinoma, or in men with trophoblastic tumors of the testis, repeated HCG assays can indicate the success of therapy or the presence of recurrence.

Chorionic gonadotropin excretion reaches its peak at the twelfth to fourteenth week of gestation, and thereafter falls to a fairly constant level of about 20,000 IU per 24 hours[15] for the rest of the pregnancy. By secreting gonadotropin, the placenta stimulates the corpus luteum to produce the steroids necessary to maintain pregnancy. As gonadotropin levels decline, the placenta begins secreting its own steroids, and the pregnancy becomes independent of ovarian protection.

PLACENTAL HORMONES

In its nine-month life, the placenta manufactures enormous volumes of active hormones. In addition to chorionic gonadotropins, three major groups have been identified: estrogens, progesterone, and a growth-hormone-like protein often called human placental lactogen (HPL).

ESTRIOL

Estriol is quantitatively the most significant estrogen. In the latter half of pregnancy, urinary estriol levels reflect the physiologic state of the fetomaternal unit. Particularly in diabetic, hypertensive, or preeclamptic women, falling estriol levels signal impending fetal damage and may suggest that delivery be accelerated, if possible.[1,22] Urinary estriol levels vary from day to day in any one woman, so serial measurements should be made to establish a baseline trend in pregnancies at risk. Thereafter, interval determinations can better be evaluated. Whatever is threatening the pregnancy affects the estriol levels. The drop in estriol excretion is not the primary event, and replacement estrogen therapy does not alter the process.[13]

PROGESTERONE

Progesterone production increases as pregnancy progresses, the greatest increment occurring after 28 weeks.[28] Urinary excretion of pregnanediol, the chief excretory metabolite of progesterone, is the most accessible index of hormonal levels. Fetal death results in diminished pregnanediol excretion, but the normal range varies widely and physiologic responsiveness is only moderate. Placental function may continue after fetal death, causing pregnanediol levels to remain high.

HUMAN PLACENTAL LACTOGEN

Human placental lactogen (HPL) is a relative newcomer to the endocrinologic scene.[30] Both functionally and structurally it resembles human growth hormone, but its physiologic actions appear to affect only the mother, and not the growing conceptus.[10] The name may be misleading, for lactogenic activity has been documented only in lower animals. In humans, the documented metabolic effects have more nearly resembled growth hormone, and other proposed names have been chorionic growth hormone-prolactin (CGP) and human chorionic somatomammotropin (HCS).[9]

The placenta manufactures 3 or 4 Gm of this hormone each day. Like growth hormone, its effects on carbohydrate, fat, and protein metabolism result in increased plasma insulin levels, reduced gluconeogenesis, increased protein synthesis, and increased levels of circulating free fatty acids. By promoting fatty acid metabolism in the mother, it may leave more glucose available for the fetus, which appears capable of using only glucose for its energy needs.[10] Radioimmunoassay can be used to measure HPL in serum, urine, amniotic fluid, or placenta, but no direct clinical applications of this procedure seem imminent.

PHYSIOLOGIC CHANGES ASSOCIATED WITH PREGNANCY

Pregnancy alters body function in many ways, so that many normal values do not apply to pregnant women who may nevertheless be perfectly healthy.

HEMATOLOGIC CHANGES IN PREGNANCY

Hemodilution

Both red cell mass and plasma volume increase with pregnancy, but plasma volume outstrips red cell production and the hematocrit tends to fall. There is considerable debate about the "physiologic anemia" of pregnancy. Many authorities consider hemoglobin values above 10 Gm per 100 ml to be normal, but this does not necessarily mean 10 Gm per 100 ml is the optimal concentration.

The body's water content increases during pregnancy, and the ability to excrete a water load diminishes. Accompanying this expansion of blood volume are increased renal plasma flow and accelerated glomerular filtration rate. This volume expansion causes hemodilution, but other factors may also contribute to the lowered hematocrit. The most serious consideration is iron deficiency, especially in women who have had several pregnancies, and low hematocrit should not be ascribed solely to hemodilution until iron deficiency has been ruled out.

Iron Deficiency

Examination of a stained blood smear is helpful in studying anemia. If iron stores are deficient, the red cells are small, pale, and frequently of variable shape. Corpuscular indices can indicate cell size and hemoglobin content, but often simple examination of the stained smear is sufficient. The smear can be stained for the presence of cells (siderocytes) containing granules of iron, which are present if the bone marrow contains adequate iron supplies. Serum iron levels do not change significantly in normal pregnancy, so demonstration of low serum iron and high serum iron-binding capacity establishes the diagnosis of iron deficiency in pregnant as well as nonpregnant women.

Megaloblastic Anemia

Certain changes are common in pregnancy but not normal. The most frequent of these is iron-deficiency anemia. Another frequent problem of pregnancy is folic acid deficiency. Since folic acid is essential for nuclear development, the rapidly growing fetus parasitizes large supplies of folic acid from the mother. Combined deficiency of iron and folic acid is very common,[2] particularly in multiparous women with poor or borderline dietary habits. In pregnancy, absorption of vitamin B_{12} becomes less effective, and fetal demands tax the maternal supply so that vitamin B_{12} deficiency may also be a problem.

Changes in Coagulation Values

The coagulation mechanism undergoes slight but consistent changes during normal pregnancy. Talbert and Langdell[29] report the greatest alteration in fibrinogen levels, which may reach 550 to 600 mg per 100 ml during the last trimester. Since fibrinogen is elevated and fibrinolytic activity is somewhat less than in the nonpregnant state,[11] some workers believe a predisposition exists toward disseminated intravascular coagulation.[26] Although no direct etiologic connection has been established, women with eclampsia or preeclampsia often have laboratory findings associated with intravascular coagulation/fibrinolysis, namely increased circulating fibrinogen degradation products, and decreased platelets.[4,5] In uncomplicated pregnancies, platelet values remain stable, and there may be slight shortening of the one-stage prothrombin time and the partial thromboplastin time.

White Cell and Other Changes

In the last half of pregnancy, the white count rises, and counts of 15,000 per cu mm are within normal limits.[24] Since the increase is largely of granulocytes, the resulting neutrophilia may suggest the presence of infection. Pregnant women are particularly prone to urinary tract infections, so neutrophilia of more than minimal degree should be investigated. Leukocyte alkaline phosphatase content rises very shortly after conception, but since the enzyme's function in the granulocytes is not understood, the significance of the elevation cannot be explained. The erythrocyte sedimentation rate may rise to as much as 30 mm per hour, probably due largely to increased plasma fibrinogen content.

ENDOCRINE CHANGES

Adrenal Steroids

Plasma cortisol levels rise during the latter half of pregnancy, but the circadian secretion pattern is only moderately altered[6] and signs of hyperadrenalism are absent. The plasma level rises because of the estrogen-induced increase in transcortin, the cortisol-binding protein which normally carries 80 per cent of the circulating hormone. Whether or not free cortisol, the metabolically active form, increases during pregnancy remains a subject of considerable debate.[17,26]

Aldosterone, the potent sodium-conserving, potassium-depleting adrenal hormone, is increased throughout pregnancy. Pregnant women do not, however, lose potassium excessively, and aldosterone secretion remains normally responsive to changes in whole body sodium,[26] even though basal levels are high. Aldosterone secretion falls in preeclampsia, declining to nonpregnant levels or below in severe eclampsia.[16] The cause and the significance of aldosterone elevation remain under scrutiny. Progesterone, present in large quantities during pregnancy, has aldosterone-inhibiting effects, so aldosterone may rise in compensation. Another possibility is that the increase may be a response to the increased amounts of renin and renin substrate that accompany pregnancy.

Thyroid Function

The most far-reaching and interesting endocrine changes relate to the thyroid gland. Pregnancy has been called a *forme fruste* of hyperthyroidism,[25] and most signs of hyperthyroidism can be found in pregnancy. Basal metabolic rate rises with pregnancy, sometimes reaching +25 per cent by the end of gestation. Since the pregnant woman is metabolizing for two and rapid tissue growth increases the metabolic rate, the rise with pregnancy is hardly surprising. Expanded blood volume and increased cardiac work load also affect oxygen consumption.

A completely different mechanism is invoked to explain the elevations in PBI and circulating thyroxine level, with lowered T_3 uptake in the second half of pregnancy. Among the serum protein alterations of pregnancy is an increase in thyroid-binding globulin. This permits increased quantities of thyroxine to be bound. Since it is the free fraction of thyroxine that is metabolically active, and the quantity of free thyroxine changes very little, increased levels of circulating hormone do not produce hyperthyroidism. This increase in thyroid-binding globulin causes a low resin T_3 uptake because more globulin is available to bind added hormone. A similar high PBI and low T_3 uptake occurs in women taking estrogen preparations as contraceptives, so thyroid function studies on young women should be interpreted with this caution in mind.

During pregnancy, thyroidal iodine uptake is increased and hormone production is augmented. This may be necessary to maintain the heightened metabolic rate of pregnancy, or perhaps the additional glandular activity simply produces the extra thyroxine that is bound to the extra thyroid-binding globulin. Changes in radioactive iodine uptake results should not cause difficulties in evaluating thyroid status during pregnancy, for radioactive iodine should not be given to women known to be pregnant. Radioactive iodine, like stable iodine and most of the antithyroid drugs, readily crosses the placenta, and management of thyroid disease in pregnancy must include appropriate observation of the newborn infant.

The increase in thyroid-binding globulin continues as long as the pregnancy continues. In the latter half of pregnancy, a fall in the previously elevated level of protein-bound iodine suggests impending abortion. The range of normal values is wide, so that a single relatively low value should not be overinterpreted. The decline precedes loss of the pregnancy, so once an individual's level has been established, the test may have predictive value. The change in thyroid function tests is an effect, not the cause, of physiologic abnormality, and treatment with thyroid hormone restores to normal neither the tests nor the pregnancy.

LIVER FUNCTION TESTS IN PREGNANCY

The most consistent pregnancy-associated alteration in conventional tests of liver function is elevation of alkaline phosphatase. In the last trimester, alkaline phosphatase levels may be double or triple the nonpregnant level, commonly reaching values to 19 or 20 King-Armstrong units.[3,21] Physicochemical and immunologic tests strongly suggest that the additional hormone derives from the placenta and is quite independent of hepatic function. Unlike thyroid-binding globulin or transcortin, alkaline phosphatase increases only in pregnant women and not in women with trophoblastic disease or those taking estrogens.[23]

Pregnancy produces increased circulating α_2 and β globulin levels, with a fall in albumin levels as great as 1 Gm per 100 ml. This may cause turbidity tests such as cephalin flocculation and thymol turbidity, which reflect proportions of albumin and globulins, to become positive. Serum protein electrophoresis quantifies these alterations. The transaminases, lactic dehydrogenase, and bilirubin are not affected by pregnancy per se, but rise in women with recurrent cholestatic jaundice of pregnancy. The intrauterine hemolysis occurring in severe hemolytic disease of the newborn does not elevate maternal bilirubin levels. Serum cholesterol levels characteristically rise in the fourth through eighth months. Since cholesterol is a precursor for progesterone and other steroid hormones, it is tempting to assign the rising cholesterol levels to increased need for steroid precursors, but net cholesterol levels result from complex interactions of hepatic, pituitary, adrenal, placental, and thyroid metabolism, so this explanation may be simplistic.

RENAL FUNCTION IN PREGNANCY

The calyceal, pelvic, and ureteral dilatation and reduced motility that accompany pregnancy probably result more from hormonal effects than mechanical obstruction. Besides increasing stasis and the risks of infection, this increased dead space, which may achieve volumes as great as 200 ml,[14] makes accurate urinary flow and clearance measurements quite difficult.

Glomerular filtration rate and renal plasma flow rise by as much as 50 per cent over nonpregnant levels. Production of nitrogenous compounds does not rise, so the increased flow lowers serum values for urea, creatinine, and uric acid. Thus, in pregnancy, findings in the "normal" or "high-normal" range constitute pathologic increases. Increasing uric acid values in later pregnancy usually signal preeclampsia.[18] Changes in sodium metabolism remain poorly understood. Net sodium content is increased over the nonpregnant state, but this may simply reflect volume change introduced by the conceptus, rather than insidious salt retention by the mother. The increased aldosterone secretion characteristic of pregnancy drops off in preeclampsia,[26] as does the glomerular filtration rate.

Glycosuria on random urine samples is so common in pregnancy that some workers question whether it means anything.[27] Glucose spilling may result from reduced tubular reabsorption or from inability to keep up with increased solute load caused by increased GFR. Investigation of random glycosuria reveals latent or gestational diabetes in many pregnant patients, and each physician must assess the test and its significance for each patient.

Bacteriuria is a common complication, and reduced upper urinary tract motility, changes in urine glucose, and alterations in potassium metabolism probably all play a role. Bacteriuria in pregnancy is particularly common among certain groups, namely women over 35, those with sickle cell trait, those with diabetes, and those in lower socioeconomic groups. Since complications of various kinds are common in these populations, the specific causal factors become difficult to unravel. Bacteriuria frequently complicates unsuspected underlying renal disease. The demonstration of bacteriuria, particularly when recurrent or resistant, should lead to thorough urinary tract and metabolic evaluation.

BIBLIOGRAPHY

1. BELING, C.G.: "Estrogens," In Fuchs, F., and Klopper, A. (eds.): Endocrinology of Pregnancy. Harper & Row, New York, 1971.
2. BENJAMIN, F., BASSEN, F.A., AND MEYER, L.M.: Serum levels of folic acid, vitamin B_{12} and iron in anemia of pregnancy. Am. J. Obstet. Gynecol. 96:310, 1966.
3. BIRKETT, D.J., DONE, J., NEALE, F.C., AND POSEN, S.: Serum alkaline phosphatase in pregnancy: an immunologic study. Br. Med. J. 1:1210, 1966.
4. BIRMINGHAM ECLAMPSIA STUDY GROUP: Intravascular coagulation and abnormal lung-scans in pre-eclampsia and eclampsia. Lancet 2:889, 1971.
5. BONNAR, J., DAVIDSON, J.F., PIDGEON, C.F., AND McNICOLS, G.P.: Fibrin degradation products in normal and abnormal pregnancy and parturition. Br. Med. J. 3:137, 1969.
6. BURKE, C.W., AND ROULET, F.: Increased exposure of tissues to cortisol in late pregnancy. Br. Med. J. 1:657, 1970.
7. GLASS, R.H., AND JESURN, H.M.: Immunologic pregnancy tests in ectopic pregnancy. Obstet. Gynecol. 27:66, 1966.
8. HENRY, J.B., LITTLE, W.A., AND CHRISTIAN, C.D.: Modified immunologic test for pregnancy. Am. J. Clin. Pathol. 42:109, 1964.
9. JAFFE, R.B.: Endocrine interactions and the placenta. Hosp. Pract. 6:71, 1971.
10. JOSIMOVICH, J.B.: "Placental lactogenic hormone," In Fuchs, F., and Klopper, A. (eds.): Endocrinology of Pregnancy. Harper & Row, New York, 1971.
11. KLEINER, G.J., MERSKEY, C., JOHNSON, A.J., AND MARKUS, W.B.: Defibrination in normal and abnormal parturition. Br. J. Haematol. 19:159, 1970.
12. KLOPPER, A.: The assessment of feto-placental function by estriol assay. Obstet. Gynecol. 23:813, 1968.
13. KLOPPER, A.: "Endocrine factors in abortion and premature labor," In Fuchs, F., and Klopper, A., (eds.): Endocrinology of Pregnancy. Harper & Row, New York, 1971.
14. LINDHEIMER, M.D., AND KUTZ, A.I.: The kidney in pregnancy. N. Engl. J. Med. 283:1095, 1970.

15. LLOYD, C.W.: "The ovaries," *In* Williams, R.H. (ed.): Textbook of Endocrinology, ed. 4. W.B. Saunders Co., Philadelphia, 1968.
16. MULROW, P.J.: "Renin-angiotensin-aldosterone and toxemia of pregnancy," *In* Fuchs, F., and Klopper, A. (eds.): Endocrinology of Pregnancy, Harper & Row, New York, 1971.
17. PETERSON, R.E.: "Cortisol," *In* Fuchs, F., and Klopper, A. (eds.): Endocrinology of Pregnancy. Harper & Row, New York, 1971.
18. POLLAK, V.E., AND NETTLES, J.B.: The kidney in toxemia of pregnancy: A clinical and pathologic study based on renal biopsies. Medicine 39:469, 1960.
19. POWELL, J., STEVENS, V.C., DICKEY, R.P., AND ULLERY, J.C.: Immunologic pregnancy testing in urine and serum. Am. J. Obstet. Gynecol. 96:844, 1966.
20. PROUT, T.: Thyroid disease in pregnancy. Am. J. Obstet. Gynecol. 96:148, 1966.
21. RICHMAN, A.: "The liver," *In* Rovinsky, J.J., and Guttmacher, A.F. (eds.): Medical, Surgical, and Gynecologic Complications of Pregnancy, ed. 2. Williams & Wilkins Co., Baltimore, 1965.
22. RIVLIN, M.E., MESTMAN, J.H., HALL, T.D. ET AL.: Value of estriol estimations in the management of diabetic pregnancy. Am. J. Obstet. Gynecol. 106:875, 1970.
23. ROBINSON, J.C., LONDON, W.T., AND PIERCE, J.E.: Observations on the origin of pregnancy-associated plasma proteins. Am. J. Obstet. Gynecol. 96:226, 1966.
24. SANDERS, M.: "Hematologic complications," *In* Rovinsky, J. J., and Guttmacher, A.F. (eds.): Medical, Surgical, and Gynecologic Complications of Pregnancy, ed. 2. Williams & Wilkins Co., Baltimore, 1965.
25. SILVER, S.: "The thyroid gland," *In* Rovinsky, J.J., and Guttmacher, A. F. (eds.): Medical, Surgical, and Gynecologic Complications of Pregnancy, ed. 2. Williams & Wilkins Co., Baltimore, 1965.
26. SIMS, E.A.H.: Pre-eclampsia and related complications of pregnancy. Am. J. Obstet. Gynecol. 107:154, 1970.
27. SIMS, E.A.H.: "The kidney in pregnancy," *In* Strauss, M.B., and Welt, L.G. (eds.): Diseases of the Kidney, ed. 2. Little, Brown & Co., Boston, 1971.
28. SOLOMON, S., AND FUCHS, F.: "Progesterone and related neutral steroids," *In* Fuchs, F., and Klopper, A. (eds.): Endocrinology of Pregnancy. Harper & Row, New York, 1971.
29. TALBERT, L.M., AND LANGDELL, R.D.: Normal values of certain factors in the blood clotting mechanisms in pregnancy. Am. J. Obstet. Gynecol. 90:44, 1964.
30. VILLEE, D.B.: Development of endocrine function in the human placenta and fetus. N. Engl. J. Med. 281:473, 1969.
31. WHITELAW, M.J., AND NOLA, V.F.: Accuracy of the immunologic pregnancy test in early pregnancy and abortion. Obstet. Gynecol. 27:69, 1966.

CHAPTER 18

Diseases Due to Inborn
Metabolic Abnormalities

A large, diverse group of diseases originates from malfunction or absence of some normally present metabolic activity. The genetic basis for many has been documented from family studies. Specific enzyme defects can be attributed to the abnormal gene in many conditions. For other familial diseases, no one molecular defect can be implicated, although the site of abnormal metabolic activity can be localized to, for example, exocrine gland function in cystic fibrosis or epithelial transport mechanisms in renal tubular disorders and hemochromatosis.

Genetically determined diseases may become apparent at any age, from birth to late maturity, depending upon the physiologic results of the abnormality. In galactosemia and phenylketonuria, early recognition of the abnormal metabolic pathway permits specific, rational therapy which prevents physiologic damage. In the lipid and glycogen storage disorders, the molecular derangement is known, but no effective therapy is known. For many other conditions, the known or unknown metabolic peculiarity cannot be corrected, but vigorous symptomatic treatment permits sufferers to lead longer, more nearly normal lives than they could without accurate diagnosis.

We have discussed some of the genetically determined diseases in other chapters. Coagulation defects are discussed in Chapter 16; hemoglobinopathies and hereditary anemias in Chapter 14; endocrine disorders and diabetes mellitus in Chapter 17; conditions relating to genetically determined blood groups in Chapter 2; and the porphyrias in Chapter 8.

DISORDERS THAT BECOME APPARENT IN EARLY CHILDHOOD

CONDITIONS THAT CAN BE TREATED EFFECTIVELY

Two genetically determined enzyme deficiencies—phenylketonuria and galactosemia—produce severe developmental abnormalities in untreated infants, but prompt diagnosis and treatment can circumvent the disastrous effects of the irremediable defect.

Phenylketonuria

Absence of the hepatic enzyme phenylalanine hydroxylase causes a condition known variously as phenylketonuria and phenylpyruvic oligophrenia. The enzyme converts phenylalanine to tyrosine, so in affected patients phenylalanine derivatives accumulate and tyrosine supplies are deficient. Since tyrosine is necessary in the manufacture of melanin, patients with phenylketonuria are less darkly pigmented than their unaffected siblings, though outright albinism does not occur. The principal problems, however, arise from the accumulation of phenylalanine and its transamination product phenylpyruvic acid.

Neurologic Effects. Phenylalanine and phenylpyruvic acid damage the central nervous system, apparently through an effect on amino acid transport leading to defective myelination.[20] Within the first few months of life, there is progressive irritability, muscular hyperactivity, seizures, and mental retardation, leading to irreversible mental deficiency within the first year. If phenylalanine intake is immediately restricted, the destructive accumulation of phenylalanine and its products can be prevented and normal neurologic development occurs. When myelination is nearly complete, the metabolic defect appears to be less destructive to the child, so that after the age of about four years, dietary restrictions are not as essential. If phenylalanine restriction is instituted later than the first few months of life, the behavioral abnormalities, hyperkineses, hypopigmentation, and skin disorders can be reversed, but the intellectual impairment is permanent.

Urinary Screening Test. Phenylalanine hydroxylase appears in the normally-maturing liver shortly after birth, so the constitutional defect does not affect fetal development. Once the child begins to ingest proteins and their constituent amino acids, the phenylalanine hydroxylase deficiency becomes apparent. The accumulating phenylalanine and phenylpyruvate spill over into the urine, and urinary tests are readily available for screening purposes. The most common screening procedure uses ferric chloride solution, which produces an olive-green precipitate in urines rich in phenylpyruvate. In another screening test, a yellow precipitate occurs when 2,4-dinitrophenylhydrazine and hydrochloric acid are added to urine which contains phenylpyruvate. These screening tests are valuable for identifying infants who need further study but the tests are not, by themselves, diagnostic.

ARTEFACTS. Ferric chloride tests may be falsely negative if the urine sample is very dilute or if the infant's protein intake is insufficient to produce the amino acid metabolite. Phenylpyruvate deteriorates within 24 hours, so the test should be run fairly promptly at a time when the child has established a good dietary intake. False-positive results may arise from the presence of acetoacetic acid, salicylates, or chlorpromazine metabolites. Since phenylpyruvic acid can be extracted with ether, the ferric chloride test can be repeated on an ether extract of suspicious urine if interfering substances are thought to be present.

Tests on the urine of newborns may be misleading, so screening procedures should preferably be done at the end of the first week of life. If there is reason for suspicion, the test should be repeated on a moderately concentrated urine sample after three or four weeks, with the child in a good state of nutrition. Ferric chloride-impregnated paper strips (Phenistix Reagent Strips) are available for easy performance of the screening test.

Serum Tests. Definitive diagnosis requires demonstration of increased blood levels of phenylalanine which can be measured by chromatographic, enzymic, or fluorometric methods. Infants with the defect may have plasma levels as high as 15 to 40 mg per 100 ml, compared with normal values no higher than 1.65 mg per 100 ml.[20] (See also Guthrie test, p. 247.)

Detection of Heterozygotes. The heterozygous carrier of one abnormal gene has certain identifiable defects but suffers no clinically apparent ill effects. These individuals have slightly elevated plasma phenylalanine levels, and administration of a phenylalanine load results in prolonged phenylalanine elevation and deficient appearance of tyrosine in the blood. Identification of the carrier state becomes clinically important primarily in problems of genetic counseling. Identification of the homozygous affected infant is far easier and far more important.

Galactosemia

Another condition causing irreversible neurologic impairment is galactosemia, specifically the form in which galactose-1-phosphate uridyl transferase is deficient. High serum and urine galactose levels also occur with deficiency of galactokinase, but these rare patients manifest early-developing cataracts as the only observed clinical problem.[39] Transferase-deficiency galactosemia has an autosomal recessive transmission, and homozygotes are unable to convert ingested galactose into metabolically usable glucose. Lactose, consisting of one galactose moiety and one glucose moiety, enters the diet primarily in milk, but numerous foods other than recognizable milk products contain this sugar, which is also used in some medications as a tablet filler.

Clinical Signs. The child who lacks galactose-1-phosphate uridyl transferase shows his intolerance very soon after ingesting milk, with vomiting and diarrhea which may lead to dehydration. If the condition is not remedied, a number of serious ill effects occur. Because the milk diet is inadequately utilized, the child suffers from malnutrition, resulting in a fatty liver which fairly quickly becomes cirrhotic. Severe hypoglycemia, both chronic and episodic, may occur, and there is albuminuria and excessive excretion of amino acids. For reasons not fully understood, cataracts develop within a few months, and severe mental retardation occurs. The cause for the mental retardation is not understood, for no morphologic defects have been identified. It appears that galactose itself exerts a deleterious effect on the developing nervous system. Interestingly enough, all of the above-mentioned problems—malnutrition, cirrhosis, hypoglycemia, renal disturbances, and cataracts—are promptly reversed when galactose intake is discontinued, but the mental changes are permanent. The importance of early diagnosis is self-evident.

Screening Tests. Galactosemia can be tentatively diagnosed if the child excretes galactose in the urine. Galactose is a reducing substance which gives a positive "sugar test" when the urine is tested with Benedict's solution or other copper-containing reagents. Since it is not glucose, it gives no reaction on tests using glucose oxidase. Thus the appearance, in the urine of an infant, of a positive nonspecific sugar test and a negative test for glucose strongly points toward galactosemia. Routine urinalysis on infants should be done using a nonspecific sugar test to avoid missing this important finding.

ARTEFACTS. One problem in diagnosing galactosemia is that galactosuria occurs only after galactose intake. If a milk-fed child is brought to the hospital with severe diarrhea, vomiting, and dehydration, he will probably be receiving intravenous feedings by the time a urine sample is collected. Since standard intravenous preparations contain glucose as their only sugar, the urine may well contain no galactose. A similar difficulty can arise if a routine screening test is done on newborn infants in the hours or days before milk feedings are begun.

The nonglucose reducing substance in urine can be identified by a variety of chemical tests, and a specific galactose oxidase test is now available. Previously it was customary to confirm a suspected diagnosis of galactosemia by performing a galactose tolerance test. Since deliberate administration of galactose may endager the small infant, this test is better avoided.

Tests of Enzyme Activity. It is now possible to document the enzymatic abnormality, for the activity of galactose-1-phosphate uridyl transferase in red blood cells can be measured directly in several ways. Defective enzymatic activity can be documented in homozygotes and also in heterozygotes with no clinical symptoms.[33] Galactosemia is reported to affect between 1 in 18,000 live births and 1 in 70,000 live births,[39] so that the number of heterozygous carriers must be fairly high. The condition is sufficiently common and preventive measures are sufficiently effective to make routine screening of newborn infants desirable. In families with known incidence of the disease, infants should have specific red cell testing as soon as possible.

CONDITIONS WITH NO PRESENTLY EFFECTIVE TREATMENT

A number of conditions are due to inborn metabolic errors for which effective treatment is not available. All of these are fairly rare and appear to be due to autosomal recessive genes.

Cystic Fibrosis

Cystic fibrosis is among the most common genetically determined diseases. Almost certainly due to a single autosomal recessive gene, it occurs every 2000 to 4000 live Caucasian births,[22] with lower rates in American Indians, American Negroes, and Orientals. A wide range of clinical problems accompanies the disease, which appears to arise from a generalized, not-yet-defined defect of exocrine gland secretion. The exocrine pancreas, the intestinal glands responsible for meconium production, the salivary glands, the sweat glands, and the mucous glands of the respiratory tract all manifest functional abnormalities. The accompanying morphologic changes are probably secondary to the deranged secretory product.

Sweat Chloride Levels. Although pancreatic insufficiency was the first symptom reliably ascribed to this syndrome, and respiratory tract disease is the usual cause of death, the abnormal composition of sweat provides the most reliable diagnostic abnormality. In cystic fibrosis, sweat sodium and chloride are four or five times higher than normal, a finding present from the first month of life, when spontaneous sweating begins. In neonates, meconium ileus is highly suggestive of cystic fibrosis, but only one affected child in six presents with this symptom.[8,22] Chloride concentration is more reliable than sodium concentration, since there is no overlap between values in affected patients and in normal individuals at any age. Mean chloride concentration in normal infants is 12 mEq per liter, rising to 39 mEq per liter in adulthood, but in one series[22] of children with cystic fibrosis, mean sweat chloride was 117 mEq per liter, with the lowest value 75. The differences are less marked, but still diagnostic, in adult patients.

Without corrective therapy, excessive sweat salinity can lead to sodium depletion and vascular collapse, especially in infants during very hot weather. Hypofunction of adrenal or thyroid glands sometimes produces high sweat chloride and sodium levels, but these revert to normal with replacement therapy and are not likely to cause clinical confusion with cystic fibrosis.

Pancreatic Abnormalities. Steatorrhea, poor fat and protein absorption, and retarded growth patterns occur early. Before age two, decreased fecal levels of trypsin and chymotrypsin may suggest the diagnosis. In older children and adults, these enzymes do not reliably appear in feces under normal conditions, but reduced enzyme production can be demonstrated in affected children after secretin stimulation. Increased viscosity of pancreatic secretions leads very early to ductal and acinar dilatation, followed by the cyst formation, tissue damage, and fibrous scarring which gave the disease its earliest name, cystic fibrosis of the pancreas.

Pulmonary Abnormalities. Most of the laboratory findings in cystic fibrosis reflect changes secondary to secretory dysfunction. Excessively viscous bronchial secretions produce progressive structural and physiologic damage. Symptoms of obstructive lung disease and increased susceptibility to bacterial pneumonia tend to occur early, and require intensive, lifelong symptomatic therapy. Staphylococcus and pseudomonas are the usual bacterial invaders, and multiple pulmonary abscesses are often found at autopsy on these children. Even without repeated acute infection, ventilatory dysfunction, generalized parenchymal damage, and pulmonary hypertension are frequent findings in older patients.

Other Findings. Mild diabetes mellitus, hypoproteinemia, and excessive fecal fat are nondiagnostic abnormalities that often accompany the disease. Serum sodium, potassium, and chloride concentrations are normal unless intercurrent illness or some precipitating event has occurred. Urine electrolytes are not significantly abnormal.

Ciliary Inhibiting Factor. Patients with cystic fibrosis have in their serum and saliva a heat-labile, nondialysable factor which disrupts ciliary function in rabbit trachea epithelium and causes oyster ciliary activity to stop. The site of origin and possible pathogenetic significance of this substance remains subject to study, but an interesting observation is that heterozygote individuals, clinically without signs of the disease, also have this factor in their serum.[3,41]

Glycogen Storage Diseases

Glycogen is a highly branched polymer of glucose, constituting the major form in which animals store this sugar. In the synthesis and degradation of glycogen, at least ten enzymes are known to be required. Enzyme deficiency states have been identified for eight of these.[14] Of the eight conditions, six have an autosomal recessive inheritance; one (Type VIII) is X-linked; and the other group, formerly known as Type VI or liver phosphorylase deficiency, is too poorly defined for accurate inheritance studies. All the deficiency states result in abnormalities of glycogen deposition or utilization or both, but the clinical presentations cover a spectrum from those (Types II and IV) in which death occurs before age two, to McArdle's disease (Type V) in which the only symptom is skeletal muscle cramps after severe exercise, and these usually develop after age 20. We will discuss only Types I,II, and III, since the others are rare indeed, although of intense interest to biochemists.

Type I (von Gierke's Disease, Glucose-6-Phosphatase Deficiency). Glucose-6-phosphatase catalyses the irreversible removal of glucose from glycogen molecules. Normally found in liver, kidneys, and intestinal mucosa, it is essential for glycogen utilization. Its absence leads to massive accumulation, largely in the liver but also in renal tubular epithelium, of structurally normal glycogen. Because the body cannot call upon its glycogen reserve, patients may suffer severe hypoglycemic episodes, and the massive glycogen deposits produce symptomatic hepatomegaly.

Definitive diagnosis rests on demonstrating increased hepatic stores of structurally normal glycogen, with absent glucose-6-phosphatase activity. Since postsurgical bleeding may be troublesome in these patients, open biopsy with direct observation of hemostasis is preferable to needle biopsy.

LABORATORY FINDINGS. Hypoglycemia, often with convulsions, occurs in infancy and is usually the initial finding. Remarkably well tolerated chronic and episodic hypoglycemia continues throughout life, and after infancy, patients with blood sugars as low as 10 mg per 100 ml[14] may be asymptomatic. Lipid metabolism is also deranged, and serum levels of free fatty acids, triglycerides, phospholipids, and cholesterol are elevated. There is an increase in circulating ketone bodies, which may possibly serve as fuel for the brain when glucose is excessively low.[29] Lactic acidemia and persistent acidosis are the rule, and glucagon or epinephrine infusion intensifies lactate elevation with very little increase in serum glucose. The glucagon test provides one of the best diagnostic tools for this disease,[40] along with measuring erythrocyte glycogen.

Despite hepatomegaly, liver function tests are variable, the transaminases often showing moderate elevation.[40] Urinary wastage of glucose, amino acids, and phosphates, simulating Fanconi syndrome, may reflect renal tubular damage from accumulated glycogen. Pronounced hyperuricemia develops very early, and severe gouty symptoms often complicate adult life. Although there may be clinical problems with bleeding and oozing, tests of hemostatic function are normal.

Type II (Pompe's Disease, α-1,4-Glucosidase Deficiency). In this disease, structurally normal glycogen accumulates in skeletal muscle, heart, and liver. Symptoms of cardiac failure and generalized hypotonia develop within the first few months, and death results, ordinarily by age two, from cardiac failure or the respiratory complications of skeletal muscle weakness. Despite the rapidly fatal course, laboratory findings are essentially normal, with no elevation of serum lipids or ketones and expected levels of blood sugar. Diagnosis is made when structurally normal glycogen and absent α-1,4-glucosidase activity are found on muscle biopsy. Enzyme deficiency can be documented in fibroblasts cultured from amniotic fluid[27] so prenatal diagnosis is possible in families known to be at risk.

Type III (Debrancher Enzyme Deficiency). Intermediate in frequency between Type I and Type II, and clinically less severe than both, is deficiency of the enzyme which controls the structure of glucose linkages in glycogen molecules. Structurally abnormal glycogen accumulates in liver, muscle, and sometimes heart. Although hepatomegaly and infantile hypoglycemic convulsions may suggest Type I disease, the disease runs a far milder course. Fasting hypoglycemia is less pronounced, and hypercholesterolemia is less severe. The blood sugar response to epinephrine or glucagon is somewhat unpredictable. Fructose and galactose infusions produce increased serum glucose, since the debrancher enzyme is not involved in this conversion. Hepatic derangement, with elevated transaminases and mild cirrhosis, may occur in childhood, but tends to regress after puberty. Survival into relatively asymptomatic adulthood often occurs, after initial growth retardation and failure to thrive during infancy and early childhood.

Conditions Affecting Lipids

Abnormalities of lipid metabolism may affect circulating lipids, tissue stores, or both. Vastly more common than lipid storage diseases are alterations of circulating lipids and lipoproteins, comprising the group of conditions formerly lumped together as *hyperlipemia*. The relative roles of genetic and environmental factors in these lipoprotein disorders remain under study. Although familial tendencies obviously exist, inheritance is unclear and exogenous influences are extremely important. These conditions are discussed in Chapter 4.

Lipid Storage Diseases. A group of rather rare diseases is characterized by excessive tissue deposits of complex lipids called sphingolipids, most of which contain ceramide (N-acylsphingosine) in a chemical linkage which determines the class of sphingolipid. The diseases vary in the class and location of accumulated material, and the clinical syndromes vary in severity. No therapies are presently available for the metabolic abnormalities, and treatment must be supportive.

GAUCHER'S DISEASE. In this most common of the lipidoses, glucosyl ceramides accumulate in reticuloendothelial cells, producing the characteristic Gaucher cell in spleen and bone marrow. These large cells have pale, fibrillar cytoplasm which contains diastase-resistant PAS-positive material. The metabolic defect is deficiency of glucosyl ceramide β-glucosidase. The deficiency almost certainly derives from an abnormal autosomal gene, but there appear to be several different mutants and the inheritance pattern is by no means clear. The different mutants produce very different clinical syndromes—the "adult" or nonneuronopathic form affects any age in a chronic, idolent manner, and the one or several conditions which affect the central nervous system begin early and pursue a rapidly deteriorating course.

Demonstration of Gaucher cells in the bone marrow usually affords presumptive diagnosis, and chromatographic identification of the cerebroside can be done from liver or spleen tissue, obtained by biopsy or splenectomy. In the chronic form, massive splenomegaly and osseous accumulations of these cells produce most of the clinical signs and symptoms. Thrombocytopenia is common; if symptomatic, response to splenectomy is usually prompt and gratifying.[46] Mild leukopenia and anemia may also occur. Bone pain is common, and patients with osseous lesions have elevated serum alkaline phosphatase. Serum acid phosphatase is reliably elevated, the enzyme activity being unaffected by L-tartrate. There are no laboratory findings specific for the accelerated infantile and juvenile forms of this disorder, and the neurologic manifestations are poorly understood.

TAY-SACHS DISEASE. The guilty metabolite in this condition is the ganglioside G_{M2}, which accumulates in ganglion cells and produces inexorable neurologic deterioration and death before the age of four or five. Originally thought to occur only in Jewish families, the gene and the disease occur in non-Jewish families as well, and should be considered in infants with psychomotor retardation and evidence of visual disorders. Definitive diagnosis is made by demonstrating deficient hexosaminidase A activity in serum, leukocytes, or cultured fibroblasts. Other findings may include elevated serum levels of lactic dehydrogenase and glutamic-oxalacetic transaminase,[36] and other storage disorders should be ruled out by evaluating acid phosphatase levels, bone marrow, and the size and configuration of spleen, liver, lungs, long bones, and the like, all of which are unremarkable in Tay-Sachs disease.

Several varieties of ganglioside disorders are known, with different enzyme deficiencies and different chemical groupings in the accumulated material.[28,36] These can be differentiated if the need arises, and sufficiently reliable tests are available so that both prenatal diagnosis[25] and heterozygote detection[36] are possible.

NIEMANN-PICK DISEASE. Less common still are the sphinogomyelin lipidoses. In this diverse group, clinical symptomatology ranges from a rapidly fatal infantile neuronopathic form to visceral involvement compatible with survival into adulthood. Type A, the acute infantile form, is the most common. In all, sphingomyelinase activity is deficient, and *mulberry-like* foam cells accumulate in the spleen, bone marrow, liver, lymph nodes, and lungs. Many other organs contain these cells but have no functional impairment. Cerebral changes in the neuronopathic forms include ganglion cell damage, patchy neuronal loss, and variably abnormal myelination as well as foam cell accumulation around blood vessels and leptomeninges. Diagnosis is by chemical analysis of foam cell-laden liver or lymph node biopsy. There are no reliable serum or hematologic findings which characterize these conditions.

Renal Tubular Disorders

The renal tubular epithelium is the site of continuous metabolic activity, resulting in absorption, secretion, and synthesis of various substances. Although some of the exact mechanisms are not understood, many individual reactions are known to occur, and there are many processes that can break down. A number of clinical disorders originate from defects of renal tubular function, although their manifestations may affect many organs.

Fanconi Syndrome. The Fanconi syndrome, as originally described, was "nephrotic-glycosuric dwarfism with hypophosphatemic rickets,"[37] but the term is often used to describe a constellation of renal tubular abnormalities which may be constitutional or acquired. The salient features are metabolic acidosis and excessive excretion of glucose, amino acids, phosphates, protein, potassium, and bicarbonate. The proximal convoluted tubules in advanced cases are narrowed (the *swan-neck* defect) and, often, shortened. The normal epithelium may be replaced by less well differentiated cuboidal cells. Since normal reabsorption of the above-named substances occurs in the proximal tubule, the morphologic and functional changes correlate well, but it is hard to pronounce which is cause and which effect.

CYSTINE METABOLISM. The familial childhood disease has been reliably associated with defective cystine metabolism, wherein remarkably high levels of cystine accumulate in intracellular fluid. The defect can be diagnosed by measuring intracellular cystine levels in circulating leukocytes or cultured fibroblasts, homozygous persons having levels 80 to 100 times normal, and heterozygotes having moderate elevation.[37] Affected children have labile fluid regulation, and may come to medical attention because of polyuria or because of dehydration and resultant fever.

LABORATORY FINDINGS. The laboratory findings, early in the disease, include glycosuria with normal blood sugar concentration; proteinuria; phosphaturia with hypophosphatemia leading to vitamin D-resistant rickets; metabolic acidosis with alkaline urine containing increased bicarbonate and associated low serum levels of CO_2; and generalized aminoaciduria with cystine present but not out of proportion to other amino acids. The erythrocyte sedimentation rate is high, and alkaline phosphatase is usually increased consequent to bone damage. As the disease progresses, renal failure supervenes, so BUN and serum creatinine rise, and serum phosphates and potassium accumulate as renal function declines.

ACQUIRED FANCONI SYNDROME. The urinary findings characteristic of Fanconi syndrome may accompany other metabolic disease, notably galactosemia, glycogen storage disease, and hereditary fructose intolerance; acquired Fanconi-like defect can follow heavy metal poisoning, renal allograft rejection, and multiple myeloma.

Cystinuria. An interesting inherited defect of renal tubular function is known as cystinuria, although cystine is only one of four amino acids excreted in excess. The other three are lysine, arginine, and ornithine, and all four are dibasic acids. The defect relates specifically to reabsorption of these four compounds, and remaining renal functions and general metabolism are normal. Cystine is the most prominent of the excreted amino acids because it is by far the least soluble, tending, at physiologic pH, to crystallize out of solutions more concentrated than 0.4 mg per ml. Since patients with this defect may excrete between 400 and 1200 mg of cystine per day, up to 3 liters of urine a day are necessary to keep the excretory load in solution.[42] As the urine becomes more acid, cystine precipitates more easily.

The chief problem in this condition is renal stones. The crystallized cystine accumulates in stones which may occur in very young patients. Progressive renal damage occurs secondary to the nephrolithiasis, and if stone formation can be prevented, the condition is compatible with a normal life span. Therapy is directed at maintaining a high urine output, preferably at relatively alkaline pH. Administration of penicillamine promotes excretion of cystine in a more soluble form, and dietary restriction of methionine reduces the amount of precursor available for metabolism to cystine.

CYSTINE CRYSTALS. Diagnosis should be suspected in young children who are first seen with renal calculi, and the condition should be considered and ruled out in every case of nephrolithiasis. The diagnosis is easily made by demonstrating cystine crystals in a concentrated acidic urine. This can be done by adding glacial acetic acid to a morning urine specimen and allowing it to chill for several hours. The cystine crystals appear as flat hexagonal plates. Patients with the homozygous condition of cystinuria nearly always have crystallizable cystine in their urine.

GENETIC TYPES. There appear to be two genes for cystinuria. One is completely recessive, so that heterozygotes cannot be detected. Another more common gene is incompletely recessive, and defective amino acid reabsorption can be detected in clinically normal heterozygotes. These heterozygotes do not excrete enough cystine to form crystals in acidified urine, but abnormal cystine excretion can be demonstrated by cyanide-nitroprusside tests on urine. The complete pattern of amino acid excretion can be observed by chromatography.

Vitamin D-Resistant Rickets with Hypophosphatemia. In vitamin D-resistant rickets, there are at least two metabolic disorders. One is excessive renal excretion of phosphates, leading to depressed serum phosphate levels. The other is decreased calcium absorption from the gastrointestinal tract. The net result of these two defects often is severe bone disease which responds only to very large doses of vitamin D, as much as 150,000 to 250,000 international units per day. The etiology of the condition is not known, since neither the phosphate defect nor the calcium defect alone can explain the syndrome, and it is difficult to link the two to a single biochemical abnormality. The inheritance appears to be fairly straightforward X-linked dominance, in which females with a single abnormal X chromosome are less markedly affected than males whose abnormal X chromosome is unopposed.

LABORATORY FINDINGS. Diagnosis depends upon demonstration of low serum phosphate levels, with normal calcium and generally high alkaline phosphatase. Virtually no calcium is excreted in the urine, while phosphate excretion is high as long as serum levels are adequate. If phosphate intake and serum levels are markedly reduced, urinary excretion diminishes also.[48] No other renal abnormalities have been demonstrated, and amino acid excretion is usually normal, although a few individual abnormalities have been noted.

The physiologic ill effects relate largely to the skeletal system and occur primarily in children. In families in which the condition is prevalent, children should be watched closely for evidence of hypophosphatemia, for this derangement appears to antedate the appearance of skeletal changes. Serum phosphate levels may be variable in children, and repeated determinations are necessary before the condition can be excluded.

Other Inborn Errors

A variety of diseases manifest themselves in urinary excretion of abnormal substances or of normal substances in abnormal amounts. Some represent primary disorders of renal function, while in others renal excretion reflects metabolic abnormalities elsewhere.

Alcaptonuria. In alcaptonuria the enzyme homogentisic acid oxidase is lacking, resulting in a build-up of homogentisic acid, a metabolite of phenylalanine and tyrosine metabolism. Homogentisic acid appears in the urine, producing a black precipitate in urinary tests for reducing substances. Alkalinized urine turns black, or urine samples may darken on prolonged standing. No renal effects occur, but after years of excessive circulating homogentisic acid, black pigment is deposited in cartilages, tendons, the sclerae, and other connective tissue. Arthritis occurs in later life. Definitive diagnosis rests on identifying the urinary substance as homogentisic acid. This can be done by paper chromatography or by enzymic methods of analysis.

Albinism. Albinism is an easily recognized defect affecting metabolism of the amino acid tyrosine. In albino patients, morphologically normal melanocytes fail to produce expected amounts of melanin, probably due to defective enzyme content. Diagnosis usually rests on clinical examination rather than on laboratory studies.

Miscellaneous Amino Acidurias. A variety of metabolic defects lead to specific amino acidurias. Most of these are very rare and cause severe mental and physical signs in affected children. Diagnosis is made by chromatographic identification of excreted amino acids. In this group are glycinuria; histidinemia; disorders of proline and hydroxyproline; and branched chain ketonuria (maple-syrup urine disease), which involves the branched chain amino acids leucine, isoleucine, and valine.

Hartnup Disease. In Hartnup disease, there are skin lesions, neurologic changes, and psychologic disorders due apparently to defective absorption, in the renal tubules and gastrointestinal tract, of amino acids with one amino group and one carboxyl group, so that uptake and metabolism of these amino acids are abnormal. The patient's development is affected by amino acid deficiencies as well as by the presence of abnormal metabolites. Diagnosis is made from the chromatographic pattern of excreted amino acids.

Renal Tubular Acidosis. Renal tubular acidosis is a serious constitutional defect that arises from defective urinary acidification. This is characterized by hyperchloremic acidosis in patients with neutral or alkaline urine. As with other conditions of hyperchloremic acidosis, there is hypokalemia, but increased serum calcium and nephrocalcinosis distinguish this disease from most cases of Fanconi's syndrome, and high serum phosphate levels distinguish it from vitamin D-resistant rickets with hypophosphatemia. Although serum bicarbonate levels are low, bicarbonate reabsorption appears to be unimpaired, and the causative defect is thought to be abnormal hydrogen ion secretion in the distal tubule.

Renal Glycosuria. Renal glycosuria is due to defective reabsorption of glucose from the tubular urine. The result is that glucose appears in the urine even though serum glucose levels are normal. Other tests of carbohydrate metabolism are unaffected, and there are no clinical symptoms.

Vasopressin-Resistant Diabetes Insipidus. Vasopressin-resistant diabetes insipidus is characterized by marked polydipsia and polyuria, with excretion of hypotonic urine. Administration of antidiuretic hormone has no effect, and the defect appears to be a constitutional inability of the distal tubular cells to respond to antidiuretic hormone. No structural or biochemical basis has been found for the disorder, and treatment consists of administration of sufficient quantities of fluids to prevent dehydration. Diagnosis is made when the symptoms of polyuria and urinary hypotonicity fail to respond to vasopressin.

DISORDERS THAT APPEAR LATER IN LIFE

Although an individual is born with a predetermined genetic complement, it may take time for the effects of certain genetic traits to become apparent. We have already considered a number of conditions that manifest themselves early in life. Another group of inherited conditions cause clinical symptoms much later. In this category we will consider disorders of uric acid, iron, and copper metabolism, which are clinically apparent as gout, hemochromatosis, and Wilson's disease, respectively.

URIC ACID METABOLISM AND GOUT

Uric acid metabolism begins, physiologically, with purines, and this is a logical point to begin the discussion. Purines are a group of compounds with a characteristic configuration of five carbon atoms, four nitrogen atoms, and various substituent groups. The nucleic acids—ribonucleic acid

(RNA) and deoxyribonucleic acid (DNA)—contain large amounts of the purines adenine and guanine. Through a complicated series of enzymically mediated steps, degradation of nucleic acids results in catabolism of the purines into uric acid, a substance that is poorly soluble at pH of 7.4 or below.

Because uric acid is poorly soluble, it may crystallize out of solution if the concentration rises within body fluids. The kidney is particularly susceptible to damage if uric acid concentration rises in acidic urine. Uric acid is freely filtrable, so the tubular urine contains all the uric acid presented to the glomerulus. The tubular epithelium resorbs virtually all the filtered uric acid, thus preventing excessive uric acid load as the urine becomes more concentrated. The uric acid present in excreted urine probably derives from active tubular secretion of the compound after its complete absorption from the filtered urine.

Uricase and Its Absence

In most mammals, the resorbed uric acid is efficiently handled by the action of the enzyme uricase, which splits it into the freely soluble compound allantoin. Allantoin is thus the excreted end product of purine metabolism, and uric acid does not accumulate. Human tissue lacks the enzyme uricase, but the kidney retains its efficiency in resorbing uric acid from tubular urine. A certain amount of recirculated uric acid is excreted through the bile into the feces, and a certain amount is excreted by tubular action into the urine. In healthy humans, balance is maintained between uric acid excreted and uric acid developed from catabolizing endogenous and dietary nucleic acids, but the balance does not allow much leeway. Males have higher urate levels than females, and various normal values are given. Values above 7.0 mg per 100 ml in men and 6.0 mg per 100 ml in women are considered by all observers to be abnormal. Since the saturation level of a solution at pH 7.4 is 6.4 mg per 100 ml, it is obvious that serious danger of uric acid deposition accompanies relatively slight elevation of serum urates.

Causes of Gout

Gout is an inherited abnormality of uric acid metabolism, in which serum urate levels are elevated and urate deposits occur in various tissues. The nature of the metabolic defect is not known, nor is the mode of inheritance understood. There is a strong possibility that at least two and possibly more constitutional abnormalities, either individually or in combination, can cause the clinical syndrome of gout. Studies have shown that the increased uric acid in the serum does not derive from increased absorption of nucleic acid from the diet.[51] Increased nucleic acid turnover, as occurs in myelo-proliferative disorders, may cause increased uric acid levels, but this excess turnover does not occur in primary gout. In patients with increased cellular turnover, the elevated serum urates cause a clearly secondary form of gout.

Metabolic Patterns. The hyperuricemia of primary gout has many possible determinants. The rates of production, of serum transport, and of excretion are all subject to various influences, both genetic and exogenous. Several enzyme defects have been defined which lead to urate overproduction, and in many patients, impaired urate excretion can be documented. Enzyme disorders account for relatively few cases of gout, leaving the large majority incompletely explained, both in biochemical, physiologic, and genetic terms. Glucose-6-phosphatase deficiency and a glutathione reductase variant can cause increased urate synthesis, and total or partial deficiency of hypoxanthine-guanine phosphoribosyl transferase (PRT, see section below on Lesch-Nyhan syndrome) produces very marked urate overproduction. Patients with the hyperlipoproteinemias that include elevated triglycerides also manifest high levels of serum urate.

The vast majority of gout sufferers can be classified by several general metabolic observations, but not explained. Attempts have been made to divide patients into those with primary urate overproduction and those with primary underexcretion; or those with normal or slightly increased urate pool and normal turnover compared with those whose total pool and turnover are markedly increased.[32] The 10 to 20 per cent incidence of urate nephrolithiasis in gouty subjects cannot clearly be correlated with urate excretion rates, although certain patients do have markedly increased excretion. Many gout sufferers consistently excrete exceptionally acid urine, which may reflect a defect in ammonium ion excretion.[52]

Serum Urate Levels. Serum uric acid levels may be high in individuals without the clinical symptoms of gout, but those individuals who do have the disease consistently have high serum urates. Only 9 per cent of gouty males in one series had uric acid levels that fell even sporadically below 7.0 mg per 100 ml.[21] In another series, the mean serum uric acid levels in gouty men was 9.2 mg per 100 ml.[50] A tendency toward hyperuricemia exists in the postpubertal male relatives of patients with gout, but no clear pattern of transmission has emerged. The incidence of gout in the United States and Northern Europe is approximately 0.3 per cent.[49] An interesting observation is that, within a given population, mean uric acid values tend to rise as social, occupational, and educational levels rise, so that the popular stereotype of gout as an aristocratic disease has some faint basis in fact.

Clinical Signs

Gout afflicts males far more frequently than females. Affected women are nearly always past the menopause. The cardinal symptom of gout is acute arthritis, and the great toe is the most frequent site of suffering. Acute attacks are invariably accompanied by sodium urate microcrystals and leukocytes in the synovial fluid, and there may be systemic leukocytosis as well. Urate crystals, in the form of monosodium urate monohydrate, deposit in soft tissue as well as joints, but these deposits, called tophi, are a late manifestation. Ordinarily, the first few attacks of gouty arthritis clear without residual changes, but repeated attacks lead to chronic joint deformities. The joints of the feet, ankles, knees, and fingers are the most commonly affected, in order of descending frequency.

Accompanying urate deposition in the joints and soft tissue may be urate precipitation in the kidneys. Excessive urate load in the blood or urine or both can cause uric acid deposition in the renal parenchyma as well as pelvic and calyceal stone formation. A glomerular defect also occurs, and progressive renal impairment is the rule in long-standing gout. As many as 30 per cent of gouty patients have renal calculi, and approximately half have albuminuria.[49] Hypertension and arteriosclerosis frequently accompany gout, and gouty patients run a higher than normal risk of developing coronary artery disease.

Laboratory Findings

Laboratory diagnosis of full-blown gout is relatively simple. The serum uric acid level is elevated, both during the acute attack and in the quiescent intervals. The hyperuricemia may not be dramatic, but values below 7.0 mg per 100 ml are rather uncommon in patients with gout. Uric acid excretion may be within the normal range of 300 to 600 mg in 24 hours or may be elevated. Before renal changes occur, the urinalysis is unremarkable and the blood urea level is normal. Gouty change and uric acid deposition may cause renal disease with consequent uremia, while moderate levels of hyperuricemia may accompany severe primary renal disease. When uric acid and urea values are both high, history usually reveals which is the primary process. Persistent marked urinary acidity is characteristic, and even alkali loading may fail to raise the urine pH. Tubular function may be moderately reduced, even in patients with minimal overt renal damage.

Secondary Hyperuricemia and Gout

Raised serum urate levels occur frequently, but gouty symptoms rarely accompany hyperuricemia arising from other metabolic problems. Secondary hyperuricemia, like primary gouty hyperuricemia, can result from increased urate production or decreased excretion. Intrinsic renal failure and diminished urate clearance due to acidosis are by far the most common causes of hyperuricemia,[30] and arthritis rarely occurs in these readily diagnosed conditions. Gouty symptoms may sometimes follow the long-standing hyperuricemia caused by certain renoactive drugs, and the over-production hyperuricemia of hematopoietic diseases or their treatment. Thiazide diuretics present particular problems, although the mechanism is not clearly understood,[32] and chronic alcohol or salicylate ingestion also produce high serum urate levels. Excessive nuclear turnover, especially in acute episodes, can increase both serum and urine urate levels, leading to renal damage and initiation or exacerbation of gouty arthritis. Leukemias, chronic hemolytic conditions, and effective cytolytic treatment of neoplasms are noteworthy for the very high urate levels they induce.

Lesch-Nyhan Syndrome

This X-linked enzyme deficiency might possibly belong in the section on inherited disorders which cause problems early in life, since affected boys start showing clinical symptoms at three or four months of age. The deficient enzyme is hypoxanthine-guanine phosphoribosyl transferase (PRT), and the measurable metabolic result is enormously increased uric acid production and uric acid excretion. Although renal damage and gouty arthritis occur when these patients reach their teens, the most striking clinical problems are neurologic and have not been clearly related to the metabolic pathways of urate and its purine precursors. The overwhelming clinical problems are compulsive self-mutilation, extreme aggressiveness, and choreoathetosis, none of which improve with allopurinol therapy. Before neurologic symptoms develop, excessive urate excretion can be documented, often by the mother who notices yellow-orange urate crystals in the diaper. Screening is possible by documenting a high ratio of urate to creatinine in a morning urine,[38] and definitive diagnosis rests on measuring PRT levels in erythrocytes and fibroblasts. Prenatal diagnosis has been successful in offspring of women known to be at risk, and these heterozygous carriers can be clearly identified by documenting enzyme levels in their cultured fibroblasts.

HEMOCHROMATOSIS

Iron is the oxygen-carrying element of hemoglobin and is thus essential for life. The normal adult body contains a total of 4 to 6 grams of iron, of which approximately 50 to 75 per cent is present as hemoglobin. Most of the remainder exists as metabolically available storage iron in the reticuloendothelial system. Small quantities are present in myoglobin and the oxygen-transport enzymes, and a few milligrams are present in the plasma, bound to iron-binding globulin, a beta globulin also known as transferrin. The total body iron may increase if dietary intake is excessive or after infusion of very large quantities of blood. Massive increase in stored iron damages the tissue in which it occurs, and dietary or parenteral iron overload results in excessive hemosiderin deposits in many organs. This condition is called *secondary hemochromatosis.*

Primary hemochromatosis is due to an intrinsic abnormality in iron metabolism. Although it appears to be constitutionally determined, the genetic transmission pattern is not clear. There is some evidence of mildly abnormal iron metabolism in relatives of patients with primary hemochromatosis, but no pattern has emerged.

Iron Regulation

The exact steps that regulate iron absorption are not known. Dietary intake is the sole source of body iron, and in healthy adult men, approximately 0.5 to 1.5 mg of iron is absorbed per day. The rate of absorption is affected by body needs, and menstruating or pregnant females absorb a higher proportion of dietary iron than do men. Iron absorption occurs in the small intestine, but the essential step of reducing the ferric form to ferrous occurs in the stomach, possibly by the action of hydrochloric acid or intrinsic factor. No pathway exists for orderly iron excretion, although a certain amount is lost each day in feces, sweat, and desquamated epidermal cells. There is no provision either for increasing iron excretion should the need arise or for conserving iron by diminishing excretion.

Iron Binding. Once iron crosses the mucosal barrier, it is transported in the blood bound to transferrin. Transferrin is capable of transporting approximately 300 micrograms of iron per 100 ml, but ordinarily only a third of its capacity is engaged. Normal serum iron levels range between 70 and 170 micrograms per 100 ml, with women having a slightly lower mean value than men. If a larger than normal proportion of transferrin is unsaturated, iron absorption is increased. This occurs in conditions of anoxia or of increased erythropoiesis.

Faulty Mechanism. In primary hemochromatosis, something goes wrong with the regulation of iron absorption. Instead of 0.5 to 1.5 mg per day, a total approximately balanced by daily excretion, 3.5 to 4.0 mg of iron enters the circulation. A net excess of 2 mg per day may appear trivial, but the simplest calculation reveals that only a year and a half would be necessary to accumulate one gram of unnecessary iron, and in 15 years, the excess would be 10 grams.

Clinical Signs

Hemochromatosis is a disease of middle-aged men, for it takes a number of decades before dangerous iron levels are reached. Approximately 80 per cent of cases become apparent after age 40,[31] and by the time the disease is full-blown, there may be 20 to 60 grams of iron in the body. Women, particularly young women, are not likely to develop the disease, since menstruation, pregnancy, and lactation demand between 10 and 35 grams of iron from the individual. Before an iron excess could accumulate in a premenopausal woman, iron absorption would have to increase enormously.

Hemosiderin. Excess iron is stored as hemosiderin, a granular material easily visible with light microscopy. Hemosiderin is normally concentrated in cells of the reticuloendothelial system and in tissue macrophages at sites of prior bleeding. To dispose of 20 to 60 grams of iron as an intracellular granular material presents a staggering problem. In hemochromatosis, hemosiderin accumulates in parenchymal cells of all organs, but especially in liver, pancreas, heart, kidneys, and endocrine glands. Hemosiderin is abundant in dermal cells, but the peculiar bronze discoloration of the skin is due both to hemosiderin and to melanin.

Hepatic Changes. Other names for primary hemochromatosis are bronze diabetes and pigmentary cirrhosis. Both these terms are appropriate, referring in part to the patient's appearance and in part to the pathologic changes wrought by the disease. The liver is almost always damaged, and a large, finely granular, rusty brown liver is the usual finding at autopsy. Liver enlargement may precede by some years the development of hepatic or other symptoms.

The liver changes include portal fibrosis and pseudo-lobule formation, and the clinical sequelae of cirrhosis are frequent. Portal hypertension and esophageal varices are less frequent in this than in other types of cirrhosis, but ascites, spider angiomas, and loss of body hair are by no means uncommon. Primary hepatic carcinoma complicates pigmentary cirrhosis even more frequently than Laennec's cirrhosis.

Other Organs. Pancreatic function is adversely affected by the accumulated hemosiderin. As many as 80 per cent of patients with the metabolic abnormality develop diabetic symptoms, although the secondary, or late, complications of diabetes are uncommon. Other tissue that may be severely damaged is that of the heart, and cardiac failure or pericardial effusion is quite common. Hemosiderin may occur in the tubular epithelial cells and can often be demonstrated in the urine. Iron stains of the bone marrow reveal a moderate increase in reticuloendothelial cells, but the quantity is much less striking than the amount of stainable iron in a sample of liver.

Laboratory Findings. The diagnostic laboratory findings in hemochromatosis relate to iron metabolism. The plasma iron level is markedly increased to 175 to 275 micrograms per 100 ml; and the iron-binding capacity is highly saturated, usually 75 to 100 per cent. The absolute level of transferrin tends to be somewhat depressed to values consistently below 300 micrograms per 100 ml. There may be hemosiderin in the urine, and if diabetes is present, blood and urine glucose levels will be high. The definitive diagnosis is made by liver biopsy, in which hemosiderin is conspicuous in parenchymal cells throughout the lobules. A similar picture may be seen in a liver with Laennec's cirrhosis and secondary hemosiderosis, but in such cases the iron pigment tends to be concentrated in a peripheral distribution.

Therapy. The treatment of hemochromatosis requires emptying the body of its excess iron. This is done by controlled phlebotomy, usually 500 to 1000 ml of blood weekly until a mild iron-deficiency state is induced. This may take several years, and the process can be accelerated by treatment with the iron-chelating agent desferrioxamine. This drug, injected intramuscularly, enhances urinary excretion of iron and can be used for a diagnostic test. In normal individuals, desferrioxamine causes urinary iron excretion to rise to perhaps ten times the baseline value, whereas in patients with iron overload, the increment in urinary iron is forty to one hundred times the original value.[18]

Relatives of patients with hemochromatosis may have increased iron absorption, increased hepatic liver stores[47] or increased serum iron levels,[9] but these findings have not served to elucidate the genetic pattern nor to permit prediction, with any success, of the likelihood of the development of later clinical problems.

Secondary Hemochromatosis. Patients who have received upwards of 50 to 100 transfusions for aplastic or hemolytic anemias are found to have excessive iron stores. Since there is no mechanism for iron excretion and hemoglobin formation is faulty, the iron accumulates. Dietary iron overload, particularly when accompanied by high alcohol intake, can also cause excessive iron stores. Initially, in these secondary conditions, the excess iron is deposited in the reticuloendothelial cells, and the site of most notable increase is in the bone marrow. If the condition progresses, however, iron may be deposited in parenchymal cells, following much the same distribution as in primary hemochromatosis. Distinction can usually be made by clinical history, especially in the case of transfusion hemosiderosis.

COPPER METABOLISM

The role of copper in normal metabolism is unclear. Most of the body's copper is present in ceruloplasmin, a blue plasma protein which has enzymic activity as an amine oxidase, but has no known physiologic function. Although copper appears to be an essential element for the development of bone, connective tissue, and central nervous system,[44] no specific effects can be ascribed to deficiency. Ceruloplasmin appears to be manufactured in the liver, the only site of active copper metabolism after it is absorbed from the upper gastrointestinal tract.

Like many other substances, copper is transported from its site of absorption to the liver partially bound to serum protein. An unbound portion also exists, and this portion is freely diffusible across the glomerular membrane into the urine. Ceruloplasmin accounts for approximately 90 per cent of the serum copper level, which is 70 to 140 micrograms per 100 ml in men and 85 to 155 micrograms per 100 ml in women.[6] The values are much lower in newborns, while children have intermediate values ranging from 27 micrograms per 100 ml to adult levels.[6] Only a small amount of copper normally appears in the urine, generally less than 100 micrograms in 24 hours.[2]

Secondary Changes. Abnormal serum copper values occur in a variety of conditions, but usually the change is secondary to other disorders. Thus, serum copper values may be low when serum proteins are low, as in nephrotic syndrome, sprue, celiac disease, and various infantile dysproteinemias.[44] Stressful conditions such as myocardial infarcts, infections, leukemia, and thyrotoxicosis may be accompanied by high levels of serum copper. Estrogens increase the level of circulating copper presumably by increasing the amount of protein to which the element is bound. With pregnancy or oral estrogen medication the serum copper may be high, and in severe cirrhosis it may also be elevated.

Wilson's Disease. The only primary condition in which disordered copper metabolism is known to play a part is Wilson's disease or hepatolenticular degeneration. There is general agreement that copper is implicated, but the nature of the defect is not understood. Serum copper levels tend to be low, but not invariably so. The serum content of ceruloplasmin, however, is consistently low. Tests for ceruloplasmin employ its enzymic properties, and the method can measure oxidation products formed or oxygen uptake. An immunologic test employing anticeruloplasmin serum is also available. Normal values average 36 mg per 100 ml for men and 41 mg per 100 ml for women, with a moderately wide range.[2] Patients with Wilson's disease have less than 20 mg per 100 ml, falling clearly below the lower limit of normal.

Clinical Signs. The manifold clinical symptoms of Wilson's disease appear due to deposition of copper in the tissues rather than to ceruloplasmin deficiency. The liver is the site of greatest abnormality, and cirrhosis is common, often occurring relatively early in childhood. Other sites of deposition are brain, kidneys, and cornea, and there are characteristic symptoms for each locus. Neurologic problems include spasticity, rigidity, or tremors, and there is a spectrum of renal abnormalities which may or may not be directly related to the presence of copper in the tissue. In the cornea, copper deposition takes the form of a greenish ring at the limbus, called a Kayser-Fleischer ring.

Biochemical Changes. Several problems arise in attempting to characterize the biochemical defect. The most favored hypothesis is that some genetically determined defect in hepatic function depresses ceruloplasmin synthesis. As ceruloplasmin is the principal site at which copper exists, failure of incorporation leaves the copper with no place to go. There seems to be rapid copper turnover between the liver and other tissues in which it is deposited. Even in the absence of morphologic change, the liver contains far more copper than normal. Tissue analysis reveals 5 to 20 mg of copper per 100 grams dry weight of liver, compared with 0.5 mg or less per 100 grams dry weight in the normal liver.[35]

Although regulation of copper absorption is not understood, it has become evident that copper absorption is increased in Wilson's disease. Serum copper values tend to be somewhat low, in the range of 38 to 80 micrograms per 100 ml.[2] Urinary excretion is increased, with 24-hour copper values of 300 to 1100 micrograms in 24 hours, upwards of 300 per cent of normal.

Renal Abnormalities. Another characteristic set of abnormalities is in renal function, and these cannot be clearly related to copper metabolism. There is decreased plasma flow and multiple abnormalities in reabsorptive function. Certain amino acids, notably cystine and threonine, are present in markedly increased quantity, and glucose, bicarbonate, uric acid, and phosphates are all present in excess. Although serum glucose levels are not much affected, low serum levels of bicarbonate, uric acid, and phosphates are commonly found. Calcium, too, may be excreted in excess, but skeletal abnormalities do not ordinarily accompany the calcium and phosphate excretion. The amino acid and bicarbonate abnormalities may simulate the renal picture found in Fanconi's syndrome, but onset in Wilson's disease is characteristically much later in life.

Genetic Pattern. Familial incidence is well established in Wilson's disease in an apparently recessive pattern. Both males and females are affected, and the disease usually becomes apparent some time in late childhood or early adulthood. Relatives of patients may have mild metabolic abnormalities; in siblings of an affected individual, demonstration of marked abnormality should be considered evidence of latent disease.

Therapy. Treatment is to prevent excess copper deposition by administering chelating agents. At present, D-penicillamine appears to offer the best results, but its effect in prolonging life cannot yet be fully evaluated.

BIBLIOGRAPHY

1. BARLOW, K.A.: Hyperlipidemia in primary gout. Metabolism 17:289, 1968.
2. BEARN, A.G.: "Wilson's disease," *In* Stanbury, J.B., Wyngaarden, J.B., and Frederickson, D.S. (eds.): The Metabolic Basis of Inherited Disease, ed. 3. McGraw-Hill Book Co., New York, 1972.
3. BOWMAN, B.H., LOCKHART, L.H., AND MCCOMBS, M.L.: Oyster ciliary inhibition by cystic fibrosis factor. Science 164:325, 1969.
4. BRADY, R.O., AND KOLODNY, E.H.: Disorders of ganglioside metabolism. Progr. Med. Genet. 8:225, 1972.
5. DAHLQUIST, A., AND SVENNINGSEN, N.W.: Galactose in the urine of newborn infants. J. Pediatr. 75:454, 1969.
6. DAMM, H.C. (ED.): Handbook of Clinical Laboratory Data. Chemical Rubber Company, Cleveland, 1965.
7. DENNY-BROWN, D.: Hepato-lenticular degeneration (Wilson's disease): two different components. N. Engl. J. Med. 270:1149, 1964.
8. DONNISON, A.B., SCHWACHMAN, H., AND GROSS, R.E.: A review of 164 children with meconium ileus seen at the Children's Hospital Medical Center, Boston. Pediatrics 37:833, 1966.
9. DREYFUS, J.C., AND SCHAPIRA, G.: "The metabolism of iron in hemochromatosis," *In* Gross, F. (ed.): Iron Metabolism. Springer Verlag, Berlin, 1964.
10. HADORN, B., JOHANSEN, P.G., AND ANDERSON, C.M.: Pancreozymin secretin test of exocrine pancreatic function in cystic fibrosis and the significance of the results for the pathogenesis of the disease. Can. Med. Assoc. J. 98:377, 1968.
11. HADORN, B., ZOPPI, G., SHMERLING, D.H. ET AL.: Quantitative assessment of exocrine pancreatic function in infants and children. J. Pediatr. 73:39, 1968.
12. HALL, W.K., CRAVEY, C.E., CHEN, P.T. ET AL.: An evaluation of galactosuria. J. Pediatr. 77:625, 1970.
13. HERS, H.G.: "Glycogen storage disease," *In* Levine, R., and Luft, R. (eds.): Advances in Metabolic Disorders. Academic Press, New York, 1964, vol. 1.
14. HOWELL, R.R.: "The glycogen storage diseases," *In* Stanbury, J.B., Wyngaarden, J.B., and Frederickson, D.S. (eds.): The Metabolic Basis of Inherited Disease, ed.3. McGraw-Hill Book Co., New York, 1972.
15. HUSKISSON, E.C., AND BALME, H.W.: Pseudo-podagra: Differential diagnosis of gout. Lancet 2:269, 1972.
16. IACOCCA, V.F., BRADDOCK, L.I., AND BARBERO, G.J.: Confirmation of the inhibitory effect of cystic fibrosis sera on oyster cilia. J. Pediatr. 79:508, 1971.
17. KALAYOGLU, M., SIEBER, W.K., RODNAN, J.B., AND KIESEWETTE, W.B.: Meconium ileus: a critical review of treatment and eventual prognosis. J. Pediatr. Surg. 6:290, 1971.
18. KEBERLE, H.: "General discussion of the therapeutic effects of desferrioxamine and calcium-D.T.P.A.," *In* Gross, F. (ed.): Iron Metabolism. Springer Verlag, Berlin, 1964.
19. KELLY, S., KATZ, S., BURNS, J., AND BOYLAN, J.: Screening for galactosemia in New York State. Public Health Rep. 85:575, 1970.

20. KNOX, W.E.: "Phenylketonuria," In Stanbury, J.B., Wyngaarden, J.B., and Frederickson, D.S. (eds.): The Metabolic Basis of Inherited Disease, ed.3. McGraw-Hill Book Co., New York, 1972.

21. LIDDLE, L., SEEGMILLER, J.E., AND LASTER, L.: Enzymatic spectrophotometric method for determination of uric acid. J. Lab. Clin. Med. 54:903, 1959.

22. LOBECK, C.C.: "Cystic fibrosis," In Stanbury, J.B., Wyngaarden, J.B., and Frederickson, D.S. (eds.): The Metabolic Basis of Inherited Disease, ed. 3. McGraw-Hill Book Co., New York, 1972.

23. MAGASANIK, B.: Regulation of the biosynthesis and interconversion of purine nucleotides. Arthritis Rheum. 8:610, 1965.

24. MAYES, J.S., AND GUTHRIE, R.: Detection of heterozygotes for galactokinase deficiency in a human population. Biochem. Genet. 2:219, 1968.

25. MILANSKY, A., LITTLEFIELD, J.W., KANFER, J.N. ET AL.: Prenatal genetic diagnosis. N. Engl. J. Med. 283:1370, 1970.

26. MILNE, M.D.: "Renal tubular dysfunction," In Strauss, M.B., and Welt, L.G.(eds.): Diseases of the Kidney, ed. 2. Little, Brown & Co., Boston, 1971.

27. NADLER, H.L.: Indications for amniocentesis in the early prenatal detection of genetic disorders. Birth Defects 7:5, 1971.

28. O'BRIEN, J.S.: Ganglioside-storage diseases. N. Eng. J. Med. 284:893, 1971.

29. OWEN, O.E., MORGAN, A.P., KEMP, H.B. ET AL.: Brain metabolism during fasting. J. Clin. Invest. 46:1589, 1967.

30. PAULUS, H.E., COUTTS, A., CALABRO, J.J., AND KLINENBERG, J.R.: Clinical significance of hyperuricemia in routinely screened hospitalized men. J.A.M.A. 211:277, 1970.

31. POLLYCOVE, M.: "Hemochromatosis," In Stanbury, J.B., Wyngaarden, J.B., and Frederickson, D.S. (eds.): The Metabolic Basis of Inherited Disease, ed. 3., McGraw-Hill Book Co., New York, 1972.

32. RASTEGAR, A., AND THIER, S.O.: The physiologic approach to hyperuricemia. N. Engl. J. Med. 286:470, 1972.

33. ROBINSON, A.: The assay of galactokinase and galactose-1-phosphate uridyl transferase in human erythrocytes: a presumed test for heterozygous carriers of the galactosemic defect. J. Exp. Med. 18:359, 1963.

34. SANDOR, G.: Serum Proteins in Health and Disease, trans. and ed. by E. Kawerau. Williams & Wilkins Co., Baltimore, 1966.

35. SCHAFFNER, F., STERNLIEB, I., BANKE, T., AND POPPER, H.: Hepatocellular changes in Wilson's disease. Am. J. Pathol. 41:315, 1962.

36. SCHNECK, L., VOLK, B.W., AND SAIFER, A.: The gangliosides. Am. J. Med. 46:245, 1969.

37. SCHNEIDER, J.A., BRADLEY, K., AND SEEGMILLER, J.E.: Increased cystine in leukocytes from individuals homozygous and heterozygous for cystinosis. Science 157:1321, 1967.

38. SEEGMILLER, J.E.: Lesch-Nyhan syndrome and the X-linked uric acidurias. Hosp. Pract. 7:79, 1972.

39. SEGAL, S.: "Disorders of galactose metabolism," In Stanbury, J.B., Wyngaarden, J.B., and Frederickson, D.S. (eds.): The Metabolic Basis of Inherited Diseases, ed. 3. McGraw-Hill Book Co., New York, 1972.

40. SPENCER-PEET, J., NORMAN, M.E., LAKE, B.D. ET AL.: Hepatic glycogen storage disease. Quart. J. Med. 40:95, 1971.

41. SPOCK, A., HEICK, H.M.C., CRESS, H., AND LOGAN, W.S.: Abnormal serum factor in patients with cystic fibrosis of the pancreas. Pediatr. Res. 1:173, 1967.

42. THIER, S.O., AND SEGAL, S.: "Cystinuria," In Stanbury, J.B. Wyngaarden, J.B., and Frederickson, D.S. (eds.): The Metabolic Basis of Inherited Disease, ed. 3. McGraw-Hill Book Co., New York, 1972.

43. TYLER, F.H.: "Urate nephropathy," In Strauss, M.B., and Welt, L.G. (eds.): Diseases of the Kidney, ed. 2. Little, Brown & Co., Boston, 1971.

44. ULMER, D.D.: "Trace elements and clinical pathology," In Stefanini, M. (ed.): Progress in Clinical Pathology. Grune & Stratton, New York, 1966, vol. 1.

45. VAN HOOF, F., AND HERS, H.G.: The subgroups of type III glycogenosis. Eur. J. Biochem. 2:265, 1967.

46. VOGEL, J.M., AND BERES, P.: Recurrent thrombocytopenia in Gaucher's disease responding to a second "splenectomy". Am. J. Clin. Pathol. 55:489, 1971.
47. WILLIAMS, R., SCHEVER, P.J., AND SHERLOCK, S.: The inheritance of idiopathic haemochromatosis: A clinical and liver biopsy study of 16 families. Quart. J. Med. 31:249, 1962.
48. WILLIAMS, T.F., AND WINTERS, R.W.: "Familial (hereditary) vitamin D-resistant rickets with hypophosphatemia," *In* Stanbury, J.B., Wyngaarden, J.B., and Frederickson, D.S. (eds.): The Metabolic Basis of Inherited Disease, ed. 3 McGraw-Hill Book Co., New York, 1972.
49. WYNGAARDEN, J.B., AND KELLEY, W.N.: "Gout," *In* Stanbury, J. B., Wyngaarden, J.B., and Frederickson, D.S. (eds.): The Metabolic Basis of Inherited Disease, ed. 3. McGraw-Hill Book Co., New York, 1972.
50. YU, T.F.: Secondary gout associated with myeloproliferative diseases. Arthritis Rheum. 8:765, 1965.
51. YU, T.F., BERGER, L., AND GUTMAN, A.B.: Renal function in gout. II. Effect of uric acid loading on renal excretion of uric acid. Am. J. Med. 33:829, 1962.
52. YU, T.F., AND GUTMAN, A.B.: Uric acid nephrolithiasis in gout. Predisposing factors. Ann. Intern. Med. 67:1133, 1967.

CHAPTER 19

NORMAL VALUES

For convenience, tables of normal data for hematology, blood chemistry, urine, and spinal fluid examinations are assembled in this section. Each of these tables also appears in the chapter devoted to the subject.

Table 2. Normal Hematologic Findings*

	Adults		Average Values for Children		
	Average	Range	Birth	1 Year	10 Years
Red blood cells in millions/mm³					
Female	4.8	4.0-5.6	5.4	4.5	4.8
Male	5.4	4.5-6.5			
Hemoglobin in Gm per 100 ml					
Female	13.9	12.0-16.0	17.0	11.4	13.0
Male	15.8	14.0-18.0			
Hematocrit in ml per 100 ml					
Female	42	36-47	54	35	39
Male	47	40-54			
Platelets in 100,000/mm³					
Male & Female	3.0	1.5-4.5	2.0	3.0	3.0
White blood cells in 1000/mm³					
Male & Female	7.0	4.0-11.0	17.0	12.0	7.5

* From Damm, H. (ed.): CRC Handbook of Clinical Laboratory Data. Chemical Rubber Co., Cleveland, Ohio, 1965. Used by permission of Chemical Rubber Co.

Table 3. Differential White Counts at Varying Ages
(Values given as per cent of total white cells)*

	Adult	Birth	1 Year	10 Years
Neutrophils	50-75	45-70	20-40	40-60
Lymphocytes	20-45	25-35	50-75	25-45
Monocytes	2-10	2-10	2-10	2-10
Eosinophils	0-6	0-6	0-6	0-6
Basophils	0-1	0-1	0-1	0-1

* From Damm, H. (ed.): CRC Handbook of Clinical Laboratory Data. Chemical Rubber Co., Cleveland, Ohio 1965. Used by permission of Chemical Rubber Co.

Table 9. Normal Blood Chemistry Values for Adults†

Substance	Serum, Plasma,* or Whole Blood*	Normal Values	Remarks
Acetone	P or S	0-1 mg/100 ml[17]	
Albumin	S	4.3-5.6 Gm/100 ml[29]	
Ammonia	WB	102 ± 23 µg/100 ml[9] (Seligson and Hirahara)[58]	Anticoagulant should not contain ammonium salts. Patient should be fasting.
		45-50 µg/100 ml[9] (Conway)	
Amylase	S or WB	80-150 units[17] (Somogyi)	A unit is 1 mg glucose per 100 ml sample after 30 min incubation.
Ascorbic acid	P	0.8-2.4 mg/100 ml[17]	Patient should be fasting.
Bilirubin	S		
Direct		0.2 mg/100 ml[61]	
Total		1.0 mg/100 ml[61]	
Calcium	S	4.5-5.75 mEq/L[17] 9.0-11.5 mg/100 ml[17]	Serum protein values may affect result.
CO_2	S or P		Heparin.
Combining power		25-33 mM/L[27] 55-75 vol/100 ml[27]	

* See footnote p. 480.
† Reference numbers in this Table refer to those given at the end of Chapter 4, pp. 141-143.

Table 9   (Continued)

Substance	Serum, Plasma,* or Whole Blood*	Normal Values	Remarks
Content: Arterial		23-31 mM/L[27]	
Venous		25-32 mM/L[27]	
Tension: Arterial		33-48 mm Hg[27]	
Venous		38-53 mm Hg[27]	
Chloride	S	95-106 mEq/L[17]	
Cholesterol	S		
Total		220 ± 50 mg/100 ml[78]	
Esters		163 ± 36 mg/100 ml[78]	
% Esterified		50-70%[61]	
Copper	S	90-150 μg/100 ml[71]	
Creatine	S	0.16-0.4 mg/100 ml[65]	
Creatine phosphokinase	S	0.2-1.42 units[73]	Unit is μ moles creatine liberated/ml serum/hr. Separate and freeze serum immediately.
Creatinine	S	0.5-1.0 mg/100 ml[65]	
Fatty acids	S		
Esterified		250-400 mg/100 ml[1] 8-20 mEq/L[17]	
Free		0.35-1.2 mEq/L[17]	
Fibrinogen	P	200-400 mg/100 ml[68]	
Globulin	S	1.3-2.7 Gm/100 ml[29]	
Glucose	WB	90-120 mg/100 ml[17] (Folin-Wu) 65-95 mg/100 ml[27] (Nelson-Somogyi) 60-105 mg/100 ml[14] (Enzymatic 46-94 mg/100 ml[42] (Ultramicro)	Whole blood diluted in water.
Icterus index	S	2 to 8 units[27]	Compared against 1:10,000 solution of potassium dichromate
Iodine	S		
Protein-bound		3.5-8.0 μg/100 ml[16]	
Butanol-extractable		3.2-6.4 μg/100 ml[27]	

---

* See footnote page 480.

Table 9   (Continued)

Substance	Serum, Plasma,* or Whole Blood*	Normal Values	Remarks
Iron	S	56-183 μg/100 ml[21]	
Iron-binding capacity	S	277-379 μg/100 ml[21]	
Lactic acid	S		Patient should be in completely basal state.
Arterial		3.1-7 mg/100 ml[27]	
Venous		5-20 mg/100 ml[27]	
Lactic dehydrogenase	S	200-450 units[27] (Wroblewski and La-Due, modified by Henry, et al.)[28]	Unit is decrease in A of 0.001/min/ml serum.
		40-78 units[28] (Wacker)[70]	Unit is increase in A of 0.001/min/ml serum.
Lipase	S	0-1.5 units[27]	Unit is ml 0.05 N NaOH needed to neutralize fatty acids in 1 ml serum.
Lipids, total	S	450-1000 mg/100 ml[27]	Patient should be fasting.
Magnesium	S	1.4-2.2 mEq/L[4,66] 1.7-2.7 mg/100 ml[4,66]	
Nitrogen (NPN)	WB	25-40 mg/100 ml[5]	Anticoagulant should not contain ammonium salts.
Osmolality	S	281-291 mOsm/kg[26]	
Oxygen			
Oxygen content	WB		Heparin. Keep sample in ice.
Arterial		15-22 vol/100 ml[17]	
Venous		11-16 vol/100 ml[17]	
Oxygen saturation	WB		Heparin. Keep sample in ice.
Arterial		98%[27]	
Venous		55-71%[27]	
pH: Arterial	WB	7.37-7.42[27]	
Venous		7.34-7.39[27]	
Phosphatase, acid	S	0.5-5[27] (Babson-Read)	Unit is amount of enzyme that liberates 1 mg of α-naphthol/hr.
		0-0.1[27] (Shinowara)	Unit is mg P/hr/100 ml serum.

* See footnote page 480.

Table 9   (Continued)

Substance	Serum, Plasma,* or Whole Blood*	Normal Values	Remarks
Phosphatase, alkaline	S	1.5-4.0[27] (Bodansky)	Unit is mg P/hr/100 ml serum.
		3.7-13.1[27] (King-Armstrong)	Unit is mg phenol/30 min/100 ml serum.
		2.2-8.6[27] (Shinowara)	Unit is mg P/hr/100 ml serum.
Phospholipids	S	150-350 mg/100 ml[17]	
Phosphorus, inorganic	S	2.6-4.8 mg/100 ml[13]	Values may rise if serum remains in contact with cells for several hours.
Potassium	S	3.8-5.1 mEq/L[25]	
Proteins (total)	S	6-8 Gm/100 ml[29]	
Electrophoretic fractions Albumin		52.0-68.0%[29]	
α_1 Globulin		2.4-5.3%[29]	
α_2 Globulin		6.6-13.5%[29]	
β Globulin		8.5-14.5%[29]	
γ Globulin		10.7-21.0%[29]	
A/G ratio		1.5-2.2[29]	
Sodium	S	138-146 mEq/L[17]	
Transaminase Glutamic-oxalacetic (SGOT)	S	12-36 units[28]	Unit is change in A of 0.001/min/ml serum.
Glutamic-pyruvic (SGPT)	S	6-53 units[17]	Units is change in A of 0.001/min/ml serum.
Urea nitrogen (BUN)	S	5-25 mg/100 ml[27]	
Uric acid	S		Separate serum from cells promptly
Males		3.0-7.0 mg/100 ml[8]	
Females		2.0-6.0 mg/100 ml[8]	

* Listed under "Remarks" is information about anticoagulants for specific procedures. If no comment is made, any effective anticoagulant is permissible.

Table 14. Normal Values for Urine

Test	Normal Values	Remarks
Addis count	WBC 1,800,000; RBC 500,000; casts (hyaline) 0–5000	Rinse bottle with 10% neutral formalin and discard excess 12-hr specimen
Albumin		
Qualitative	Negative	Single specimen
Quantitative	10–100 mg/24 hr	24-hr specimen
Aldosterone	2–23 μg/24 hr	24-hr specimen; keep refrigerated.
Amino acid nitrogen	100–290 mg/24 hr	24-hr specimen; collect in thymol; refrigerate
Ammonia	700 mg/24 hr	24-hr specimen
Amylase	2–50 Wohlgemuth u/ml	Single specimen
Amylase, total in 24 hr	6–30 Wohlgemuth u/ml Up to 5000 Somogyi u/24 hr	24-hr specimen
Bence-Jones protein	Negative	First morning specimen
Bilirubin	Negative	Single specimen
Blood, occult	Negative	Single specimen
Calcium		
Sulkowitch	Positive 1 +	Single specimen
Quantitative	30–150 mg/24 hr	Average diet
	100–250 mg/24 hr	High-calcium diet; 24-hr specimen
Catecholamines	Less than 230 μg in 24 hr	24-hr specimen; use 1 ml conc. H_2SO_4 for preservative
Chloride	110–250 mEq/24 hr	24-hr specimen
Coproporphyrin	50–200 μg/24 hr. Children: 0–80 μg/24 hr	24-hr specimen in 5 Gm of Na_2CO_3
Creatine	Less than 100 mg in 24 hr, or less than 6% of creatinine. Pregnancy: up to 12% of creatinine. Children under 1 yr: may equal creatinine. Children over 1 yr: up to 30% of creatinine	24-hr specimen
Creatinine	Females: 0.8–1.7 Gm/24 hr Males: 1–1.9 Gm/24 hr	24-hr specimen

Table 14.   (Continued)

Test	Normal Values	Remarks
Estrogens	Females: 4–60 μg/24 hr Males: 4–25 μg/24 hr	24-hr specimen; refrigerate
Fishberg concentration test	Specific gravity: 1.022 to 1.032	Collect specimens at 7,8 and 10 A.M.
Fishberg dilution test	Volume of 40 ml in first hour with specific gravity 1.001 to 1.003	Collect 4 hourly specimens after drinking 1200 ml of water
Glucose Qualitative	Negative	Single specimen
Quantitative	Less than 100 mg/100 ml	24-hr specimen
Gonadotropic hormone, pituitary	10 to 15 mouse uterine u/24 hr _	24-hr specimen; collect with toluene
17-Hydroxycortico-steroids	Females: 2–8 mg/24 hr Males: 3–10 mg/24 hr	24-hr specimen; tranquilizers interfere
5-Hydroxyindoleacetic acid	2–9 mg/24 hr	24-hr specimen; tranquilizers interfere
Indican	4–20 mg/24 hr	24-hr specimen
17-Ketosteriods	24-hr excretion:	24-hr specimen
Lead	0.021–0.038 mg/liter	24-hr specimen
pH	4.8 to 7.8	Single specimen
Phenylpyruvic acid	Negative	Single specimen
Phosphorus	0.9–1.3 Gm/24 hr	24-hr specimen
Porphobilinogen	Negative	Single specimen
Potassium	25–100 mEq/24 hr	24-hr specimen
Pregnanediol	Children: negative. Females: 1–8 mg/24 hr. Males: 0–1 mg/24 hr	24-hr specimen; refrigerate
Pregnanetriol	Children: Less than 0.5 mg/24 hr. Females: 0.5–2 mg/24 hr. Males: 1.0–2.0 mg/24 hr	24-hr specimen; refrigerate
Protein Bence-Jones	Negative	First morning specimen
Qualitative	Negative	Single specimen
Quantitative	10–100 mg/24 hr	24-hr specimen

17-Ketosteriods excretion:

Age	Females	Males
10	1–4 mg	1–4 mg
20–30	4–16 mg	6–26 mg
50	3–9 mg	5–18 mg
70	1–7 mg	2–10 mg

Table 14.   (Continued)

Test	Normal Values	Remarks
Serotonin	*See* 5-Hydroxyindoleacetic acid	
Sodium	About 110 mEq/24 hr	24-hr specimen
Specific gravity	1.002–1.030 1.015–1.025	Single specimen 24-hr specimen
Sugars	Negative	Single specimen
Urea clearance	Maximum: 75 ml Standard: 54 ml	Serum and urine
Uric acid	0.5–1.0 Gm/24 hr	24-hr specimen
Urobilinogen		
Semiquantitative	Up to 1 Ehrlich u/2 hr	2-hr specimen; collect between 1 and 3 P.M.
Quantitative	1.0–4.0 mg/24 hr	24-hr specimen; collect in dark container with 5 Gm of Na_2CO_3
Vanilmandelic acid	0.7–6.8 mg/24 hr	24-hr specimen in 3 ml 25% H_2SO_4; omit fruit and coffee 2 days before test
Volume	Adults: 1000-1500 ml/24 hr (about 15–21 ml/kg body wt) Children: 3 to 4 times as much as adults per kg of body wt	

Table 15.   Normal CSF Values for Children and Adults

	Adults	Infants and Young Children
Quantity (Total)	100-150 ml	Varies with size
Appearance	clear	clear
Pressure	75-200 mm H_2O	50-100 mm H_2O
Cells	0-5	0-20
	All lymphocytes	All lymphocytes

Table 16.   Normal Values for Some Commonly Measured
Substances in Cerebrospinal Fluid

	CSF Level	*Compared with Plasma Level*
pH	7.32-7.35	Very slightly lower
Glucose	45-85 mg/100 ml	50-80 per cent
Protein	15-45 mg/100 ml	0.2-0.5 per cent
A/G Ratio	8:1	3-4 times higher
Chloride	110-125 mEq/liter	115-125 per cent
Urea nitrogen	10-15 mg/100 ml	Same

Index

NOTE: Page numbers in *italics* refer to illustrations and tables.